Medication Administration

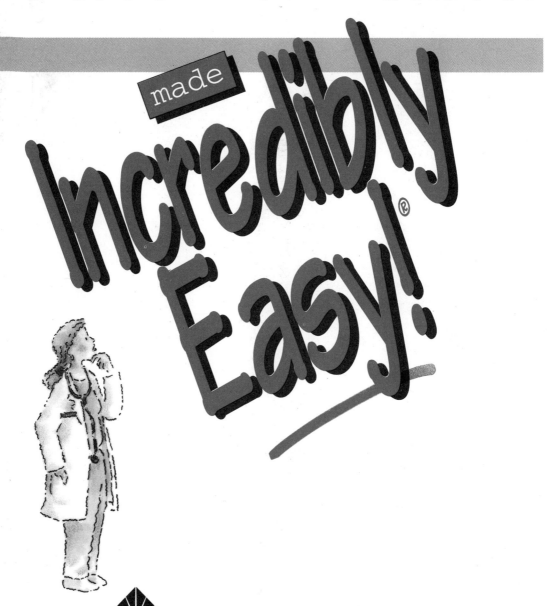

made

Incredibly Easy!®

LIPPINCOTT WILLIAMS & WILKINS
A **Wolters Kluwer** Company

Philadelphia • Baltimore • New York • London
Buenos Aires • Hong Kong • Sydney • Tokyo

Staff

Publisher
Judith A. Schilling McCann, RN, MSN

Editorial Director
David Moreau

Clinical Director
Joan M. Robinson, RN, MSN

Senior Art Director
Arlene Putterman

Art Director
Mary Ludwicki

Clinical Editors
Denise D. Hayes, RN, MSN, CRNP (project manager);
Collette Bishop Hendler, RN, CCRN; Jana L. Sciarra,
RN, MSN, CRNP; Beverly Ann Tscheschlog, RN, BS

Editors
Julie Munden (senior editor), Ty Eggenberger, Kevin
Haworth, Carol H. Munson

Copy Editors
Kimberly Bilotta, Amy Furman, Shana Harrington,
Marcia Ryan, Pamela Wingrod

Designer
Lynn Foulk

Illustrator
Bot Roda

Digital Composition Services
Diane Paluba (manager), Joyce Rossi Biletz (senior
desktop assistant), Richard Eng (desktop assistant)

Manufacturing
Patricia K. Dorshaw (senior manager), Beth Janae
Orr (book production coordinator)

Editorial Assistants
Danielle J. Barsky, Beverly Lane, Linda Ruhf

Indexer
Barbara Hodgson

Library of Congress Cataloging-in-Publication Data
Medication administration made incredibly easy.
      p. ; cm.
      Includes index.
      1. Drugs—Administration. 2. Nursing.
      [DNLM: 1. Drug Administration Routes. 2. Drug Therapy—
      nursing. 3.Pharmaceutical Preparations—administration &
      dosage. WB 340 M4887 2003] I. Lippincott Williams &
      Wilkins. II. Title.

RM147 .M434 2003
615'.6—dc21
ISBN 1-58255-222-3 (pbk. : alk. paper)   2002013628

Contents

Contributors and consultants

Elizabeth A. Archer, RN, EdD
Assistant Professor
Baptist College of Health Sciences
Memphis

Cheryl L. Brady, RN, MSN
Adjunct Faculty
Kent State University
Liverpool, Ohio

Michelle Byrne, RN, MS, PhD, CNOR
Independent Nurse Consultant
Acworth, Ga.
Clinical Instructor
North Georgia College and State University

Lawrence Carey, PharmD
Senior Medical Information Specialist
CoMed Communications
Philadelphia

Nan S. Carey, RN, MSN
Assistant Professor
Baptist College of Health Sciences
Memphis

Rebecca Sue Chamberlain, RN, MSN, CRNP
Pediatric Nurse Practitioner
Children's National Medical Center
Washington, D.C.

Laurie Donaghy, RN
Emergency Room Charge Nurse
Nazareth Hospital
Philadelphia

M. Susan Emerson, RN, PhD, BC, ANP, ACNP, CNS
Clinical Assistant Professor—Nurse Practitioner
University of Missouri—Kansas City School of
Nursing

Susan K. Poole, BSN, MS, CNSN, CRNI
Senior Director, Professional Services
Option Care, Inc.
Bannockburn, Ill.

Gail A. Viergutz, MS, ANP-C
Nurse Practitioner—Urgent Care/Emergency
Ministry Health Care—St. Michael's Hospital
Stevens Point, Wis.

Marilyn J. Vontz, RN, PhD
Nurse Educator
Bryan School of Nursing
Lincoln, Nebr.

Foreword

Accurate administration of medications is one of the most important skills nurses bring to the health care arena. Students have reported that dispensing medications, especially those that are injectable, is one of the most stressful experiences they face as they begin their nursing education. They need a text that provides content in a nonthreatening manner that makes medication administration easy to learn.

Practicing nurses encounter an ever-increasing number of new drugs with new equipment and routes of delivery. *Medication Administration Made Incredibly Easy* provides an excellent resource to guide student learning and for practicing registered nurses and licensed practical nurses who must maintain their clinical expertise and professional judgment. This book is a well-written, accurate, and complete text that presents material in a humorous, understandable manner. The content is thoroughly up-to-date—addressing the latest in medication administration information.

Part I presents the fundamentals of medication administration, including essential concepts, such as drug names and routes, how drugs act in the body, important considerations, the nursing process applied to medication administration, legal and ethical issues, medication orders and typical errors, dosage calculations, and documenting medications.

Part II provides an excellent overview of drug administration methods and routes. This section includes every route utilized in medicine today, such as topical routes through skin and mouth mucous membranes, including buccal and sublingual; eye, ear, and nasal routes; respiratory and gastric routes; rectal and vaginal routes; and the typical injection routes, such as subcutaneous, intradermal, intramuscular, and intravenous. Epidural, intrapleural, intraperitoneal, intra-articular, and intraosseous routes are also addressed.

Part III addresses specific routes used for chemotherapy and parenteral nutrition. A major advantage of this text is the way in which various learning styles are incorporated into the delivery of content. Each chapter includes a summary of key points with definitions of key terms. Key concepts are presented with numerous illustrations providing visual interpretations of the material. Content is made easy to follow through abundant use of bullets and checklists that focus on key points. A major strength of the text is the logos and icons used to address important information including:

Memory joggers give you helpful, effective ways to remember the more difficult concepts.

Ages and stages highlights important pediatric and geriatric concerns.

Peak technique shows how to administer specific drugs.

No place like home gives tips for patient's and their families about the medication regimen.

Danger zone alerts the reader to dangerous situations and provides prevention and intervention tips.

Gear up provides detailed instructions for types of drug delivery equipment.

Write it down features essential points to document for each medication administered.

The best part of the text is the incorporation of humor throughout—making it fun to learn a topic that's typically intimidating. You'll learn essential information you'll need in everyday practice and have a good time in the process. The text clearly fulfills its title promise, demonstrating how learning medication administration can be made to be incredibly easy.

Juanita Fogel Keck, RN, CNS, DNS
Associate Professor and Chair, Adult Health Department
Indiana University School of Nursing
Indianapolis

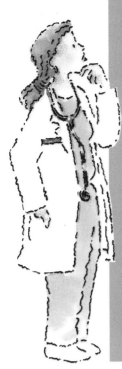

Part I   Fundamentals of medication administration

Essential concepts

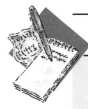

Just the facts

In this chapter, you'll learn:

♦ the basics of medication administration

♦ drug administration routes

♦ key concepts of pharmacokinetics and pharmacodynamics

♦ dosage and administration considerations.

A look at medication basics

When you care for patients in your day-to-day nursing practice, one of the most crucial skills you bring to the bedside is your ability to administer medications. From legal, ethical, and practical standpoints, medication administration is much more than simply a delivery service. It's a highly technical skill that requires you to exercise wide-ranging knowledge, analytical skill, professional judgment, and clinical expertise. Indeed, some would consider the safe, effective administration of medications the foundation of your success as a professional nurse.

To deliver medications accurately, you need a sound working knowledge of:
• drug terminology
• the routes by which drugs are delivered
• the effects the drugs produce after they're inside the body.

Pharmacology is the scientific study of the origin, nature, chemistry, effects, and uses of drugs. This chapter reviews some concepts basic to pharmacology—and essential to your ability to administer drugs wisely—starting with the most basic of all: drug names.

The name game

The typical drug has three or more names:
• The *chemical name* describes the drug's atomic and molecular structure.

- The *generic name* is a shorter, simpler version of the drug's chemical name.
- The *trade name* (also known as the brand name or propriety name) is the name selected by the drug company that sells it. Trade names are protected by copyright laws. (See *What's in a name?*)

A class act

Drugs that share similar characteristics are grouped together into pharmacologic classes, or families. For example, the class known as beta-adrenergic blockers contains several drugs with similar properties.

Drugs can also be grouped according to their therapeutic class, which classifies drugs according to their therapeutic use. For example, thiazide diuretics and beta-adrenergic blockers are both antihypertensives, but they belong to different pharmacologic classes because they share few characteristics.

Routes of administration

A drug's administration route influences the quantity given and the rate at which the drug is absorbed and distributed. These variables, in turn, affect the drug's action and the patient's response. Routes of administration that involve the GI tract are known as *enteral routes*. Those that don't involve the GI tract are known as *parenteral routes*. Parenteral routes can be useful for treating a patient who can't take a drug orally. Compare the advantages and disadvantages of the following routes.

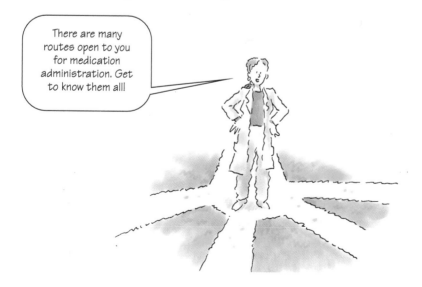

What's in a name?

Most drugs have three names—chemical, generic, and trade—as the example below demonstrates. Some drugs may have more than one trade name. The best way to avoid confusion is to use the generic name when speaking or writing about a drug.

Chemical name

> 7-chloro-1,3-dihydro-1-methyl-5-phenyl-2H-1,4-benzodiazepin-2-one

Generic name

> diazepam

Trade name

> Valium

Topical route

The topical route is used to deliver a drug via the skin or a mucous membrane. The advantages of delivering drugs by this route include:
- easy administration
- few allergic reactions
- fewer adverse reactions than drugs administered by systemic routes.

You can make a real mess of it

Delivering precise doses can be difficult with the topical route. Also, these medications can be messy to apply — and even messier for your patient to wear! They may stain the patient's clothing and bed linens, they may have a distinctive smell, and they may get on you as well.

Ophthalmic administration

Ophthalmic administration involves drugs, such as creams, ointments, and liquid drops, that are placed in the conjunctival sac or directly onto the surface of the eye. Intraocular inserts and collagen shields can be used to deliver drugs to the eye as well. For all types of ophthalmic administration, take care to avoid contaminating the medication container or transferring organisms to the patient's eye.

Convenience at a price

Ocusert Pilo, one type of intraocular insert, supplies pilocarpine to the ciliary muscles to treat glaucoma. Because this eye medication disk releases the drug for an entire week, it's more convenient than eyedrops. However, intraocular inserts cost much more than eyedrops, and they may be uncomfortable. Also, the drug may be absorbed systemically, causing adverse effects.

Wielding the shield

Collagen shields that have been presoaked in a drug solution can be applied to the eye to treat corneal ulcers and severe iridocyclitis (inflammation of the iris and ciliary body). Collagen shields may prove more effective than injections of collagen beneath the conjunctiva, where the substance is poorly absorbed.

Otic administration

Otic administration involves drugs that are placed directly into the ear. Solutions placed into the ear can be used to treat infection or inflammation of the external ear canal, produce local anesthesia, or soften built-up cerumen (earwax) for removal.

Bring otic solutions to room temperature before administering them because cold solutions can cause pain or vertigo.

Nasal administration

Nasal administration involves drugs that are placed directly into the patient's nostrils. Medicated solutions can be placed into the patient's nostrils from a dropper or as an atomized spray from a squeeze bottle or pump device.

Bypassing the first-pass effect

The highly vascular nasal mucosa allows systemic absorption while avoiding first-pass metabolism by the liver (the liver changes the drug to a more water-soluble form for excretion before it enters circulation).

Respiratory route

Drugs that are both lipid-soluble and available as gases can be administered into the respiratory tree. The respiratory tree provides an extensive, highly perfused region for enhanced absorption. Smaller doses of potent drugs can be given by this route to minimize their adverse effects. Because this route is easily accessible, it provides a convenient alternative when other routes are unavailable.

Emergency!

In emergencies, some injectable drugs, such as atropine, lidocaine, and epinephrine, can be given directly into the lungs via an endotracheal tube. A drug administered into the trachea is absorbed into the bloodstream from the alveolar sacs. Surfactant, for example, is administered to premature neonates via the trachea to improve their respiratory function. And atropine can be administered to patients with symptomatic bradycardia and no vascular access to increase their heart rate.

Breathing easy? Not so fast!

A major disadvantage of the respiratory route is that few drugs can be given this way. Other disadvantages include:
• difficulty in administering accurate doses — or full doses, if the patient isn't cooperative
• nausea and vomiting when certain drugs are delivered into the lungs
• tracheal or bronchial mucosa irritation, causing coughing or bronchospasm
• possible infection from the equipment used to deliver drugs into the lungs.

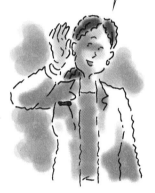

Did you hear that good advice? Bring otic solutions to room temperature.

Memory jogger

How about an **ale** to remember the emergency medications that can be administered through an endotracheal tube?

A   atropine
L   lidocaine
E   epinephrine

Buccal, sublingual, and translingual routes

Certain drugs are given buccally (in the pouch between the cheek and teeth), sublingually (under the tongue), or translingually (on the tongue) to prevent their destruction or transformation in the stomach or small intestine. Drugs given by these routes act quickly because the oral mucosa's thin epithelium and abundant vasculature allow direct absorption into the bloodstream.

Cheeky checklist

These routes can be used if the patient can take nothing by mouth, can't swallow, or is intubated. What's more, the drugs have no first-pass effect in the liver, and they don't cause GI irritation. Only drugs that are highly lipid-soluble may be given by these routes, and they may irritate the oral mucosa.

Oral route

Oral administration is usually the safest, most convenient, and least expensive method. For that reason, most drugs are administered to patients who are conscious and able to swallow.

Down in the mouth

The oral route does have some disadvantages:
• It produces variable drug absorption.
• Because it moves drugs through the liver, first-pass metabolism may take place.
• Drugs can't be given orally in most emergencies because of their unpredictable and relatively slow absorption. (See *Enteral administration: Why absorption varies.*)

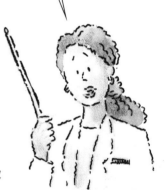

Here's a quick oral exam — What route is the safest, most convenient, and least expensive? The oral route!

Enteral administration: Why absorption varies

A drug that's administered enterally—orally or by gastric tube—can undergo variable rates of absorption due to:
• changes in the pH of the GI tract
• changes in intestinal membrane permeability
• fluctuations in GI motility
• fluctuations in GI blood flow
• food in the GI tract
• other drugs in the GI tract.

- Oral drugs may irritate the GI tract, discolor the patient's teeth, or taste unpleasant.
- Oral drugs can be accidentally aspirated if the patient has trouble swallowing or is combative.

Gastric route

The gastric route allows direct instillation of medication into the GI system of patients who can't ingest the drug orally. A variety of tubes can be placed for instillation. Oily medications and enteric-coated or sustained-release tablets or capsules can't be administered by this route.

Rectal and vaginal routes

You may instill suppositories, ointments, creams, or gels into the rectum or vagina to treat local irritation or infection. Some drugs applied to the mucosa of the rectum or vagina can be absorbed systemically. Drugs may also be delivered to the rectum in a medicated enema or to the vagina in a medicated douche.

The up side

Drugs administered through the rectal or vaginal routes don't irritate the upper GI tract, as some oral medications do. Also, these drugs avoid destruction by digestive enzymes in the stomach and small intestine.

The down side

However, there are some disadvantages to the rectal and vaginal routes:
- The rectal route is usually contraindicated when the patient has a disorder affecting the lower GI tract, such as rectal bleeding or diarrhea.
- Drug absorption may be irregular or incomplete with these routes.
- The rectal route usually can't be used in an emergency.
- Rectal doses of some drugs may need to be larger than oral doses.
- Because rectal administration typically stimulates the vagus nerve, this route may pose a risk for cardiac patients.
- Drugs given rectally may irritate the rectal mucosa.
- Administering a drug by either the rectal or vaginal route may cause discomfort and embarrassment for the patient.

Intradermal route

Intradermal drug administration is used mainly for diagnostic purposes when testing for allergies or tuberculosis. To administer drugs intradermally, inject a small amount of serum or vaccine between the skin layers just below the stratum corneum. Because this route results in little systemic absorption, it produces mainly local effects.

Don't get too deep

You must be sure not to inject the substance too deeply. If you do, you'll have to reinject it, causing added stress, cost, and delay of treatment for the patient.

Subcutaneous route

When using the subcutaneous (S.C.) route, you inject small amounts of a drug beneath the dermis and into the subcutaneous tissue, usually in the patient's upper arm, thigh, or abdomen. Patients with diabetes use this technique to give themselves insulin. The drug is absorbed slowly from the subcutaneous tissue, thus prolonging its effects. What's more, this route requires no venipuncture and no I.V. access site.

Tissue issues

There are disadvantages to the S.C. route:
• S.C. injection may damage skin tissue.
• The S.C. route can't be used when the patient has occlusive vascular disease and poor perfusion because decreased peripheral circulation delays absorption.
• The S.C. route can't be used when the patient's skin or underlying tissue is grossly adipose, edematous, burned, hardened, swollen at the common injection sites, damaged by previous injections, or diseased.

Implants eliminate noncompliance

Aside from injection, another method of S.C. administration is to implant pellets or capsules beneath the skin that contain small amounts of a drug. From the dermis, the medication seeps slowly into the tissues. Goserelin, one such implant, is inserted into the upper abdominal wall to manage advanced prostate cancer. With the contraceptive Norplant, six silicone capsules that contain levonorgestrel are inserted beneath the skin of the woman's upper arm. They provide contraception for 5 years.

Because S.C. implants require no patient action after they're in place, they eliminate the problem of noncompliance. Their major drawback is the need for minor surgery to insert or remove them.

Intramuscular route

The I.M. route allows you to inject drugs directly into various muscle groups at varying tissue depths. You'll use this route to give aqueous suspensions and solutions in oil and to give medications that aren't available in oral form. The effect of a drug administered by the I.M. route is relatively rapid, and aqueous I.M. medications can be given to adults in doses of up to 5 ml in some sites. The I.M. route also eliminates the need for an I.V. site.

Intramuscular miscues

Despite the advantages, there are many disadvantages to the I.M. route:
• A drug delivered I.M. may precipitate in the muscle, thereby reducing absorption.
• The drug may not absorb properly if the patient is hypotensive or has a poor blood supply to the muscle.
• Improper technique can cause accidental injection of the drug into the patient's bloodstream, possibly causing an overdose or an adverse reaction.
• The I.M. route may cause pain and local tissue irritation, damage bone, puncture blood vessels, injure nerves, or break down muscle tissue, thus interfering with myoglobin — a marker for acute myocardial infarction.

> When delivering drugs I.M., you have to be strong in technique.

Intravenous route

The I.V. route allows injection of substances directly into the bloodstream through a vein. Appropriate substances include drugs, fluids, diagnostic contrast agents, and blood or blood products. Administration can range from a single dose to an ongoing infusion delivered with great precision.

In the I.V. league

Because the drug or solution is absorbed immediately and completely, the patient's response is rapid. Instant bioavailability (the drug's availability for target tissues) makes the I.V. route the first choice for giving drugs during an emergency to relieve acute or long-term pain. This route has no first-pass effect in the liver and avoids damage to muscle tissue caused by irritating drugs. Because absorption into the bloodstream is complete and reliable, large drug doses can be delivered at a continuous rate.

This road can be bumpy

Life-threatening adverse reactions may arise if I.V. drugs are administered too quickly, if the flow rate isn't monitored carefully

Reviewing specialized infusions

If drug therapy needs to take a direct route to a specific site in the patient's body, you may use one of the specialized routes of drug administration as shown in the chart below.

Epidural infusion	• The drug is injected into the epidural space, outside or above the dura mater. • The drug is absorbed into cerebrospinal fluid and works directly on the central nervous system. • Epidural anesthesia or analgesia is given through a special catheter and is considered safe and versatile. It may be tailored to affect a specific area of the body from the legs up to the upper abdomen. • The drug infused through an epidural catheter must be preservative-free to prevent serious reactions to the preservative. • Epidural catheters should be labeled "for epidural use only" to prevent the accidental injection of other drugs into the epidural space.
Intrapleural infusion	• The drug is injected into the pleural cavity. • The drug crosses the pleural membrane and enters the pleural space, where it works locally at the disease site. • Chemotherapy is an example of a drug given by this type of infusion to minimize systemic effects and increase drug effects on the tumor.
Intraperi-toneal infusion	• The drug is injected into the peritoneal cavity. • The drug or solution crosses the peritoneal membrane and enters the peritoneal space, where it works locally. • This administration route is used for peritoneal dialysis, in which the peritoneum functions as a diffusible semipermeable membrane. • Fluid or electrolyte imbalances can be corrected, toxins removed, and normal renal excretion facilitated using this route. The drug is injected into the synovial cavity of a joint to suppress inflammation, prevent contractures, and delay muscle atrophy.
Intra-articular infusion	• This route is most commonly used to treat rheumatoid arthritis, gout, systemic lupus erythematosus, osteoarthritis, and other joint disorders. • Corticosteroids, anesthetics, and lubricants are most commonly administered into the shoulder, elbow, wrist, finger, knee, ankle, or toe joints. • This route is used sparingly because of the risk of infection.
Intraosseous infusion	• The drug is injected into the rich vascular network of a long bone for rapid absorption. • Drugs and solutions administered through bone marrow are absorbed as rapidly as those administered I.V. • With a special intraosseous access needle, this route has been used successfully in children and adults for emergency infusions when normal vascular access isn't possible.

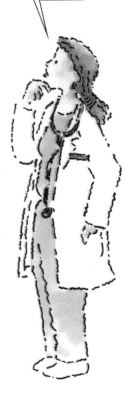

I need a specialized route. Which one shall I choose?

enough, or if incompatible drugs are mixed together. Also, the I.V. route increases the risk of complications, such as extravasation, vein irritation, systemic infection, and air embolism. Follow the I.V. administration guidelines in chapter 14, Intravenous administration, to help pave your way to success.

Specialized infusions

Under certain circumstances, drug infusion may take place directly at the site of intended activity. Using specialized catheters and devices, drugs and solutions can be delivered to an organ or its blood vessels to manage emergencies, treat disease, infuse tumors, or relieve pain. These infusions may be given by the epidural, intrapleural, intraperitoneal, intra-articular, or intraosseous routes. (See *Reviewing specialized infusions*, page 11.)

Pharmacokinetics

A solid understanding of *pharmacokinetics* — the movement of a drug through the body — can help you to predict your patient's response to a prescribed drug regimen and anticipate potential problems. Any time you give a drug, a series of physiochemical events takes place in the patient's body and includes four basic processes: absorption, distribution, metabolism, and excretion. (See *What happens after drug administration.*)

Absorption

Before a drug can act on the body, it must be absorbed into the bloodstream. How well a patient's body absorbs a drug depends on several factors. These include the drug's:
• physiochemical properties
• form
• route of administration
• interactions with other substances in the GI tract
• various patient characteristics, especially the site and the condition of the absorbing surface.
    These factors can also determine the speed and amount of drug absorption.

Becoming bioavailable

When taken orally, some drug forms, such as tablets or capsules, may have to disintegrate before free particles are available to dissolve in the gastric juices. Only after dissolving in these juices can

What happens after drug administration

Drug disposition begins as soon as a drug is administered. The drug proceeds through pharmacokinetic, pharmacodynamic, and pharmacotherapeutic phases. This chart shows the various phases, the activities that occur during them, and the factors that influence those activities.

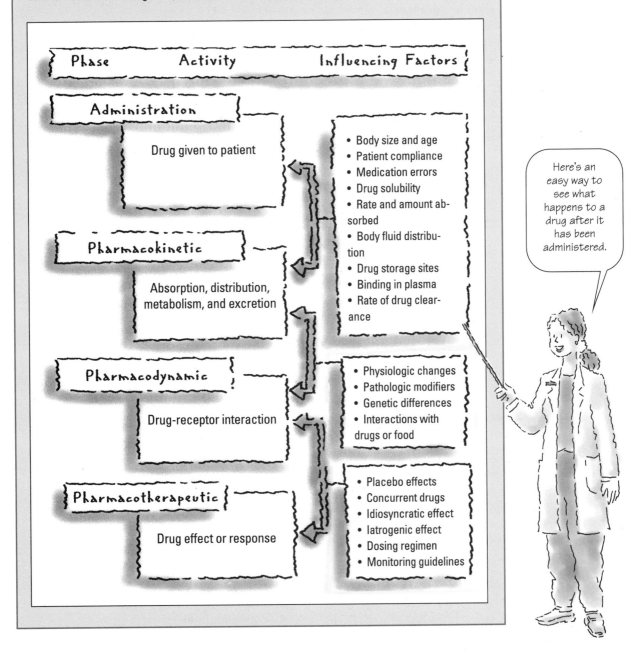

Phase	Activity	Influencing Factors
Administration	Drug given to patient	• Body size and age • Patient compliance • Medication errors • Drug solubility • Rate and amount absorbed • Body fluid distribution • Drug storage sites • Binding in plasma • Rate of drug clearance
Pharmacokinetic	Absorption, distribution, metabolism, and excretion	
Pharmacodynamic	Drug-receptor interaction	• Physiologic changes • Pathologic modifiers • Genetic differences • Interactions with drugs or food
Pharmacotherapeutic	Drug effect or response	• Placebo effects • Concurrent drugs • Idiosyncratic effect • Iatrogenic effect • Dosing regimen • Monitoring guidelines

Here's an easy way to see what happens to a drug after it has been administered.

the drug be absorbed, circulate in the bloodstream, and thus become bioavailable. A bioavailable drug is one that's ready to produce a physiologic effect.

Timing is everything

Some tablets have enteric coatings, which delay disintegration until after the tablets leave the acidic environment of the stomach. Others, such as liposome capsules, have special delivery systems that release the drug only at a specific osmotic pressure. Oral solutions and elixirs, which don't have to disintegrate and dissolve to take effect, usually are absorbed more rapidly.

If the patient has had a bowel resection, anticipate slow absorption of any oral drug you administer. And remember that a drug given I.M. must first be absorbed through the muscle before it can enter the bloodstream. Rectal suppositories must first dissolve to be absorbed through the rectal mucosa. Drugs administered I.V.—thereby placed directly into the bloodstream—are completely and immediately bioavailable.

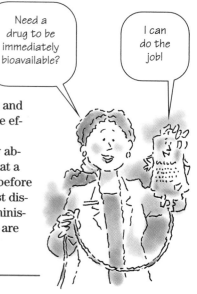

Need a drug to be immediately bioavailable?

I can do the job!

Distribution

When a drug enters the bloodstream, it's distributed to body tissues and fluids through the circulatory system. To better understand drug distribution, think of the body as a system of physiologic compartments defined by blood flow. The bloodstream and highly perfused organs—such as the brain, heart, liver, and kidneys—make up the central compartment. Lesser perfused areas form the peripheral compartment, which is subdivided into the tissue compartment (viscera, muscle, and skin) and the deep compartment (fat and bone).

Highly perfused tissues receive the drug before lesser perfused areas do. Each compartment then stores portions of the drug, releasing it as plasma drug levels decline. (See *How the body stores a drug*.)

Leaping lipid barriers

Distribution also depends partly on a drug's ability to cross lipid membranes. Some drugs can't cross certain cell membranes and thus have limited distribution. For instance, antibiotics have trouble permeating the prostate gland, abscesses, and exudates.

It's got to be free

Distribution can also be affected if the drug binds to plasma proteins, especially albumin. Only a free, unbound drug can produce an effect at the drug receptor site, so such binding greatly influences the drug's effectiveness and duration of action.

How the body stores a drug

The body can store a drug in fat, bone, or skin. Knowing the characteristics of each drug storage compartment will help you understand how distribution can affect a drug's duration of action.

Fat storage
A drug that dissolves easily in lipids migrates to adipose tissue (what we commonly think of as fatty tissue). Because this tissue lacks receptors for drug action, the drug remains inactive there. Eventually, it's released by fat cells to exert its pharmacologic effect. With some drugs, this slow, prolonged action is an advantage. For example, slow release of anesthetic barbiturates provides effective anesthesia during surgery. With other drugs, such prolonged action can be dangerous.

Bone storage
Bone acts as a storage compartment for certain drugs. Tetracycline, for example, is distributed throughout bone and may eventually crystallize there. In a growing child, this can cause tooth discoloration. Lead and some chemicals can also accumulate in bone, resulting in prolonged exposure to toxins.

Skin storage
Storage of drugs in the skin typically causes photosensitivity. Tetracycline and amiodarone are examples of drugs that are stored in the skin.

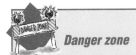

Danger zone

Dosing dilemma

Some drugs—such as digoxin, gentamicin, and tobramycin—are poorly distributed to fatty tissue. Therefore, dosing based on actual body weight in a highly obese patient may lead to overdose and serious toxicity.

Go lean
When administering such drugs, calculate the dose based on lean body weight, which you can estimate from actuarial tables that give average weight ranges for various heights.

Disease disrupts distribution

Certain diseases impede drug distribution by altering the volume of distribution—the total amount of drug in the body in relation to the amount in plasma. Heart failure, dehydration, and burns are example of such disorders. If the patient has heart failure, expect to increase the dosage because the drug must be distributed to a larger fluid volume. On the other hand, if the patient is dehydrated, expect to decrease the dosage because the drug will be distributed to a much smaller fluid volume. (See *Dosing dilemma.*)

Metabolism and excretion

Most drugs are metabolized in the liver and excreted by the kidneys. The rate at which a drug is metabolized varies with the individual. Some patients metabolize drugs so quickly that their blood and tissue levels prove therapeutically inadequate. Others metabolize drugs so slowly that even ordinary doses can produce toxic results.

Slow or fast? Here's some help...

Drug metabolism may be faster in smokers than in nonsmokers because cigarette smoke contains substances that induce production of hepatic enzymes. Also, a diet high in fat or carbohydrates may slow the metabolism of certain drugs, whereas a diet high in protein may speed metabolism.

Hepatic diseases, or diseases that interfere with hepatic blood flow or transport of drugs to the liver, may affect one or more of the liver's metabolic functions. Thus, in patients with hepatic disease, drug metabolism may be either increased or decreased. All patients with hepatic disease must be monitored closely for drug effects and toxic reactions.

The kidneys can be key

Some drugs, such as digoxin and gentamicin, are eliminated almost unchanged by the kidneys. Thus, inadequate renal function causes the drug to accumulate, producing toxic effects. Some drugs can block renal excretion of other drugs, thereby allowing them to accumulate and enhancing their effects. In contrast, some drugs can promote renal excretion of other drugs, thus diminishing their effects.

Different escape routes

Although most drugs are excreted by the kidneys, not all are. Some are excreted hepatically, via the bile and into stool. A few drugs leave the body in sweat, saliva, and breast milk. Certain volatile anesthetics—for example, halothane—are eliminated primarily by exhalation. When natural excretion mechanisms fail, as in drug overdose or renal dysfunction, many drugs can be removed through dialysis.

Underlying disease

Underlying disease can have a marked influence on drug action and effect. For example, acidosis may cause insulin resistance. Genetic diseases, such as glucose-6-phosphate dehydrogenase (G6PD) deficiency and hepatic porphyria, may turn drugs into toxins. As a result, patients with G6PD deficiency may develop hemolytic anemia when given sulfonamides or certain other drugs.

It's in your genes

A genetically susceptible patient can develop an acute porphyria attack if given a barbiturate.

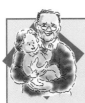

Ages and stages

Age-old influence

The patient's age has an important influence on a drug's overall action and effect. Older adults usually have decreased hepatic function, less muscle mass, and diminished renal function. Consequently, they need lower doses and sometimes longer dosage intervals to avoid toxicity.

Neonates have underdeveloped metabolic enzyme systems and inadequate renal function, which can also lead to toxicity. They need highly individualized dosages and careful monitoring.

Toxic conditions

Also, patients with highly active hepatic enzyme systems (rapid acetylators, for example) can develop hepatitis when treated with isoniazid because of the rapid intrahepatic build-up of a toxic metabolite.

Sphere of influence

Other conditions that may influence a patient's response to drug therapy include infection; fever; stress; starvation; hypersensitivity; sunlight; exercise; variations in circadian rhythm; GI, renal, hepatic, cardiovascular, and immunologic function; alcohol intake; pregnancy; lactation; immunization; and barometric pressure. (See *Age-old influence*.)

Dosage considerations

You must consider many issues when planning and monitoring a patient's dosage regimen. They include the drug's half-life; the patient's age, height, and weight; the time required to establish a steady-state dose in the patient's body; the level of drug in the patient's blood during therapy; and the degree of tolerance or dependence that develops.

Half-life

The *half-life* of a drug is the time it takes for half of the drug to be eliminated by the body. Factors that affect a drug's half-life include its rate of absorption, metabolism, and excretion. Knowing how long a drug remains in the body helps determine how frequently a drug should be taken.

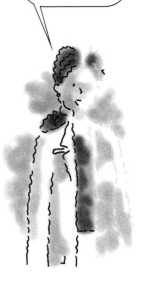

The demands on my time can make me feel like half my life has been eliminated — remember a drug's half-life is the time it takes the body to eliminate it by half.

Steady-state dosing

Doses of drugs taken at regular intervals eventually establish a steady state in the patient's body. The *steady state* is the point at which drug input equals drug output. (See *Reaching a steady state.*)

Patient characteristics

The doctor needs to know the patient's current age, weight, and height when calculating the dosage for many drugs. Body measurements should be in metric units (weight in kilograms; height in centimeters), and all data should be recorded in the patient's chart. The chart should also include current laboratory data, especially renal and liver function studies, so the doctor can adjust the dosage as needed.

Blood level

The level of drug in a patient's blood helps to indicate whether the dosing regimen has achieved its therapeutic goals. Usually, drug level is measured in plasma or serum. However, it can be measured in other fluids as well, such as cerebrospinal fluid and saliva.

Keeping things in the right range

By correlating the drug level in a patient's blood with the dosing times and the patient's response, doctors and clinical pharmacists can gain valuable information about the minimum effective concentration (MEC), the minimum toxic concentration (MTC), and the therapeutic range of a drug.

Minimally speaking

The MEC is the blood level needed for the drug to be effective in most patients. The MTC is the lowest blood level at which significant adverse reactions usually occur. The therapeutic range is bordered at the bottom by the MEC and at the top by the MTC. The time during which the blood level remains between these values is the drug's duration of action.

Longer lasting, less toxic

One goal of therapy is to extend the duration of action while avoiding the minimum toxic concentration. Regular monitoring of the patient's blood level can help. Shortly after a drug is administered, its peak level can be measured. Just before the next dose is administered, the trough (lowest) level can be measured. (See *Understanding therapeutic range.*)

Reaching a steady state

A drug that's given only once is eliminated from the body almost completely after five half-lives. A drug that's administered at regular intervals, however, reaches a steady concentration (or steady state) after about five half-lives. Steady state occurs when the rate of drug administration equals the rate of drug excretion.

Understanding therapeutic range

The minimum effective concentration (MEC) and the minimum toxic concentration (MTC) represent the lower and upper borders of the therapeutic range. The graph below shows peak and trough drug levels and how they relate to drug administration and therapeutic range. The time when the curve remains between the MEC and the MTC represents the drug's duration of action. Determining a drug's blood level helps the doctor and pharmacist make drug therapy decisions.

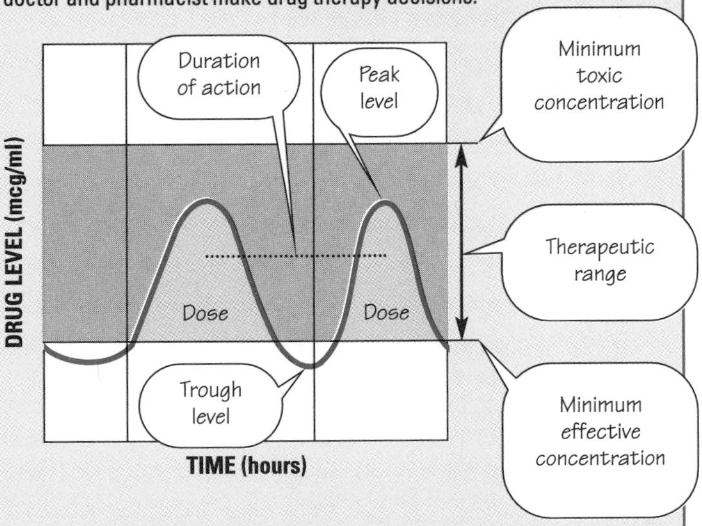

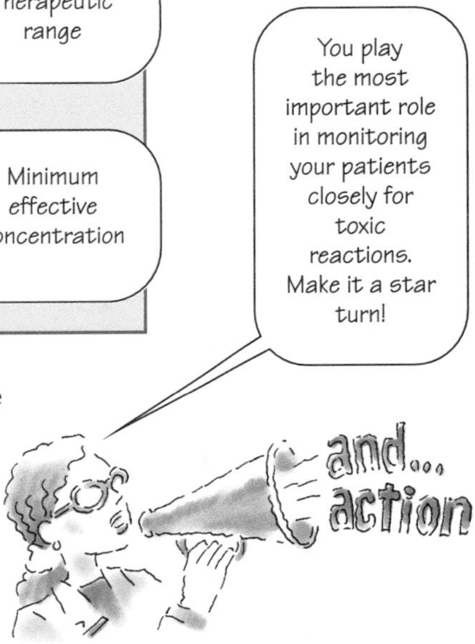

DRUG LEVEL (mcg/ml)

Duration of action

Peak level

Minimum toxic concentration

Therapeutic range

Dose

Dose

Trough level

Minimum effective concentration

TIME (hours)

You play the most important role in monitoring your patients closely for toxic reactions. Make it a star turn!

For many drugs, the blood level correlates with the anticipated therapeutic response. However, because commercial assay methods aren't available for most drugs, you play a critical role in monitoring patients for toxic reactions.

and...
action

Tolerance and dependence

Tolerance refers to a patient's decreased response to a repeated drug dose. It differs from *dependence*, which refers to a patient's physical or psychological need for a drug. For example, an alcohol-dependent patient not only needs increasing quantities of alcohol to achieve the same effects (tolerance), he also risks physical and psychological withdrawal symptoms if he stops using alcohol (dependence).

Hasn't got time for the pain

A patient with cancer who receives a narcotic analgesic for severe pain can develop tolerance and dependence. However, the psychological aspects differ from those of the substance abuser. The patient with cancer is usually concerned with maintaining a reasonable level of pain relief, whereas the substance abuser seeks the euphoric effects of the drug.

Administration considerations

Many practical aspects of drug administration influence the effectiveness of prescribed therapy, such as:
- the form of a drug
- its route of administration
- the timing of administration
- proper storage.

Drug form

Some tablets and capsules are too large to be swallowed easily by patients who are seriously ill. For these patients, request an oral solution or elixir of the drug. Remember, however, that a liquid form is more easily and completely absorbed than a tablet, so it produces higher blood levels than a tablet.

A change for the better

If you're giving a drug known to cause toxic reactions (such as digoxin), the increased amount absorbed from its liquid form could cause toxicity. Always ask the prescriber or a pharmacist whether a change in drug form requires a change in dosage. (See *Major administration routes and drug forms.*)

> Remember the liquid form of a drug produces higher blood levels than a tablet.

Administration route

Routes of administration aren't therapeutically interchangeable. For example, phenytoin is readily absorbed orally but slowly and erratically absorbed when given I.M. In contrast, vancomycin must be given parenterally because oral administration yields inadequate blood levels for treating systemic infections. However, it can be given orally to treat antibiotic-associated pseudomembranous colitis because it concentrates in stool.

Major administration routes and drug forms

The table below shows the major administration routes and the drug forms available for each.

Route	Form	Route	Form
Oral (solid)	Capsule Powder Tablet	Vaginal	Foam Gel Solution Suppository Tablet
Oral (liquid)	Elixir Emulsion Solution Suspension Syrup	Topical (ear, eye, nose, skin)	Aerosol Cream Lotion Ointment
Parenteral	Solution		Paste Patch
Rectal	Solution Suppository		Powder

Timing

Sometimes giving an oral drug during or shortly after a meal decreases the amount of drug absorbed. This decrease isn't clinically significant with most drugs and may in fact be helpful with irritating drugs, such as aspirin or ibuprofen. However, many penicillins and tetracyclines shouldn't be scheduled for administration at mealtimes because certain foods can inactivate them. If you're in doubt about the effect of food on a certain drug, consult a pharmacist.

Storage

Storing a drug improperly can alter its potency. Most drugs should be stored in tightly capped containers and protected from direct sunlight and extremes of temperature and humidity, which can cause them to deteriorate. Some may require special storage conditions such as refrigeration.

Pharmacodynamics

Pharmacodynamics is the study of the interactions between drugs and living tissues and serves as the basis of drug treatment. The pharmacodynamic phase of drug administration encompasses both drug action and drug effect.

Drug action

After absorption, drug molecules migrate to target tissues or organs, interacting with receptors to cause the drug action. After this series of complex physical or chemical reactions, the drug action in turn alters the function of the target cell, causing the drug effect. Depending on the range of cellular receptors affected by a drug, its effects can be local, systemic, or both.

Think local...

Local drug effects are specific to a limited number of receptors. For example, famotidine—a drug given for peptic ulcers—acts solely by blocking histamine receptors in the parietal cells of the stomach, thus limiting drug action and effect to one area of the body.

...act global

In contrast, a systemic drug effect is generalized and affects diverse organ systems. For example, diphenhydramine also blocks histamine receptors, but it does so throughout the body. A systemic drug effect may be the desired therapeutic response, or it may be an adverse reaction.

Drug-receptor interactions

Each drug is selectively active and attracted to a specific receptor within the body. A certain portion of the drug molecule interacts or combines with the receptor to produce a pharmacologic effect. Although a drug can't force a cell or tissue to assume a new function, it can modify the cell's function or environment in a way that interrupts, replaces, or potentiates a physiologic process.

Copycats

Some drugs interact with receptors or enzymes to alter cell function. The drug can either agonize or antagonize the receptor site.

An agonist mimics the activity of the hormone or other natural chemical that normally binds to the receptor site. This brings about the drug's effect.

Binding and blocking

In contrast, an antagonist drug binds to a receptor, thereby preventing binding by other molecules. For example, acetylcholine receptor blockers, such as atropine, are antagonists because they prevent the access of acetylcholine to the acetylcholine receptor. This results in reduced effects of acetylcholine.

Engaging with enzymes

A drug may also interact with enzymes to stimulate or depress certain biochemical reactions. For example, neostigmine, which is used to treat myasthenia gravis, interacts with the enzyme acetylcholinesterase to prevent acetylcholine destruction. Thus, acetylcholine accumulates in the tissues, thereby enhancing cell activity and increasing gastric contractions and gastric acid secretion.

Enzymes enhance our activity.

A more general approach

Some drugs lack structural specificity; that is, they act through general effects on cellular membranes and processes. By penetrating cells or accumulating in cell membranes, these drugs interfere physically or chemically with either a cell's function or its basic metabolism.

Typically, such drugs alter a cell's physical or chemical environment to produce a systemic effect. For instance, if you administer sodium bicarbonate I.V. to a patient with severe diabetic ketoacidosis, the drug alters the cellular environment by restoring normal pH. This change, in turn, improves cell function. Other drugs that act nonspecifically on the cell environment include osmotic diuretics, stool softeners, skin protectants, cathartics, plasma expanders, and chemical antidotes.

Outcome of drug action

The location and function of a drug's receptors determine the outcome of drug action. Drugs that interact with common receptors throughout the body have widespread effects, as in chemotherapy. Obviously, this poses a danger if the drug causes a toxic reaction.

On the other hand, drugs that interact with specific receptors in highly differentiated cells (cells that physically and functionally change as they form different body structures, such as nerve and muscle cells) produce a safe, predictable response. For example, controlled doses of radioactive iodine, which has a strong affinity for receptor sites in the thyroid gland, effectively treat hyperthyroidism.

Scoring direct hits or exerting influence

The outcome of drug action also depends on whether the drug affects target organs and tissues directly or indirectly. Theophylline, which is used to treat asthma, directly modifies bronchodilator receptors in the lungs to improve ventilation. Such a direct effect promotes a rapid clinical response.

In contrast, levodopa exerts an indirect action on tissues. A dopamine precursor, it breaks down into dopamine after crossing the blood-brain barrier. To slow the peripheral breakdown of levodopa and increase its availability for transport to the brain, the doctor may prescribe it in combination with carbidopa. Although effective, this approach produces a slower therapeutic response than would result if dopamine could be supplied directly.

Dose-response relationship

Drug levels at the receptor site also affect the outcome of drug action. The patient's response to a particular drug reflects the size of the administered dose. Typically, as the dose increases, the pharmacologic response increases gradually and continuously until receptor sites become fully occupied by the drug. At this point, increasing the dose won't enhance the response, but it will increase the risk of adverse reactions.

It can be a relative relationship

Because all drugs can elicit more than one response, the dose-response relationship isn't an absolute. In small doses, for example, morphine may calm an irritable bowel. In larger doses, it acts as an opioid analgesic. Furthermore, adverse reactions can occur with therapeutic doses. For example, in some patients, morphine can cause respiratory depression when given in doses large enough to effectively control pain.

> Administering drugs is a balancing act. To get the desired response, know the proper dose.

Drug potency and efficacy

A drug's action also depends on its potency and efficacy. *Potency* refers to the amount of drug needed to produce a desired response. By comparing the required doses of two comparable drugs, you can determine which one is more potent. For example, when giving tetracycline, you need to administer 1,000 to 2,000 mg/day to achieve a therapeutic effect, compared with just 100 to 200 mg/day of doxycycline. Because doxycycline achieves comparable effects at a lower dosage, it's considered more potent.

Efficacy refers to the effect achieved when the dose-response curve reaches its plateau. For example, at its plateau, morphine relieves a greater degree of pain than aspirin does. To assess a drug's efficacy, however, you must also consider the occurrence and severity of adverse reactions. A drug that's likely to cause severe adverse reactions before reaching its plateau has reduced efficacy. Efficacy also decreases if the plateau falls short of the maximum drug amount needed for effective treatment.

Adverse reactions

As you know, an adverse reaction is an undesirable or harmful response to a drug that can occur in any patient. It can range from a mild reaction that disappears when the drug is withdrawn to a severe reaction that progresses to a chronic, debilitating disease — or death. The patient's response to a given drug and his risk for adverse reactions depend on many factors.

Adverse reactions can be predictable or unpredictable. Predictable reactions are usually dose related; unpredictable reactions typically result from patient sensitivity. Although some predictable reactions can be prevented, others can't be prevented because they're closely tied to the drug's therapeutic effects.

You should see these coming

Administering an excessive drug dose can cause one of two types of predictable reactions — an excessive therapeutic effect or drug accumulation. An excessive therapeutic effect usually occurs with drugs that require precise, individualized dose calculations. For example, a patient with diabetes who receives too much insulin will have an excessive drop in blood glucose level. Accumulation can occur with certain chemotherapeutic drugs. If these drugs accumulate around hair follicles, they can damage the follicles, causing alopecia (hair loss).

Giving a drug too rapidly can also cause predictable adverse reactions. For example, rapid administration of I.V. aminophylline can cause hypotension and circulatory collapse.

Second to none

Most drugs produce a secondary pharmacologic action in addition to a therapeutic effect. In some cases, this secondary action is an undesirable but predictable adverse reaction. For example, morphine may help control a patient's pain, but it may also cause constipation and respiratory depression. Occasionally, a doctor prescribes a drug specifically for its secondary action. For example, minoxidil is used mainly as an antihypertensive, but it may be prescribed in topical form to treat alopecia.

Give too high a dose? I see adverse reactions in your patient's future!

Patients can be full of surprises

When first exposed to a drug, a patient's immune system may identify the drug, its metabolite, or a drug contaminant as a dangerous foreign substance that must be neutralized or destroyed. This initial exposure sensitizes the immune system, which then mobilizes to fight the drug if the patient receives another dose of the same or a similar substance. If that happens, the patient has a hypersensitivity reaction.

This unpredictable adverse reaction is a type of allergic reaction. Allergic reactions range in severity from mild (type IV hypersensitivity) to life-threatening (type I hypersensitivity). Mild allergic reactions include contact dermatitis, as from a topical medication; life-threatening reactions include anaphylactic shock, as from penicillin.

Even more surprising

Another type of unpredictable reaction occurs in patients who are highly susceptible to a drug's primary or secondary actions. Such increased susceptibility may stem from altered pharmacokinetics, which leads to an excessively high serum level or increased receptor sensitivity. In these patients, even a normal therapeutic dose may trigger an adverse reaction.

Idiosyncratic reactions are also unpredictable. For example, phenobarbital, a sedative-hypnotic, may cause nervousness and excitability in some patients. Idiosyncratic reactions may have a genetic basis.

Iatrogenic reactions

Sometimes a drug produces an iatrogenic reaction—a disorder unrelated to the condition for which the drug was given. The reaction may be predictable or unpredictable. Typically, it involves a blood dyscrasia, liver or kidney dysfunction, or a skin condition. In a pregnant patient, it may cause teratogenic (physical defects caused in utero) changes in the fetus.

Making the wrong call

Misdiagnosis is a potentially serious consequence of an iatrogenic reaction. When confronted with the new disorder, the doctor may mistakenly treat it instead of stopping the drug.

Drug interactions

Some drugs interact when given together, neutralizing their therapeutic effects or causing an adverse reaction. (See *Types of drug interactions.*) Other drugs can interact with certain foods or alter

Types of drug interactions

Several types of drug interactions can occur, including indifference, additive, synergistic, and antagonistic. To lower the patient's risk of these drug interactions, make sure you know all of the drugs he's receiving, including herbal and over-the-counter drugs.

Interaction	Characteristics
Indifference	• This is the most common type of drug interaction. • Both drugs promote the action of the most active component of the combination. • Interaction doesn't alter the therapeutic effect of either drug or produce unpredictable adverse effects.
Additive interaction	• The total effect of the two drugs together equals the sum of the drugs' separate effects. • Some additive interactions are intended and desirable; for instance, aspirin and codeine may be prescribed together to enhance pain relief. • Unplanned additive interactions can have adverse effects, causing extreme sedation or other dangerous conditions.
Synergistic interaction	• One drug increases the other's effects, causing a total effect greater than the sum of the drugs' separate effects. • Like an additive interaction, synergism can be beneficial or harmful.
Antagonistic interaction	• One drug interferes with the other's actions, negating its therapeutic value. • An example is levodopa and pyridoxine (vitamin B_6) administered simultaneously; normally, levodopa reduces stiffness, rigidity, and other symptoms of Parkinson's disease, but because pyridoxine antagonizes it, the patient may not receive levodopa's therapeutic actions.

the results of laboratory tests. Interactions involving I.V. drugs can present their own unique problems.

Make a list...and check it twice!

To reduce the risk of interactions, find out if the patient is taking other drugs — prescribed, over-the-counter, or herbal — before you give a new one. These also include:
• home remedies
• nonprescription drugs
• vitamin and mineral supplements
• medicines borrowed from family members or others
• recreational drugs (must be specifically addressed).

Be especially careful when giving drugs to an older adult. Many older patients take multiple drugs, and their age makes them more sensitive to drug effects. As a safeguard, make it a habit during the initial health history to ask the patient which drugs, nutritional supplements, and herbal remedies he's taking.

Food for thought

Food can delay or reduce the absorption of an oral drug, thereby reducing its therapeutic effects. With acidic foods, however, the food enhances drug absorption by stimulating gastric acid secretion.

By the same token, some drugs can alter the metabolism of nutrients in food. For instance, a drug taken with a certain food may bind with the food and impair vitamin and mineral absorption.

Lab test interference

Certain drugs can cause misleading laboratory test results. For example, the calorimetric method used to measure serum creatinine levels can't differentiate between creatinine and a noncreatinine chromogen contained in many cephalosporins, such as cefazolin and cefoxitin. Therefore, if the patient is receiving a cephalosporin, you should stay alert for a falsely elevated creatinine level.

Similarly, iron supplements can skew the results of stool guaiac tests, and ascorbic acid can cause inaccurate urine glucose test results.

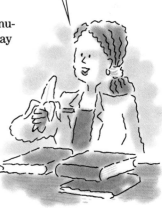

Food can interact with the drugs you administer as much as other drugs can.

I.V. drug incompatibility

Mixing incompatible I.V. drugs can cause undesired physical or chemical reactions or can interfere with the pharmacologic action of one or both drugs.

Flush first before switching drugs

Color changes, gas formation, cloudiness, or precipitation can result. One drug may inactivate the other; worse yet, the drugs may interact in a way that harms the patient. That's why you must always flush the line with normal saline solution before and after infusing many drugs.

Stop that reaction

To avoid I.V. drug incompatibility, don't combine drugs you're not sure you can combine safely. Also, before you give an unfamiliar drug or drug combination, consult a pharmacist or the manufacturer's recommendations. For general guidelines, check a drug compatibility chart.

If the patient's I.V. fluid contains multivitamins or other additives, confirm compatibility before administering drugs through the same line. If you can't easily access the patient's peripheral veins, consider asking the doctor to place a central line or to replace the peripheral line with a multi-lumen catheter so you can administer incompatible drugs simultaneously.

By following these recommendations and using careful practice methods based on sound knowledge, you can provide safe, effective drug administration for the patients who are relying on you.

Adsorption

Some I.V. drugs adhere to plastic containers, syringes, and administration sets. This adherence, known as adsorption, can reduce drug availability or cause precipitation. Diazepam, for instance, forms a precipitate after prolonged contact with polyvinyl chloride infusion sets. For this reason, you should administer I.V. diazepam directly into a large vein. If that isn't feasible, administer it by slow injection through a running I.V. line. Use the port closest to the I.V. insertion site.

Photolysis

Some I.V. drugs are discolored when exposed to light. The change doesn't always reflect chemical breakdown, but you should consult a pharmacist before administering a drug that has changed color.

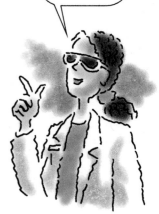

Want to hear a bright idea? If the I.V. drug you're about to give is discolored, consult a pharmacist first.

Quick quiz

1.   Which type of drug interaction occurs when one drug increases the other's effect, causing a total effect greater than the sum of the drugs' separate effects?
    A.   Antagonistic interaction
    B.   Additive interaction
    C.   Synergistic interaction
    D.   Adverse reaction

Answer: C. A synergistic interaction occurs when one drug increases the other drug's effects. This interaction results in a total effect that's greater than the sum of the drugs' separate effects.

2. Which branch of pharmacology deals with the study of interactions between drugs and living tissues and serves as the basis of drug treatment?

    A.   Pharmacokinetics
    B.   Pharmacodynamics
    C.   Steady-state dosing
    D.   Bioavailability

Answer: B. Pharmacodynamics is the study of the interactions between drugs and living tissues and serves as the basis of drug treatment. It encompasses drug action and drug effect.

3. Which administration route requires you to inject a small amount of a drug beneath the dermis?

    A.   Intradermal route
    B.   Topical route
    C.   I.M. route
    D.   S.C. route

Answer: D. When using the S.C. route, you inject small amounts of a drug beneath the dermis and into the subcutaneous tissue.

4. You're caring for a patient who is experiencing a decreased response to pain medication. This patient is most likely experiencing:

    A.   tolerance.
    B.   addiction.
    C.   dependence.
    D.   drug-receptor interaction.

Answer: A. Drug tolerance refers to a patient's decreased response to a repeated drug dose.

Scoring

★★★ If you answered all four questions correctly, excellent! You're on the route to greatness!

★★ If you answered two or three correctly, you're getting the essentials! You used the key concepts to unlock the door to understanding!

★ If you answered fewer than two correctly, don't worry! Go back and review this chapter, and soon you'll be pharmaco-dynamite!

2

Applying the nursing process

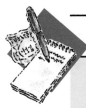

Just the facts

In this chapter, you'll learn how to:

♦ assess your patient before medication administration

♦ form nursing diagnoses for drug-related problems

♦ plan outcome criteria and interventions

♦ implement the nursing process for drug administration

♦ evaluate the patient's response to drug therapy.

Putting the nursing process into action

Administering medications safely and accurately is a complex process that requires technical competence, sound judgment, critical thinking, and meticulous attention to detail. If you administer a drug incorrectly, you could harm or even kill a patient.

Stepping up to success

That's why you need to follow the nursing process any time you administer a drug regimen. This five-step system promotes:
- thorough assessment
- appropriate nursing diagnoses
- effective planning
- thoughtful interventions
- continual evaluation.

Using this systematic approach to guide your nursing decisions helps to ensure accuracy and therapeutic success each time you deliver a drug.

Assessment

When preparing to administer a drug, you'll first need to assess the patient. Naturally, if you're responding to an emergency, your assessment will be brief, possibly involving no more than checking the patient's allergies. Typically, however, you'll want to collect a range of important information in your assessment.

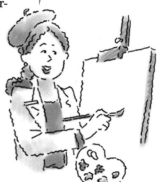

Paint a complete picture of your patient — include medical history, allergies, drug history, socioeconomic status, sensory and cognitive barriers, and clinical status.

Your mission begins after admission

In general, you'll start collecting assessment data right away — just after admission. Gather subjective and objective data so you can build a comprehensive, pertinent picture of the patient's condition. Doing so will verify the accuracy of any drug orders, and will also allow you to evaluate the patient's response to drug therapy.

Whenever possible, obtain your assessment information directly from the patient. When necessary, you can also obtain information from a family member or close friend. In addition, remember to check the patient's previous medical records for pertinent information.

Details, details, details

Your assessment should include details about the patient's medical history, allergies, drug history, socioeconomic status, sensory and cognitive barriers, and clinical status. Ask specific questions about the patient's background and current condition. To assess the patient's clinical status, perform a physical examination and review relevant laboratory or diagnostic test results.

Medical history

When investigating the patient's medical history, note chronic diseases or disorders he reports; for each one, record the:
- date of diagnosis
- initial prescribed treatment
- current treatment
- treating doctor.

Allergies

Next, find out whether the patient has any allergies to drugs, foods, or other substances. For drug allergies, make sure you record:
- the drug involved
- the patient's description of the reaction he had to it

- how, when, and where the reaction occurred
- factors that might have contributed to the reaction, such as tobacco, alcohol, stimulants, illicit drugs, or a change in diet.

This gives the patient's doctor and other health care providers the information they need to assess and maintain the patient's safety when ordering and administering drugs.

Allergy or fallacy?

As the patient describes what he considers to be an "allergic" reaction, listen carefully. Is he describing a true drug allergy? Did he develop such common signs as a rash, itching, tightness in his chest, or trouble breathing? If not, then he may not have had an allergic reaction but an adverse drug effect or a drug interaction. Or perhaps he simply disliked the drug's intended effects.

Don't forget food

Make sure to ask about food allergies as well because they may affect the patient's drug therapy. For example, an allergy to shellfish may affect the use of contrast agents or other drugs that contain iodine or shellfish by-products. They may be contraindicated, or the patient may need to be premedicated with an antihistamine. Likewise, an allergy to eggs may affect the use of vaccines, which commonly contain components derived from chick embryos. (See *Food interference*.)

Drug history

Next, gather as much information as possible about drugs the patient currently takes. Whenever possible, ask open-ended questions about his drug history. Doing so allows the patient to provide information in his words — information that closed-ended questions might overlook. (See *Elements of a drug history*, page 34.)

Make sure to include questions about over-the-counter (OTC) drugs, herbal remedies, weight-loss formulas, and prescription drugs in your assessment. Also, ask about lifestyle drugs, such as alcohol and caffeine, and about aspects of the patient's diet that could affect his drug therapy. Do your best to find out whether the patient uses illegal drugs as well. As you gather information about the patient's drug use, assess his cognitive status and his ability to adequately carry out a therapeutic drug regimen.

Get it on record

For each prescription and OTC drug the patient takes, record the following information:
- his reason for using the drug
- his understanding of the prescribed dosage

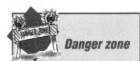

Danger zone

Food interference

Even foods can alter the effects of some prescribed medications. For example, if the patient takes warfarin, he shouldn't vary the amount of green, leafy vegetables he normally eats. Vitamin K reduces the anticoagulation effect of warfarin by increasing the synthesis of clotting factors. Therefore, it's important to teach the patient to maintain a consistent daily intake of green, leafy vegetables.

Elements of a drug history

When taking a drug history, be sure to include the following details.

General data

Allergies	• Drugs • Foods
Medical history	• Previous illnesses • Current illnesses
Habits	• Diet • Tobacco • Stimulants such as caffeine • Illegal drugs
Socioeconomic characteristics	• Age • Educational level • Occupation • Health insurance • Lifestyle and beliefs • Ethnic, cultural, racial background • Support systems • Marital status • Childbearing status • Attitudes toward health and health care • Use of the health care system • Pattern of daily activities
Sensory and cognitive barriers	• Senses of vision, hearing, touch • Memory and orientation

Drug data

General	• Prescription and over-the-counter drugs and supplements • Knowledge of drugs taken
Prescription	• Reasons for use • Dosages • Pattern and route of administration • Effectiveness and adverse effects
Over-the-counter (including herbal preparations)	• Reasons for use • Frequency of use • Effectiveness and adverse effects

No place like home

Assessing a patient's monitoring performance

If the patient is responsible for performing a special monitoring procedure as part of his drug therapy, make sure you assess his ability to do it correctly. For example, if he has diabetes, make sure he knows when and how to check his blood glucose levels. If he takes digoxin, make sure he can take his radial pulse accurately. And if he takes warfarin, make sure he knows how, where, and when to have his clotting time checked.

Ensuring success
By assessing the patient's ability to perform these important tasks—and by making sure the results are within acceptable limits—you can help ensure the success of his drug therapy.

- how he determines the drug's effectiveness (if appropriate)
- the route by which he takes the drug
- the schedule he uses to take the drug
- what the patient knows about, and how he responds to, adverse effects caused by the drug
- the patient's understanding about drug-related problems for which he should contact his doctor.

Prescription drugs

When talking with the patient about his prescription drugs, discuss the effects that his drug therapy has on him, and find out whether new symptoms or unexpected adverse reactions have developed. Make special note of the patient's pattern of drug administration and monitoring procedures he's supposed to perform; this may offer insight into why a drug regimen may not be yielding the expected result. (See *Assessing a patient's monitoring performance.*)

Uncovering conflict

Careful attention to the patient's medical history can uncover one of the most important problems with drug therapy—conflicting and incompatible drug regimens. The risk of this problem is especially high if the patient doesn't have a family doctor to oversee and coordinate his care. Instead, if he sees several specialists for several different health problems, one doctor may prescribe a regimen that's incompatible with an existing regimen already prescribed by another doctor—and never know about the conflict.

> Are conflicting drug therapies using your patient as a boxing ring? Stop the fight!

Pharm aid

Besides reviewing all of the problems for which the patient sees different doctors—and making note of the drugs they've prescribed—ask the patient where he has his prescriptions filled. Chances are, even if he sees several doctors, he gets all his medications from one pharmacist. By contacting that pharmacist, you may be able to obtain a detailed list of drugs the patient takes, even though several different doctors have prescribed them.

If your assessment uncovers what you believe to be conflicting or overlapping drug regimens, you'll need to notify the doctors involved. Then, take time to teach the patient about the importance of sharing all of his drug information with all of his prescribers.

Over-the-counter drugs

A comprehensive drug history should also include questions about all OTC drugs the patient takes. Many OTC drugs can alter the effects of prescribed drugs. For example, aspirin potentiates the anticoagulant effects of warfarin.

Under-standing what's over-the-counter

Keep in mind that OTC drugs include a wide range of products, including:
- analgesics
- nutritional supplements
- herbal remedies (see *Heads up for herbal interactions*)
- homeopathic remedies
- various sprays and cleaning agents—for example, contact lens disinfectants.

The patient may not think of these as drugs, so you may need to name some categories of drug products to prompt him to give you complete and accurate information.

How much?

Dosage and frequency of use may be just as important as the type of OTC product the patient takes. For instance, one aspirin tablet taken once daily may have no effect on concomitant drug therapy; however, a higher dosage (such as that used for arthritis) could profoundly influence therapy.

Recreational drugs

Carefully consider the patient's use of nontherapeutic drugs, including:
- alcohol
- tobacco
- caffeine

Danger zone

Heads up for herbal interactions

Some herbal remedies may exert druglike effects that can interact with the patient's prescribed medications. Below are some herbal interactions to watch for.

Herb	Possible effects
Aloe	Increased digoxin effects
Arnica	Decreased antihypertensive effects
Bee pollen	Decreased hypoglycemic effects
Black cohosh	Increased antihypertensive effects
Capsicum	Decreased antihypertensive effects and toxic reaction with monoamine oxidase (MAO) inhibitors
Cat's claw	Increased anticoagulant and antihypertensive effects
Chamomile	Increased anticoagulant effects
Chondroitin	Increased anticoagulant effects
Dandelion	Increased antihypertensive, diuretic, and hypoglycemic effects
Garlic	Increased anticoagulant effects
Ginger	Increased anticoagulant effects
Ginkgo	Increased anticoagulant effects
Ginseng	Increased hypoglycemic effects and toxic reaction with MAO inhibitors
Goldenseal	Increased antihypertensive and digoxin effects
Kava	Increased central nervous system (CNS) depressant effects
Lavender	Increased CNS depressant effects
Melatonin	Increased hypoglycemic effects
St. John's wort	Increased digoxin effects
Yohimbe	Increased antidepressant and sedative effects

Watch out for these herbs in combination with prescription drugs.

- marijuana
- cocaine
- heroin.

These drugs can profoundly influence the patient's health — and the effects of prescribed drug therapy.

Collecting the facts

If the patient uses alcohol, note the frequency of use, the amount consumed each day, and the type consumed. Document the intake of stimulants, such as caffeine, because they significantly affect the cardiovascular and nervous systems. Record the type of stimulant used, the frequency of intake, and the amount consumed.

If the patient uses tobacco, document:
- the number of years he has used it
- the kind of tobacco he smokes (cigarettes, cigars, or a pipe) or chews
- the quantity of cigarettes, cigars, pipe tobacco, or chewing tobacco he uses each day
- the brand of tobacco he smokes or chews.

Encouraging honesty

You may have difficulty soliciting information from the patient about the use of illegal drugs. Be sure you ask about it in a nonthreatening, nonjudgmental manner. If you suspect that the patient may use these drugs, encourage him to discuss it honestly, emphasizing that these drugs have profound effects that may result in serious drug interactions. If the patient admits to using an illegal drug, you should document the drug used, the amount and frequency of use, and the route of administration.

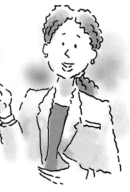

Illegal drug use is a difficult subject. Be sure to use a nonjudgmental approach.

Socioeconomic status

Note the patient's age, educational level, occupation, and insurance coverage. These characteristics may play a significant role in his ability to understand, comply with, and provide feedback about a therapeutic drug regimen. The patient's age also suggests whether you should include other people in your care plan, such as parents or other family members, and the appropriate intellectual level at which to teach the patient.

Knowing the patient's educational background and occupation may help you select appropriate interventions, plan a drug regimen that fits his daily routine, and devise methods to enhance compliance. The patient's insurance status may help you anticipate the need for financial assistance and counseling. Keep in mind that a lack of money is a common reason for noncompliance with drug therapy. (See *Noncompliance in elderly patients*.)

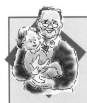

Ages and stages

Noncompliance in elderly patients

For many older patients, the most crucial aspect of drug therapy is compliance. Noncompliance in older patients is so prevalent that most nurses consider it a top priority when planning nursing care. Convincing an older patient to follow a drug regimen faithfully can be quite a challenge.

Reasons for noncompliance
Keep in mind that older patients may have many reasons for noncompliance:
• Financial limitations can make it difficult or impossible for patients to pay for their medications.
• Sensory changes, such as poor vision or declining motor abilities, can make it hard for them to physically manage drug therapy.
• Cognitive changes (such as memory dysfunction) can make it easy for the patient to forget his medication.
• Psychological obstacles—for example, a belief that medications indicate frailty or sickness—can make the patient less willing to cooperate with prescribed therapy.
• Adverse reactions can make it harder for the patient to feel comfortable taking his medication.

Compounding the problem
Naturally, the danger is that noncompliance will render a treatment unsuccessful. The doctor may then increase the drug dose or prescribe an additional drug, which only compounds the risk of adverse reactions.

Bring the patient's background to the foreground

Evaluate other aspects of the patient's life that could influence the success of his drug therapy, such as his support systems, marital status, childbearing status, attitudes toward health and health care, use of the health care system, and daily activity patterns.

For example, an 18-year-old single parent who dropped out of high school, is currently on medical assistance, and has no family support will require more teaching and support to achieve compliance than a 40-year-old affluent professional who has family support, can understand why he needs a drug, and can readily pay for it.

Sensory and cognitive barriers

As you assess the patient, pay attention to sensory or cognitive problems that could affect his drug therapy. For example, impaired vision could raise the risk that he'll take the wrong drug or wrong dosage. Impaired sensation in his fingers could interfere with his ability to break a scored tablet or open a medicine bottle. Impaired hearing could keep him from understanding your instructions.

The patient's cognitive abilities directly influence his ability to understand his drug therapy and to take the actions needed for compliance. During your interview, note whether he's alert and oriented and interacts appropriately. Can he think clearly and express his thoughts coherently? Check his short-term and long-term memory. He'll need both to follow a specified drug regimen.

Is it time to call a team meeting?

If you determine that the patient has a cognitive deficit, assess whether he'll be able to carry out the prescribed drug regimen. If not, you'll need to work with the patient's care team to implement other arrangements to ensure that he receives the prescribed therapy.

Clinical status

After completing the patient history, perform a physical examination to assess body systems that may be affected by a drug the patient is taking. Every drug affects at least one body system.

Good intentions, bad reactions

Typically, the effect represents the prescribed action of the drug, but sometimes a drug may affect the intended body system or another body system in adverse ways. For example, chemotherapy drugs destroy cancer cells, but they also affect normal cells. As a result, patients may lose their hair or develop nausea, diarrhea, or both. Thus, you'll want to examine the patient not only for the influence of intended drug effects, but also for known adverse reactions.

What's next?

After you've identified patient problems in your physical assessment, you'll use this information to plan and implement interventions aimed at resolving the problem and preventing complications related to the problem. For example, a plan for your patient with diarrhea will probably include pharmacologic interventions such as the administration of an antidiarrheal agent like Imodium, along with a clear liquid diet to prevent dehydration and electrolyte imbalances secondary to diarrhea.

Testing — one, two, three

Don't forget to check the patient's laboratory and diagnostic test results before and after drug therapy begins. Data compiled before the patient begins taking a drug give you valuable baseline information. Data gathered during and after therapy can help you evaluate the effects — and the success — of therapy. For example, if the patient has an infection, baseline tests will reveal a high white blood cell (WBC) count. After antibiotic therapy, however, the same tests will show the WBC count declining and eventually returning to normal. Diagnostic tests can help you pinpoint adverse drug effects as well.

Nursing diagnosis

Using information gathered during your assessment, your next step is to write one or more nursing diagnoses for each potential or actual drug-related problem you discovered. Nursing diagnoses provide a common language to convey the nursing care plan the patient needs.

Communicating clearly

To enhance communication among all nurses using nursing diagnoses, the North American Nursing Diagnosis Association (commonly called NANDA) has developed and sanctioned a set of nursing diagnosis labels based on human response patterns. When you create a nursing diagnosis for the patient, you do so by analyzing the data you collected, identifying the patient's specific signs or symptoms (defining characteristics), and determining the probable cause of those signs or symptoms (related factors or risk factors). (See *Writing a nursing diagnosis*, page 42.)

Planning

Nursing diagnoses provide the framework for planning outcome criteria (patient goals) and interventions. Outcome criteria express the desired patient behaviors or responses that should result from nursing care. It should be patient-centered, measurable, objective, concise, realistic, and attainable through nursing management and also express expectations of patient behavior that will occur over a specific time frame. (See *Writing outcome criteria*, page 43.)

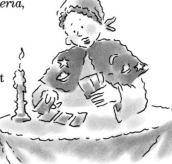

You don't need to see the future to write outcome criteria. Make it measurable, objective, and realistic.

Achieving your patient goals

After you develop outcome criteria for the patient, your next step is to identify interventions needed to help him reach the desired behavior or goals. Nursing interventions can be classified as:
• dependent—dictated by doctors' orders involving drugs, treatments, activity levels, diet, and so on

Writing a nursing diagnosis

To write a nursing diagnosis, consider the patient's signs and symptoms (defining characteristics), the probable cause of those characteristics (related factors or risk factors), and the diagnostic label that best fits your findings.

A case of noncompliance

Taking a noncompliant patient as an example, you would write the following:

Defining characteristics

The noncompliant patient typically has defining characteristics that include:
• behavior that indicates failure to follow a regimen, supported by direct observation or a statement by the patient or an informed observer
• failure on objective tests
• evidence of the development of complications
• worsening of symptoms
• failure to keep appointments
• failure to progress
• inability to set or maintain mutual goals.

Related factors

The noncompliant patient typically has related factors that include:
• lack of knowledge
• lack of necessary resources
• denial of a health problem
• misinterpretation of information
• belief that treatment measures are ineffective or unnecessary.

Diagnostic label

Based on these traits, an appropriate nursing diagnosis is: *Noncompliance, failure to keep appointment related to lack of necessary resources.*

• independent—based on the nursing process and professional judgment
• interdependent—actions you perform in collaboration with other health care professionals, such as physical therapists, social workers, dietitians, and doctors.

Administering a prescribed drug on time is a dependent intervention. Altering a drug schedule to accommodate a patient's daily routine is an independent intervention. Asking a doctor to change a patient's medication to minimize an adverse reaction is an interdependent intervention.

Writing outcome criteria

The essential components of outcome criteria appear below, along with examples for each component.

Content area
This component describes the subject on which the patient focuses or the response to be elicited. For example:
- *the action of digoxin*
- *taking a pulse.*

Action verb
In this component, you describe how the patient will achieve the topic of the content area. For example:
- *explain* the action of digoxin
- *demonstrate* taking a pulse.

Time frame
Here you give a target date for the patient to complete the outcome criterion. For example:
- *explain* the action of digoxin *after the teaching session*
- *demonstrate* taking a pulse *before discharge.*

Criterion modifiers
Finally, add the component that specifies the subject, action, or time of the criterion. For example:
- *explain* the major action of digoxin *after the initial teaching session*
- *demonstrate* taking a pulse *before discharge with a degree of accuracy* within 4 beats of the pulse taken by a nurse.

No one said it was an easy job

Appropriate interventions may require you to administer drugs or to teach patients about drug actions, adverse effects, scheduling, how to avoid or respond to a drug reaction, and ways to administer drugs. The care plan you devise may be shaped by legal and ethical concerns and by the unique needs of certain groups of patients, such as pediatric, geriatric, pregnant, or breast-feeding patients.

Implementation

During the implementation step of the nursing process, you put your interventions into action and provide care for the patient as described in the nursing care plan. By following the care plan and gearing your actions toward the outcome criteria, you'll contribute to implementing the proposed interventions effectively.

For drug therapy, implementation includes all aspects of medication administration:

- working with the doctor
- giving drugs as prescribed
- calculating dosages
- preparing drugs
- using appropriate administration techniques
- modifying techniques for patients with special needs, such as pediatric, geriatric, pregnant, and breast-feeding patients
- staying alert for medication errors
- documenting drugs given
- teaching patients about drugs
- evaluating the effectiveness of drug therapy.

As needed, give the patient written instructions to take home with him.

Evaluation

In the final step of the nursing process, you systematically compare the patient's therapeutic goals with his actual response to drug therapy. This comparison helps you determine whether or not the outcome criteria have been met and how you should modify subsequent interventions.

For example, say the patient had a headache; 1 hour after taking a p.r.n. analgesic, his headache resolved. In this case, the outcome criterion was met. If the headache had lingered or worsened, the outcome criterion wouldn't have been met. You would then need to reassess the patient; the resulting new data may invalidate your original nursing diagnosis or may suggest new nursing interventions. Your reassessment may suggest a need to reevaluate the cause of the patient's headache, or it may suggest that the patient needs a higher dose or a different analgesic.

You'll be the one with all the answers

To fully evaluate the effectiveness of a patient's drug therapy, you need to know the answers to these questions:

- What therapeutic effects should the drug produce?
- By what mechanism of action does the drug work?
- What adverse reactions is the drug known to cause?
- Which drug-drug or food-drug interactions are known to alter the drug's therapeutic effects?
- Which adverse reactions to drugs, if any, has the patient experienced in the past?
- How is the drug administered?
- What should the patient know about the drug?

• Which conditions might affect the patient's ability to follow the prescribed drug regimen?
• Which therapeutic effects has the drug produced for the patient? If none, or if the effects have been insufficient, which issues may be involved?
• Which nursing interventions should be applied to resolve these problems and foster the outcome criteria?

Evaluation enables you to design and implement a revised care plan, to reevaluate outcome criteria continuously, and to replan until each nursing diagnosis is resolved. As a result, the patient gets the most benefit from his drug therapy.

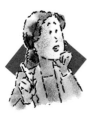

Quick quiz

1. When you prepare to administer a drug, you'll first need to assess the patient. You should obtain your assessment data from:

    A.   a close friend.
    B.   the patient's family.
    C.   the doctor.
    D.   the patient.

Answer: D. Whenever possible, obtain your assessment information directly from the patient. When necessary, you can also obtain information from a family member or close friend.

2. Which sign or symptom indicates that the patient most likely experienced an allergic reaction to a medication?

    A.   Rash
    B.   Nausea
    C.   Diarrhea
    D.   Sore throat

Answer: A. If the patient experienced an allergic reaction to a medication, he'll describe the following signs and symptoms: rash, itching, chest tightness, and difficulty breathing. If the patient doesn't describe these signs and symptoms, he most likely experienced an adverse reaction or a drug interaction.

3. The patient uses the herbal remedy aloe. Aloe can increase the effects of which drug?

    A.   Coumadin
    B.   Phenelzine
    C.   Digoxin
    D.   Vitamin K

Answer: C. Aloe can increase the effects of digoxin.

4.   You alter the patient's drug schedule to accommodate his daily routine. This is an example of which type of intervention?
    A.   Interdependent
    B.   Independent
    C.   Dependent
    D.   Collaborative

Answer: B. Independent nursing interventions are based on the nursing process and professional judgment. Altering the patient's drug schedule to accommodate his daily routine is an independent intervention.

5.   Which is considered a desirable characteristic of properly written outcome criteria?
    A.   Subjective
    B.   Nurse-centered
    C.   Measurable
    D.   Detailed

Answer: C. Outcome criteria should be measurable, patient-centered, objective, concise, realistic, and attainable through nursing management.

Scoring

☆☆☆   If you answered all five questions correctly, excellent! You processed the nursing process like a pro!

☆☆   If you answered three or four correctly, you're definitely applying yourself! Self-diagnosis will show a job well done!

☆   If you answered one or two correctly, don't worry! Review this chapter for a quick assessment, and implement another try.

3

Legal and ethical concerns

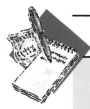

Just the facts

In this chapter, you'll learn:

♦ about drug control laws

♦ how to protect yourself from liability

♦ about the patient's right to refuse treatment

♦ about your ethical obligations.

A look at legal and ethical concerns

When you administer a drug, your focus is on doing it accurately, so the patient receives the most benefit from his therapy. However, while the patient's welfare is always your chief concern, it's not your only concern when you're administering drugs. You also need to consider your own welfare. That's because drug administration — perhaps more than any other aspect of nursing practice — has significant legal and ethical overtones that you can't ignore.

A risky business

Indeed, drug administration is legally one of the most risky tasks you perform as a nurse. This chapter reviews the key legal issues involved in drug delivery (including I.V. therapy) and the best ways to protect yourself from legal problems.

Drug control laws

The legal system has much to say about drugs and how they're defined, handled, prescribed, and administered. (See *A drug defined*, page 48.) In general, what you need to know about drugs and their administration is contained in a set of federal and state or provincial laws.

> ## A drug defined
>
> Legally speaking, a drug is defined as a substance listed in an official national, state, or provincial formulary. It may also be defined as a substance other than food that affects body structure or function and that can be used to diagnose, mitigate, treat, or prevent disease.
>
> ### A prescription description
> A prescription drug is one that isn't available for public purchase. Instead, it must be prescribed by a person licensed to authorize its use. The drug requires a prescription because a national, state, or provincial government has determined that the drug is or may be unsafe when used without qualified medical supervision.

Federal laws

Two important federal laws govern the use of drugs in the United States:
• The Comprehensive Drug Abuse Prevention and Control Act, which incorporates the Controlled Substances Act, categorizes drugs by their abuse potential and regulates the production, possession, and handling of those most likely to be abused.
• The Food, Drug, and Cosmetic Act restricts interstate shipment of drugs not approved for human use, and outlines the process for testing and approving new drugs.

Assuming control of controlled substances

Under federal law, you're responsible for the proper storage of controlled substances on the nursing unit, including the maintenance of detailed records of each dose dispensed and the remaining quantities. You're also obligated to report discrepancies in medication counts of controlled substances. Become familiar with your facility's policy for reporting such discrepancies.

State and provincial laws

At the state or provincial level, pharmacy practice acts are the main laws affecting drug distribution and use. These laws give pharmacists (and sometimes doctors in Canada) the sole legal authority to prepare, compound, preserve, and dispense drugs. The term *dispense* refers to the process of taking a drug from the pharmacy supply and giving or selling it to another person. This differs from *administering* a drug, which is the process of getting the drug into the person's body.

Act accordingly

Your state or provincial nurse practice act contains the legal guidelines regarding the administration of medications by nurses. Most nursing, physician, and pharmacy practice acts include a:
• definition of the tasks that belong uniquely to the profession
• statement that anyone who performs such tasks without being a licensed or registered member of the defined profession is performing an illegal act. (See *Protecting your license.*)

In some states and provinces, certain tasks overlap. For example, in the United States, both nurses and doctors can provide bedside care for the sick and, in Canada, both doctors and pharmacists can prepare medicines. In recent years, with the development of advanced practice roles in nursing—for example, nurse practitioners and nurse anesthetists—the act of prescribing and dispensing medications has been legally extended to many of these professionals as well.

Protecting yourself from liability

When you have a nursing license, you're legally required to be familiar with any drug you administer. A licensed practical nurse (LPN) or licensed vocational nurse (LVN), after taking a pharmacology course or becoming authorized to administer drugs, assumes the same legal responsibility as a registered nurse with respect to medication administration. (See *Great expectations*, page 50.)

Know your stuff

To guard against lawsuits, you must fulfill your legal obligations. That means being thoroughly familiar with the drugs you administer and knowing when not to follow a medication order. It also means documenting your actions, the patient's response to the medication, and incidents related to patient care, including errors made by you or your colleagues.

Executing drug orders

Think of drug orders as classifiable into one of three groups. They can be:

 correctly written orders

 ambiguous orders

 apparently erroneous orders.

Protecting your license

According to the law in many states, if you're a nurse and you prescribe a drug, you're practicing medicine without a license. If you go into the pharmacy or drug supply cabinet, measure out doses of a drug, and put the powder into capsules, you're practicing pharmacy without a license.

For either action, you can be prosecuted, lose your license, or both, even if no harm results. In most states and Canadian provinces, to practice a licensed profession without a license is, at minimum, a misdemeanor.

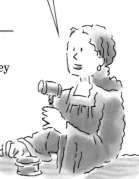

I sentence you to be familiar with every drug you administer. It's the law!

Great expectations

When it comes to drug administration, the law encourages you to use precaution. For example, you're expected to:
• refuse to administer the drug if the order is illegible, confusing, or otherwise unclear
• ask the doctor or other facility-sanctioned person to clarify a confusing order rather than trying to interpret it yourself
• know the drug's safe dosage limits, indications, contraindications, risk of toxicity, and possible adverse effects
• know which drug allergies the patient has experienced
• know other drugs the patient is taking to anticipate and avoid interactions
• properly store controlled substances and maintain accurate records on them.

Naturally, you can simply administer a medication order that you agree is appropriate and correct. However, if you think a medication order is vague, ambiguous, or confusing, then you must clarify it. Your health care facility should have guidelines for this procedure.

Clearing away the confusion

When dealing with ambiguous drug orders, your health care facility may require you to try each of the following actions until you receive a satisfactory resolution of your concern:
• Obtain clarification from the prescriber. If he's unavailable, ask the provider "on call" or the prescriber's supervisor or director.
• Consult a reliable drug reference.
• Request assistance from your charge nurse and, if needed, the nursing supervisor.
• Consult your facility's pharmacist.
• If you're unable to satisfactorily resolve the situation through any means noted above, contact the clinical administrator of your health care facility and explain your problem.

In a holding pattern

If you think a medication order is clearly erroneous and could potentially cause serious harm or injury to the patient, and you have exhausted attempts to clarify the order for accuracy and appropriateness, you have the legal authority to hold the drug. (However, your duty with respect to that order doesn't end here.)

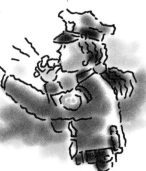

Remember you have the legal authority to hold a drug order when you think it could be harmful to the patient.

You may feel it prudent to hold a drug order because:
- the dosage or route is incorrect
- it's contraindicated by the patient's condition or may produce significant interactions with other medications or substances (for example, beta-adrenergic blockers administered to a patient with severe bronchial asthma or advanced heart block)
- its administration is outside your scope of practice
- you conscientiously object to giving it—as long as your state or province has enacted a right-of-conscience law excusing medical personnel from participating in certain practices, such as abortion or sterilization procedures.

Consider this

Suppose the doctor orders propranolol 20 mg P.O. q.i.d. for the patient. You know that this patient has a history of bronchial asthma and that propranolol is contraindicated for patients who have bronchial asthma. The prudent course of action may be to hold the drug and consult the doctor about an alternate order.

Here's another one

The doctor orders a medication to be given by I.V. bolus, commonly known as I.V. push. This requires special training, and if you haven't received this training, you aren't qualified to independently administer it. An appropriately trained nurse should give it, or she may supervise you in its administration if allowed by your facility's training guidelines. Occasionally, the prescriber may need to administer a drug personally.

It doesn't just end there...

Any time you refuse to carry out a medication order, you have a legal obligation to:
- notify the prescribing health care provider
- notify your immediate supervisor so she can make other arrangements, such as assigning another nurse or clarifying the order
- document that the drug wasn't given, your reason for not giving it, and whom you notified.

Under no circumstances may you simply elect to ignore an order, taking no further action.

Dispensing drugs

Recall the distinction between administering and dispensing medications. Occasionally, you may need to give a medication that isn't available on your unit. If you're working the night or weekend shift and a pharmacist is unavailable, what should you do?

Tales of dispense

Health care facilities should have written policies describing the procedure for obtaining medications from in-house pharmacy supplies after hours, including which staff are authorized to do so and under what circumstances. Usually, this is done by supervisory nursing staff, typically for in-house administration of the medication.

At times, it may also be necessary to dispense a small supply of a medication to the patient for home use, as at the time of discharge from a facility on a weekend or holiday, when pharmacies are closed. Again, you need to follow your facility's policy. Dispensing outside these guidelines or by unauthorized persons is in violation of the law. Not only are you liable for any harm or injury a patient experiences as a result of your action, you may also be prosecuted for exceeding your scope of practice.

Documenting incidents

The term *incident* refers to an event that's inconsistent with the ordinary routine of your health care facility, regardless of whether or not an injury occurs as a result. Whether you're a registered nurse, an LPN, an LVN, a staff nurse, or a nurse-manager, you have a legal duty to report any incident about which you have firsthand knowledge.

To err is human; to document is absolutely necessary

If you make an error in giving a drug or if a patient reacts adversely to a properly administered drug, you should assess the patient's condition and render necessary care. Also, immediately notify the appropriate staff who can assist in rectifying the problem, such as the prescriber, your nursing supervisor, and the pharmacist.

Then document the incident thoroughly. In the patient's chart, document the reaction and medical or nursing interventions applied. Also, complete an incident report that identifies what happened, the names and functions of all personnel involved, and what actions were taken to protect the patient after the error was discovered. If you made an error, you can be held liable, and appropriate documentation is critical in this evaluation. (See *Why file an incident report?*)

Completing an incident report

Most health care facilities require an incident report in response to a patient injury, patient complaint, medication error, or injury to an employee or visitor. To be useful, the incident report must be completed thoroughly and accurately, and it must be filed promptly.

Why file an incident report?

An incident report is a document on which you record pertinent facts about a medication error or an injury to a patient, visitor, or staff member. It serves to:
• inform facility administrators about the incident so they can monitor the facility's patterns and make necessary changes to prevent similar incidents in the future (risk management)
• alert facility administrators to a possible need for further investigation and to notify the facility's insurance company about the possibility of a liability claim (claims management).

Think of it as long-term insurance
Even when an incident doesn't warrant further in-house investigation, the report serves as a contemporary, factual statement of the event and helps identify witnesses in case a lawsuit is filed months or even years later.

If you're the staff member with firsthand knowledge about an incident at the time of its discovery, you should complete an incident report. When you do so, include only the facts—no opinions or irrelevant data. If information is second-hand, place it within quotation marks and identify the source.

Filling out a good report

In general, an incident report should include:
- the identities of persons involved along with any witnesses
- a description of what happened and the consequences to the person involved—include sufficient information so the administrators of your health care facility can determine whether the matter needs further investigation
- other relevant facts.

An incident report shouldn't include:
- opinions (for example, your thoughts about the patient's prognosis)
- conclusions or assumptions (for example, guessing at the particulars of events you didn't witness)
- speculation (for example, your theories on who might be responsible)
- suggestions (for example, your ideas on how to prevent the incident from happening again).

Including such statements in an incident report could seriously hinder the defense in any lawsuit that arises from the incident.

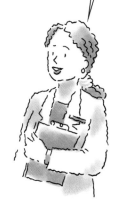

As nurses, we can be held liable for our errors. Good documentation is crucial.

This is an initial report; investigations to follow...

Remember that an incident report serves only to notify administrators that an incident has occurred. In effect, it says, "Administration: Note that this incident happened and decide whether you want to investigate it further." Such items as detailed statements from witnesses and descriptions of remedial action are normally part of an investigative follow-up; don't include them in the incident report itself. After completing an incident report, sign and date it, and give it to your supervisor.

Avoiding problems with incident reports

Be careful that your facility's reporting system doesn't raise the risk of improper incident reporting. For example, some health care facilities require nursing supervisors to correlate reports from witnesses and then to file a single report. The problem with this policy is that it creates added opportunities for misinterpretation.

Inviting trouble

Some incident report forms invite inappropriate conclusions and assumptions by asking, "How can this incident be prevented in the future?" If your facility's reporting system or forms contain such legal pitfalls, alert the administration to them.

Also, remember that most health care facilities don't want you to write "incident report filed" in your nurse's notes. Doing so damages the confidentiality of the report.

Covering up only leads to bigger problems

It may seem intimidating to document on an official incident report the details of an error you committed. However, it's your duty to file such a document immediately. Making a mistake is serious and may result in corrective action by your health care facility and legal action by the patient. However, the potential consequences of trying to cover up an error are worse. Failure to report an incident can result in serious employment concerns, even termination, and can expose you to increased malpractice liability — especially if your failure to report the incident causes injury.

Keep in mind that the likelihood of an incident report being used against you is slight. Your health care facility wants you and other nurses to report incidents and to keep proper records. However, if an incident results from your gross negligence or irresponsibility or is one of a series of incidents in which you've been involved, your health care facility may take action against you. That may also happen if the patient is injured because of your error.

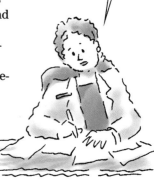

Avoid mentioning incident reports in your nurse's notes. It damages confidentiality.

When a patient refuses treatment

Any mentally competent adult (parent or legal guardian, in the case of minors or persons declared mentally not competent) may legally refuse treatment, including drugs, provided he's fully informed about his medical condition and about the possible results of his refusal.

As a nurse, you may find it hard to accept a patient's decision to refuse treatment, knowing that negative outcomes are a real possibility — especially in refusals of life-saving treatment. But as a professional, you must respect that decision. Laws and court rulings give almost all patients the right to refuse treatment. (See *When a patient says no.*)

Refusing to take "No" for an answer

You can challenge a patient's right to refuse treatment if you believe the patient is incompetent or if compelling reasons exist to overrule his wishes. The courts consider a patient incompetent when he lacks the mental ability to make a reasoned decision such as when he's delirious.

When a patient says no

Before you can perform any type of treatment, including administering a medication, your patient must consent. If he refuses, take the following steps:

• Tell him the risks created by not having the treatment.

• If the patient understands the risks but still refuses, notify your supervisor and the prescriber.

• Record the patient's refusal in your nurse's notes.

• Ask the patient to complete a release form that documents his refusal of treatment. An example appears below. This signed form indicates that the appropriate treatment would have been given had the patient consented to it. The form protects you, the patient's doctors, and your health care facility from liability for not providing treatment.

• If the patient refuses to sign the release form, document his refusal in your nurse's notes.

• For additional protection, your facility's policy may require you to have the patient's spouse or closest relative sign a second release form. Document whether the spouse or relative signs the form.

Refusal of treatment release form

I, _____Brandon Smith_____, refuse to allow anyone to _____insert an I.V. catheter_____ (insert treatment). The risks attendant to my refusal have been fully explained to me, and I fully understand the results of this treatment and that if the same is not done, my chances for regaining normal health are seriously reduced and that, in all probability, my refusal of such treatment or procedure will seriously endanger my life.

I hereby release _____Tower Memorial Hospital_____, its nurses, and employees, together with all doctors in any way connected with me as a patient, from liability for respecting and following my express wishes and direction.

Juanita Ramerez, RN	_Brandon Smith_
WITNESS	PATIENT OR LEGAL GUARDIAN
_2/10/03_	_36_
DATE	AGE OF PATIENT

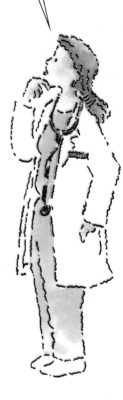

Take these steps when a patient refuses treatment.

The courts also recognize several compelling circumstances that justify overruling a patient's refusal of treatment. They include:

• when refusing treatment endangers the life of another. For example, a court may overrule a pregnant woman's objection to treatment if it endangers her unborn child's life.

• when a parent's decision to withhold treatment threatens a child's life. For example, a court may overrule parents' religious objections to their child's treatment when the child's life is in danger.

• when, despite refusing treatment, the patient makes statements indicating that he wants to live. For example, some Jehovah's Witnesses who oppose blood transfusions say or imply that they won't prevent the transfusions if a court takes responsibility for the decision.

• when public health interests outweigh the patient's right. For example, the law requires that school-age children be immunized against many childhood illnesses before they can attend school.

Your ethical obligations

The rights and responsibilities you carry as a licensed nurse are supported and regulated by legal principles. However, these principles aren't the sole source by which you guide your practice. Ethical principles play a major role as well.

Nursing ethics represents the application of moral principles and values to your professional practice. These principles and values focus on the duties and obligations that you have to yourself, your patients, and your professional colleagues. Value conflicts can occur when you have a different opinion than that of a patient, a doctor, or a colleague about what actions to take in a particular situation. Resolving these differences of opinion can be considerably more complex than simple adherence to a law.

Quality assurance

Ethical conflicts always have existed in nursing, but they've become more prominent these days, largely because of quality-of-life issues. Rapidly advancing technology has resulted in the prolongation of life, the quality of which may vary. As a nurse, you may encounter situations in which your ethical opinions conflict with aspects of patient care.

Moral principles

In the realm of patient care, including drug administration, six moral principles are important to consider when you're trying to make an ethical decision. These principles include:
- autonomy
- paternalism
- truthfulness
- beneficence
- fidelity
- respect for property.

Give me liberty

Autonomy refers to the right of every person to make rational decisions about one's life. Your belief in autonomy fosters respect for the patient's decisions. You must assess each patient and consider the patient's decision regarding medication administration.

Paternal instinct

Paternalism results when someone decides what is best for another person. For example, if a terminally ill patient refuses a dose of pain medication because he's worried that he'll get too sleepy and you convince the patient to accept it, downplaying its sedative effects, you may be practicing justified paternalism. In this case, you would consider the patient's pain relief as justification for your actions. Anyone acting paternalistically toward a patient must consider whether the action is justifiable.

To tell the truth

Truthfulness refers to being honest. You display truthfulness by not withholding information. You should answer all questions honestly and provide or seek further information if necessary.

Reaping the benefits

Beneficence refers to the concept that nursing actions always should cause beneficial effects, never harmful ones. All nursing procedures are based on the principle of beneficence. You always should plan and implement actions that assure safe outcomes for the patient and avoid negative consequences, which might cause harm. For example, you must read drug labels repeatedly, double-check dosage calculations, and compare the patient's identification band to the name on the medication order.

High fidelity

Fidelity requires you to be faithful and truthful and to keep promises made to yourself, your patients, patients' families, your coworkers, and your employer. Don't make a promise to a patient without being absolutely sure that you can keep it.

R-E-S-P-E-C-T, find out what it means

Respect for property refers to the safekeeping of the patient's personal possessions. If the patient brings medications to your facility, for example, policy may dictate that you take them from the patient at admission and store them to prevent double dosing or undesirable drug interactions. However, the patient must first consent to the storage and you must return the medications to him at discharge. Likewise, medications ordered from the pharmacy become the patient's personal property even though you keep them in the medication cart and you administer them to the patient.

Be of a questioning mind

For each of these six characteristics, ask yourself the following questions when analyzing an ethical issue:
• What is morally right and therefore should be done?
• What benefits and harms would result from this action?
• Who would benefit or be harmed?

Placebos

A common area of ethical concern for many nurses involves *placebos*. A placebo is a benign substance — such as a glucose pill or saline solution injection — given to ease nonspecific, often psychosomatic symptoms when the patient thinks he's receiving an actual treatment. Placebos are also given as part of certain drug experiments, in which no one knows which study subjects are receiving the experimental treatment and which are receiving a placebo.

Can the truth be counterproductive? Ahh, ethics...

The ethical problem presented by a placebo is that it requires you to withhold information from the patient, which violates the principle of truthfulness. Typically, doctors and nurses don't tell the patient he's receiving a placebo because doing so reduces the chance of achieving the desired effect. The success of a placebo stems from the patient's belief that he's receiving a treatment.

Health care professionals who administer placebos should comply with the following guidelines:
• Use a placebo only after careful diagnosis.
• Use only an inert substance.
• Answer questions as truthfully as possible.
• Honor the patient's request if he specifically asks not to receive a placebo.

• Never give a placebo when another treatment is indicated or before exploring all treatment options.
• When taking part in a drug experiment that uses placebos, make sure the patient understands the experiment and has given informed consent in writing.

Taking a principled approach

Clearly, legal and ethical principles combine to provide substantial guidelines for all areas of nursing practice, especially drug administration. By following federal and state laws and making ethical decisions, you'll reduce the risk of errors — and the risk of legal action if you do make an error.

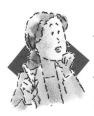

Quick quiz

1. An incident is best described as an:
   A. event that's inconsistent with facility policy that causes injury to the patient.
   B. event that's consistent with facility policy that causes injury to the patient.
   C. event that's inconsistent with facility policy, whether an injury occurs as a result.
   D. event that results in a patient complaint.

Answer: C. The term incident refers to an event that's inconsistent with the ordinary routine of your facility, whether an injury occurs as a result.

2. The courts are compelled to overrule a patient's refusal of treatment when:
   A. parents refuse treatment for their child based upon religious beliefs.
   B. refusing treatment endangers the patient's life.
   C. a parent's decision to withhold treatment threatens the child's life.
   D. the patient's doctor insists on the treatment.

Answer: C. The courts may overrule the patient's refusal of treatment if the parent's decision to withhold treatment threatens a child's life.

3. Moral principles are important to consider when trying to make an ethical decision. Which moral principle requires you to be faithful and truthful and to keep promises made to your patients?

    A.   Autonomy
    B.   Beneficence
    C.   Paternalism
    D.   Fidelity

Answer: D. Fidelity requires you to be faithful and truthful and to keep promises made to yourself, your patient, your patients' families, your employer, and your coworkers.

4.   A doctor prescribes propranolol 10 mg P.O. q.i.d. for the patient. The patient has a history of asthma, which is a contraindication of propranolol. You should:

    A.   administer the drug according to the doctor's order.
    B.   don't give the drug and consult the doctor about an alternative order.
    C.   don't give the drug and notify your nursing supervisor.
    D.   give the drug as ordered, but inform your supervisor about your concerns.

Answer: B. Because propranolol is contraindicated in patients with asthma, the appropriate course of action is to not give the drug and to consult the doctor about an alternative order.

Scoring

☆☆☆   If you answered all four questions correctly, excellent! You're a legal eagle and an ethical...well, nothing rhymes with ethical!

☆☆   If you answered two or three correctly, there's no reason for concern — legal, ethical, or understanding-wise! You met all the obligations of this chapter!

☆   If you answered fewer than two correctly, it's time to lay down the law! Go back and review this chapter; after all, we feel a certain liability for your understanding.

Medication orders and errors

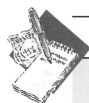

Just the facts

In this chapter, you'll learn:

♦ the different types of medication orders

♦ proper administration procedures

♦ various drug delivery systems

♦ common medication errors.

Working with medication orders

In the state where you practice nursing, a number of different health care professionals may be legally permitted to prescribe, dispense, and administer medications — such as doctors, nurse practitioners, dentists, podiatrists, and optometrists. Aside from nurses in advanced practice roles, nursing's primary focus with respect to medications is their administration.

On the front lines

That means you're almost always on the front line when it comes to patients and their medications. It also means that you bear a major share of the responsibility for avoiding medication errors. These days, when most nurses are busier than ever, that's a tough assignment. It's also why you need to know and practice certain drug-related procedures until they become second nature.

This chapter reviews the most important methods for avoiding medication errors. You'll need to:

• understand the various types of medication orders you may receive

• consistently employ the 5 rights of medication administration

• know your facility's procedural safeguards and drug delivery systems

• rapidly recognize situations that increase the risk of a medication error.

Types of medication orders

In an outpatient setting, the process of ordering a medication is rather simple. A prescriber typically writes the order on a prescription pad and gives it to the patient. The patient then takes the written prescription and has it filled at a pharmacy.

This is where it gets tricky (and where you come in)

In an inpatient setting, however, the process may be somewhat more complex. Several types of medication orders can be used for inpatients, including:

- standard
- single (or one-time)
- stat
- p.r.n.
- standing
- verbal
- telephone.

Standard orders

A standard order is a prescription that remains in effect indefinitely or for a specified period. The prescriber either writes the order—along with instructions, such as for diet, X-rays, and laboratory work—on the order sheet in the patient's chart or enters the order into a computer. The order is then printed out on a computer-generated patient record.

Let's follow this order

The order must specify the name of the medication, dosage, route of administration, frequency, duration (if time limited), and indication (if p.r.n.) (See *Components of a medication order.*) For example, the order might be written this way:

"Amoxil 500 mg P.O. q 8 hr × 10 days."

It's your job to schedule administration times based on the order, your facility's policies, and pertinent characteristics of the medication itself, such as onset and duration of action and whether it's to be given with or without food.

If a standard order doesn't specify a termination time, then the order usually remains in effect until the prescriber writes another order to replace or discontinue it. For some types of drugs, however, the amount of time covered by the order may be limited by facility policy. For instance, narcotic orders may have a controlled delivery time of 3 days. Some antibiotics may have a controlled

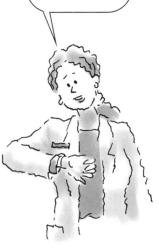

It's time I looked at the standard orders and scheduled administration times for my patients.

Components of a medication order

For a hospitalized patient, a prescriber either writes a medication order on an order sheet in the patient's chart or enters the order into the computer system. An example of a written order is shown below.

Component list

Whether written or entered into the computer, all drug orders must contain the following information: the patient's full name, date and time of the order, name of the drug being ordered, dosage form, dose amount, administration route, time schedule for administration, and prescriber's signature or computer code.

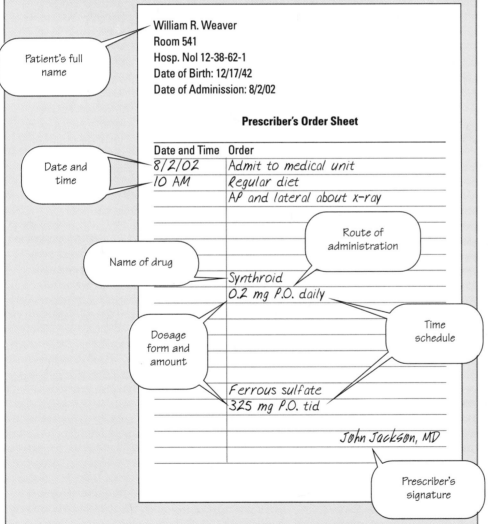

William R. Weaver
Room 541
Hosp. Nol 12-38-62-1
Date of Birth: 12/17/42
Date of Adminission: 8/2/02

Patient's full name

Prescriber's Order Sheet

Date and Time	Order
8/2/02	Admit to medical unit
10 AM	Regular diet
	AP and lateral about x-ray

Date and time

Route of administration

Name of drug

Synthroid
0.2 mg P.O. daily

Dosage form and amount

Time schedule

Ferrous sulfate
325 mg P.O. tid

John Jackson, MD

Prescriber's signature

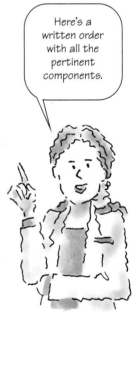

Here's a written order with all the pertinent components.

delivery time of 7 days. If the patient still needs the drug after the termination date has passed, the prescriber must write another order.

The same is true for postoperative medications; the prescriber must rewrite standard orders for all medications that are to continue after surgery.

Single (one-time) orders

When a medication is to be given only once, a prescriber writes what's called a single order. For example, he may order one injection of tetanus toxoid for a patient with a puncture wound who received a primary tetanus toxoid series more than 5 years earlier.

Stat orders

If a patient needs a medication right away for an urgent problem, a prescriber writes a stat order. For example, he may order an immediate single dose of an antianxiety drug to calm an acutely agitated patient. For a patient with acute chest pain, he may write a stat order for nitroglycerin (sublingual, spray, or I.V. form).

P.R.N. orders

The term "p.r.n." comes from a Latin phrase that means "as the occasion arises." A p.r.n. order allows you to give a medication when the patient needs it for a specified problem, such as pain, fever, or constipation. Naturally, you should exercise sound professional judgment in determining when and how often to administer a drug p.r.n. (See *Stick with the purpose*.)

Any time you administer a p.r.n. medication, explain your reason for giving it in the patient's record. Also, describe its degree of effectiveness.

Standing orders

Also known as protocols, standing orders are derived from guidelines created by health care providers for use in specific settings, for treating certain diseases or sets of symptoms. Some units of a health care facility (such as the coronary care unit) routinely employ standing orders. For example, the unit may have standing orders for morphine sulfate to treat chest pain and anxiety, for lidocaine to treat ventricular tachycardia, and for furosemide to treat pulmonary congestion.

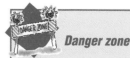
Danger zone

Stick with the purpose

Sometimes a p.r.n. order specifies a reason for giving the drug. For example, the prescriber may order "acetaminophen 650 mg P.O. q 4 hr, p.r.n. for a temperature above 101.3° F (38.5° C)."

Although acetaminophen can be used to treat various problems, in this case, your facility may allow you to give it only for the purpose stated in the medication order. In other words, under such a policy, you couldn't give the acetaminophen ordered above if the patient complained of a headache but had no fever.

Does a standing order need an order? Yes.

Standing orders specify which drugs you're permitted to administer and under which circumstances. They must still be individually reviewed and ordered for each patient by his provider. That is, there must be an order to enact the standing orders. They may also provide guidelines or algorithms for making dosage adjustments. For example, you may need to change the dosage of a heparin infusion based on your patient's anticoagulation studies.

A good test of your skills

Standing orders require considerable judgment and expertise on your part in assessing a patient's need for a drug and in detecting any dose-related adverse reactions that could occur. No standing order should be automatically implemented without a careful review regarding its appropriateness for a given patient at a given time.

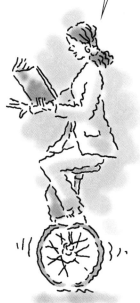

Implementing a standing order is a chance to show off your considerable nursing expertise.

Verbal and telephone orders

Medication orders given orally rather than in writing are known as verbal orders. Whenever possible, avoid them. Because miscommunications can occur and you'll lack a written record of the order.

You're now entering the danger zone

The danger of miscommunication rises even higher when a prescriber gives a verbal medication order over the telephone. A bad connection, commotion on either end, and the lack of nonverbal communication cues can easily result in medication errors if you fail to clarify exactly what the prescriber wants.

If possible, use a fax machine to obtain a written order, instead of taking a verbal order over the phone. (See *Telephone order accuracy*, page 66.)

An emergency? Make it a repeat performance...

In urgent situations, you may not be able to avoid verbal orders. Repeat the order aloud so the prescriber can verify that you understood it. For example, your patient goes into hypoglycemic or insulin shock and the doctor tells you to immediately prepare 50 ml of 50% glucose for I.V. administration. To verify the order, show the doctor the label on the empty glucose vial and say the drug's name out loud as you hand him the syringe. That way, he can confirm the accuracy of the drug and its dose.

Danger zone

Telephone order accuracy

If you have to take a medication order over the telephone, follow these steps to help ensure its accuracy:
• Have another nurse listen in on the call to confirm that she heard the same order you did.
• Repeat the name of the ordered drug to the prescriber to verify that you heard it correctly. Have the prescriber spell the drug name, if necessary.
• Repeat the individual digits of the dose ordered. For instance, you could say, "You ordered one-five milligrams of meperidine, is that right?" The prescriber can then confirm the amount or correct it with something like, "No, I ordered fifty, five-zero, milligrams of meperidine."
• Write out the order, noting that it was a telephone order, then sign and date it.
• Administer the medication as ordered.
 The prescriber must cosign your written order within the time allotted by your facility.

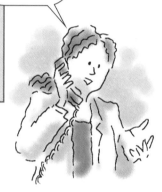

Let me repeat that. 5 mg morphine I.V. push....

It may be verbal, but still get a signature

Anytime you accept a verbal order, it's your responsibility to ensure the accuracy of the communication. This holds true even in an emergency. Ask the prescriber to spell the drug's name if you aren't sure what it is. Afterward, write and sign the order that was given to you verbally by the prescriber. Then have the prescriber sign your written copy as soon as possible. Your facility should have a policy that specifies a time frame allotted for a prescriber to sign a verbal order.

Administration procedures

Making sure you understand a medication order is just the start of your responsibilities when it comes to administering medications correctly. Next, you have to make your own judgment about the correctness of the order based on your knowledge of the medication and your understanding of the patient's condition.

The order looks good, now what?

If you're convinced that a medication order is appropriate for the drug and the patient involved, your next step is to prepare the drug correctly for administration. (See *Orders into action.*)

After you transcribe the medication order onto a working document, go to a quiet area to prepare the medication for delivery. Then follow the 5 rights of medication administration.

Orders into action

After you receive a written medication order, transcribe it onto a working document approved by your health care facility. For example, your facility may want you to use a medication administration record (MAR), a medication Kardex, medication cards or tickets, or a computer printout.

Stepping away from errors
Each time you copy a medication order, you introduce the possibility of making an error. Make sure you follow these steps:
- Read the order carefully.
- Concentrate on copying it correctly.
- Check it when you're finished.

Don't rely on memory
Next, prepare the medication from the approved copy. Never prepare a medication from memory or from your personal worksheets or notes.

To reduce the risk of overlooking a medication order, your facility may require you to periodically check all MARs against the original order sheets.

The 5 rights

Following a tried-and-true set of safeguards known as the 5 rights can quickly and easily help you avoid the most basic and common sources of medication error. Each time you administer a medication, confirm that you have the:

 right drug

 right dose

 right patient

 right time

 right route.

Right drug

Always compare the name of an ordered drug with the name printed on the container label. Take your time and do this carefully; drugs with similar-sounding and similar-looking names may have very different indications and effects.

Sounds like...

For example, Celexa (citalopram) and Celebrex (celecoxib) sound quite similar. However, Celexa is a selective serotonin reuptake inhibitor used to treat depression. Celebrex is a nonsteroidal anti-in-flammatory drug used to treat osteoarthritis and rheumatoid arthritis. Other similar-sounding drugs may raise a similar risk of mix-ups.

Make sure you aren't unwrapping any surprises

When a medication is individually wrapped in single doses, check the name when removing it from the drawer and again when un-wrapping and giving the drug to the patient. Always mention the drug name and the reason you're giving it before actually giving it to the patient.

From the mouth of the patient

Besides carefully checking the ordered drug name against the container label, also check the patient's reaction to the drug as you try to administer it. If he says, "I usually take one pink pill, but you've given me two yellow pills," stop what you're doing and recheck the order. Perhaps you'll simply explain to the patient that the pink pill contains 10 mg of the drug and the yellow ones contain 5 mg each.

Or perhaps you'll discover that you're giving the patient the wrong medication. Either way, you must carefully follow up on any comment a patient makes about changes in a medication—before you administer it.

Don't just blindly throw a pill in my mouth.

Always gauge your patient's reaction while administering medications.

Right dose

The growing use of unit-dose medications (in which a single dose of medication is wrapped and labeled for individual use) has greatly reduced the risk of giving a patient the wrong drug dose. Also, many commercially prepared medications are available in various tablet sizes, decreasing the number of calculations you have to do to determine the dosage.

Even so, you still need to know how and when to perform the appropriate dose calculations. (See *Keeping calculations correct*.) For more calculations, see chapter 5, Measurement systems and dosage calculations.

The buddy system

Whenever possible, double-check all your calculations with another nurse or with a pharmacist. Many hospitals require these double-checks when your dosage calculations involve children's medications or drugs with narrow safety margins, such as heparin and insulin.

Danger zone

Keeping calculations correct

A recent study of 200 equation-based prescribing errors found that more than half resulted from calculation mistakes. To help keep your medication calculations correct, use these safeguards:
• Think about whether a dosage seems right, given the patient's diagnosis and the drug involved.
• If your calculation indicates that you need more than one or possibly two dosage units to prepare a prescribed dose, double-check the calculation.
• If your calculation indicates that you need a small fraction of a dosage unit to prepare a prescribed dose, double-check the calculation.
• Be especially careful when calculating with decimal points because a mistake can increase or decrease the intended dose many times over.
• Minimize the possibility of confusion anytime you have to write down a dose that contains a decimal point by putting a zero in front of a decimal point that has no other number in front of it. In other words, write 0.25 mg rather than .25 mg, which someone could easily mistake for 25 mg. Likewise, never write a zero after a dose that includes a decimal point. In other words, don't write 0.250 mg for a dose of 0.25 mg.
• Never break an unscored tablet to prepare a calculated dose because you won't get an exact amount. Instead, ask a pharmacist for a form of the drug that you can measure accurately.

Know your role on the team

No matter what, never take it upon yourself to alter the drug dosage specified in a prescriber's order. Say, for example, that a doctor orders 75 mg of meperidine for postoperative pain. You give the medication after the patient's surgery, but he says he still has intense pain. Your conclusion may be that 75 mg of meperidine isn't enough, and that 100 mg would probably do the trick. But that doesn't give you the authority to change the dose.

Instead, consult with the doctor and obtain a new standard order. However, if the prescriber's original medication order specifies a range of dosages, then you must determine the most appropriate dose for the patient—within that range.

Right patient

To reduce the risk of medication errors, never assume that the patient in a labeled bed is indeed the patient named on the label. Instead, always check the patient's ID bracelet carefully against the medication administration record (MAR) before giving any medication.

Roll call

As an additional check, also ask the patient to tell you his name. (Don't say something like, "You're John, right?" because the patient could misunderstand you, could be confused, or could be a different John than the one scheduled for a medication.)

Right time

The considerations that make an administration time the "right" time may be therapeutic, practical, or both. For therapeutic purposes, the right time is one that appropriately maintains the level of drug in the patient's bloodstream. For practical purposes, the right time is one that's convenient for the staff and the patient. Naturally, therapeutic goals take precedence over practical ones.

Working around the clock

To meet therapeutic goals, you may need to space the delivery of some medications evenly around the clock. Doing so helps to maintain a consistent level of the drug in the patient's bloodstream. If you don't have a particular need to space the drug delivery over 24 hours, you can space it over the patient's waking hours to avoid disrupting his sleep.

For some drugs, you may need to measure the patient's therapeutic response before determining whether it's the right time to give another dose. For example, you should check the patient's apical pulse rate (determined by cardiac auscultation for 1 minute) before giving digoxin, and you should assess the patient's respiratory rate before giving morphine.

The perfect plan

Besides maximizing the therapeutic effect, giving medications at specified, evenly spaced intervals provides some practical benefits. For one thing, it allows you to plan administration times that don't interfere with meals or especially busy times on the nursing unit. For example, instead of scheduling twice-daily administration times at 8 a.m. and 6 p.m., which are common times for shift changes, schedule them at 9 a.m. and 7 p.m. instead.

Another practical benefit of standardized administration times is that they establish a habit in the patient's mind. This may make it easier for him to keep taking the medication appropriately when he gets home.

If it's on the schedule, you need to be on time

Regardless of the reasons behind the administration times you establish for the patient, you'll need to follow those times carefully. In fact, many facilities consider it a medication error if you fail to give a medication within 30 minutes before or after its scheduled administration time.

Right route

Always pay careful attention to the administration route specified in the medication order and on the product's label. Also, make sure the ordered form of the drug is appropriate for the intended route. Only drugs labeled "for injection" should be used for injections of any kind.

Before you give the drug, consider whether the amount ordered is appropriate for the route by which you're preparing to give it. For example, 10 mg is an appropriate amount of morphine sulfate to give by the intramuscular route to relieve pain in an adult. If the patient will be receiving it by the I.V. route, however, the equivalent dose would be more like 2 to 4 mg. If he's taking the drug orally, he'll need more than 10 mg to achieve the same effect.

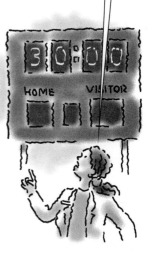

The clock's ticking. Always give your meds within 30 minutes (before or after) of the scheduled time.

Different routes

Remember that the route by which you give a drug affects the rate at which it gets absorbed into the patient's bloodstream. Because certain forms of a drug may be intended for specific routes, be careful not to interfere with a drug's action by changing routes or circumventing the chemical preparation. For example, you wouldn't want to crush an enteric-coated tablet or open a sustained-release capsule. (See *Working with sustained-release drugs*, page 72.)

Different speeds

You can also help increase the speed at which topical nitroglycerin enters a patient's bloodstream by spreading it over a larger skin area and covering it with plastic wrap.

On the other hand, you can decrease the rate of absorption and effectiveness of a drug. For example, if a patient chews or swallows a sublingual drug, such as sublingual nitroglycerin, the rate of absorption and effectiveness will be decreased.

Procedural safeguards

The 5 rights of medication administration afford you a basic level of protection against medication errors. However, most experts consider them the minimum requirement. Here are some additional measures you should take to help avoid medication errors.

Working with sustained-release drugs

A growing number of drugs are being formulated to exert an effect over many hours. The components of each drug dose dissolve at different rates, thus releasing the drug gradually but continuously into the patient's bloodstream. Convenient for staff and patients, sustained-release drugs require fewer doses per day and provide steadier control over symptoms.

Easy identification
Sustained-release drugs are supplied as plain tablets, coated tablets, and capsules filled with tiny granules. They may be identified by an SR (for sustained release) after the drug name, or they may have one of a number of prefixes attached to the name that suggests an extended effect. Some common examples include Quinaglute Dura-Tabs, Dimetapp Extentabs, Chlor-Trimeton Repetabs, and Desoxyn Gradumets. You may also see such names as Spansules and Gyrocaps.

Don't split, crush, or chew
Never split or crush a sustained-release drug. Warn the patient not to chew the drug. And never open a sustained-release capsule to mix the granules into foods or beverages. All these actions could alter the drug's absorption rate, put too much drug into the patient's bloodstream too quickly, or reduce the drug's overall effect.

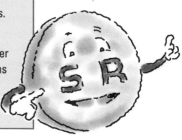

Remember, sustained-release drugs like me should never be split, crushed, chewed, or opened. You'll alter my effects for sure!

Storage and preparation

Follow these guidelines when storing and preparing drugs:
• Store and handle drugs carefully to maintain their stability and potency. Remember that some drugs can be altered by temperature, air, light, and moisture; make sure you follow all drug-specific precautions. Some drugs may need to be kept in brown bottles. Some I.V. bags may need to be covered with foil to block the light during infusion.
• Always keep drugs in the containers in which the pharmacy dispensed them. Cap all containers tightly. If you see small cylinders in a container, they probably serve to absorb moisture and keep the product fresh; don't remove them.
• Store drugs at room temperature unless you're instructed to refrigerate them. Refrigeration causes moisture to form and could alter some drugs through condensation.
• As required by law, keep narcotics and controlled substances under double lock.

Out of date? Out of the question!

• Always note a drug's expiration date—the date after which it loses some amount of potency. Never administer an outdated drug or one that looks or smells unusual.
• If the original package looks like someone may have tampered with it, don't give the drug; instead, return it in its package to the pharmacy for an investigation.

• Check the medication label three times — when you take it from the shelf or drawer, before putting it into the medication cup, and before returning the container to the shelf or drawer — to make sure you're giving the prescribed medication. For a unit-dose medication, check the label just after obtaining the medication and again before discarding the wrapper.
• You may need to reconstitute a drug dispensed as a powder just before you administer it. If medication is left over after you remove your dose, label the container with the date, time, strength, and your initials or signature.
• Never administer a drug that wasn't labeled properly after reconstitution.
• Discard any drug that will reach its expiration date before another dose is scheduled.
• If you find an unlabeled syringe with medication inside, discard it.
• Let a refrigerated drug reach room temperature before administering it, unless you're instructed otherwise.

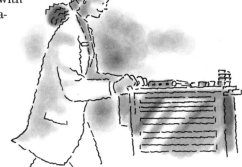

Be smart! Always stay with the cart.

Administration

Follow these guidelines when administering drugs:
• Before administering a medication based on new orders, review the patient's medication history for known allergies or other problems.
• If you know a patient has a drug allergy, make sure his chart clearly displays the allergy.
• When you deliver drugs to a patient's room, stay with the medication cart. Never leave without locking the cart and taking it back to the medication room or its usual storage place.
• Assess the patient's physiological and psychological condition before administering any medication.
• Stay with the patient until he takes the medication to verify that he took it as directed.
• Never leave medication doses at a patient's bedside unless you have a specific order to do so. (See *Handling orders for bedside medications*, page 74.)
• Administer only medications you've prepared personally or that the pharmacist prepared.
• Don't open individually prepared doses (unit-dose medications) until you're at the bedside and you've confirmed the patient's identity.
• When administering an oral drug, urge the patient to drink a full glass of water, if appropriate. Doing so helps move the medication

---

Handling orders for bedside medications

If a medication order specifies that you should leave a drug at the patient's bedside for self-administration, label the drug with:
• patient name
• drug name
• dosage
• any instructions the patient needs.
   Drugs commonly left at the patient's bedside include antacids and nitroglycerin tablets.

Supervision requires a super nurse
In most health care facilities, you're responsible for supervising a patient whose drugs are left at the bedside. For example, you must know how many nitroglycerin tablets the patient took, the exact times of self-administration, the degree of relief he obtained, and any unusual reactions he had to the drug. Record this information in the patient's chart, and report it to the prescriber.

---

out of the esophagus and into the stomach. It also dilutes the drug, thus reducing the chance of gastric irritation.

Write it down!

• Document drugs immediately after you administer them. Delayed charting, especially of p.r.n. medications, can result in repeated doses. Documenting before giving a medication can lead to missed doses.
• Record your observations of the patient's positive and negative responses to the medication. For instance, if you give an antibiotic to a patient with pneumonia, chart such positive responses as decreased sputum, reduced fever, and easier breathing to confirm the drug's effectiveness. Also chart such adverse reactions as skin eruptions or gastric upset. Severe adverse reactions may prompt the prescriber to substitute another drug.

Drug delivery systems

Yet another area of medication administration that you'll need to master is the dispensing system. Your facility may use one of several systems by which you can obtain ordered drugs from the pharmacy. In each one, you serve a vital coordinating function between the prescriber and the pharmacist.

Systems analysis

Common drug delivery systems include:
• unit-dose system
• automated systems

• individual prescriptions.

Regardless of the delivery system used by your facility, the doctors, nurses, and pharmacists must collaborate to make it work effectively.

Drug delivery systems require teamwork!

Unit-dose system

In a unit-dose system, the pharmacist dispenses a supply of wrapped, labeled individual doses of all forms of drugs: oral, injectable, and I.V. solutions with additives. The pharmacist usually dispenses sufficient drugs and I.V. solutions to last 24 hours; he may also prepare trays of medications for you to administer at specified hours.

Keep it under wraps

The pharmacist may prepare unit doses or purchase them commercially. He usually places each patient's drugs in an individual drawer of a portable medication cart. Keep the drugs in their labeled wrappers until you actually administer them. The unit-dose system reduces the likelihood of drug administration errors.

Automated systems

In essence, an automated drug delivery system is a computerized version of the unit-dose system. A pharmacist fills an electronic drug-dispensing unit and keeps it locked. The unit then delivers individually wrapped and labeled medications when you request them. A computer records all drug transactions on electronic tape and furnishes requested printouts.

To avoid the possibly disastrous effects of computer downtime, facilities that use automated dispensing systems must have a backup plan for dispensing medications and documenting their delivery.

Freeing time for patients

An automated system greatly simplifies record keeping because the computer can monitor and track drugs from the original inventory to patient billing. It saves staff time and may allow you to spend more time teaching and consulting with patients. (See *Understanding automated drug delivery*, page 76.)

Individual prescriptions

In an individual prescription system, a pharmacist fills a prescription using a container that's been labeled for a particular patient. You then administer the drug to the patient directly from the container. Because the drug is designated for a particular person, this system reduces the risk that you'll give a drug to the wrong patient. However, the system is cumbersome and slow because the medication order must travel from you to the pharmacy and back to you again.

Common medication errors

Besides following your facility's policies faithfully, you can help prevent medication errors by studying common ones and avoiding the slip-ups that allowed them to happen.

Similar names

As you read earlier, drugs with similar-sounding names can be easy to confuse. Keep in mind, however, that even different-sounding names can look similar when written out rapidly by hand on a medication order: Soriatane and Loxitane, for example, both of which are capsules. Any time a patient's drug order doesn't seem right for his diagnosis, call the doctor to clarify the order. (See *Avoiding med mix-ups.*)

A case of mistaken identity

Drug names aren't the only kinds of words you can confuse. Patient names can cause trouble as well if you fail to verify each person's identity. This problem can be especially troublesome if two patients have the same first name.

Consider this clinical scenario. Robert Brewer, age 5, was hospitalized for measles. Robert Brinson, also age 5, was admitted after a severe asthma attack. The boys were assigned to adjacent rooms on a small pediatric unit. Each had a nonproductive cough. When Robert Brewer's nurse came to give him an expectorant, the child's mother told her that Robert had already inhaled a medication through a mask.

The nurse quickly figured out that another nurse, new to the unit, had given Robert Brinson's medication (acetylcysteine, a mucolytic) to Robert Brewer in error. Fortunately, no harmful adverse effects ensued. Had the nurse checked her patient's identity more carefully, however, no error would have occurred in the first place.

Understanding automated drug delivery

An automated drug delivery system may free you from doing some of what you currently do by hand. For example, you may no longer have to transcribe medication orders or procure and store drugs.

The responsibility stays the same
However, keep in mind that an automated system doesn't relieve you of the responsibility for noting medication orders and administering medications properly. It also can't take your place in unusual patient circumstances, in which a computer can't render your professional judgments.

Checking ID

Always check each patient's full name. Also, teach each patient (or parent) to offer an ID bracelet for inspection and to state a full name when anyone enters the room with the intention of giving a medication. Also, urge patients to tell you if an ID bracelet falls off, is removed, or gets lost. Replace it right away. (See *Reducing medication errors through patient teaching.*)

Allergy alert

After you've verified your patient's full name, take time to check whether he has drug allergies — even if he's in distress.

Here's a reenaction of an allergic reaction

Consider this real-life example. A doctor issued a stat order for chlorpromazine (Thorazine) for a distressed patient. By the time the nurse arrived with it, the patient had grown more distressed and was demanding relief. Unnerved by the patient's demeanor, the nurse gave the drug without checking the patient's MAR or documenting the order — and the patient had an allergic reaction to it.

Anytime you're in a tense situation with a patient who needs or wants medication fast, resist the temptation to act first and docu-

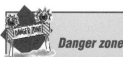

Danger zone

Avoiding med mix-ups

Many nurses have confused an order for morphine with one for hydromorphone (Dilaudid). Both drugs come in 4-mg prefilled syringes. If you give morphine when the doctor really ordered hydromorphone, the patient could develop respiratory depression or even arrest.

Consider posting a prominent notice in your medication room that warns the staff about this common mix-up. Or try attaching a fluorescent sticker printed with "not morphine" to each hydromorphone syringe.

No place like home

Reducing medication errors through patient teaching

You aren't the only one who is at risk for making medication errors. Patients are at an even higher risk because they know so much less about medications than you do.

Clearly, patient teaching is a crucial aspect of your responsibility in minimizing medication errors and their consequences — especially as more patients receive outpatient rather than inpatient care.

Teaching tips
You can help minimize medication errors by:
- teaching the patient about his diagnosis and the purpose of his drug therapy
- providing the patient with his drug information in writing
- asking if he takes over-the-counter medications at home in addition to his prescribed drugs
- asking about herbal remedies and other nutritional supplements
- telling the patient what kinds of drug-related problems warrant a call to his doctor
- urging the patient to report anything about his drug therapy that concerns or worries him.

ment later. Skipping that crucial assessment step could easily lead to a medication error. (See *Safe alternative*.)

Order errors

Many medication errors stem from compound problems—a mistake that could have been caught at any of several steps along the way. For a medication to be administered correctly, each member of the health care team must fulfill the appropriate role. The doctor must write the order correctly and legibly. The pharmacist must evaluate whether the order is appropriate and then fill it correctly. And the nurse must evaluate whether the order is appropriate and then administer it correctly.

Chain reaction

A breakdown anywhere along this chain of events can lead to a medication error. That's why it's so important for members of the health care team to act as a real team, checking each other and catching any problems that arise before those problems affect the patient's health. Do your best to foster an environment in which professionals can double-check each other.

For example, the pharmacist can help clarify the number of times a drug should be given each day, he can help you label drugs in the most appropriate way, and he can remind you to always return unused or discontinued medications to the pharmacy.

Clear the confusion

You must clarify any doctor's order that doesn't seem clear or correct. You also must correctly handle and store any multi-dose vials obtained from the pharmacist. Additionally, store drugs in their original containers to avoid errors. (See *Container confusion.*)

Administer only those drugs that you've prepared personally; never give a drug that has an ambiguous label or no label at all. Here's an actual example of what could happen if you do.

Label liability

A nurse placed an unlabeled cup of phenol (used in neurolytic procedures) next to a cup of guanethidine (a postganglionic-blocking agent). The doctor accidentally injected the phenol instead of the guanethidine, causing severe tissue damage to a patient's arm. The patient needed emergency surgery and developed neurologic complications.

Obviously, this was a compound problem. The nurse should have labeled each cup clearly, and the doctor shouldn't have given an unlabeled substance to a patient.

Danger zone

Safe alternative

A patient who is severely allergic to peanuts could have an anaphylactic reaction to Atrovent aerosol given by metered-dose inhaler. Ask the patient or his parents whether he's allergic to peanuts before you administer this drug.

If you find that he has such an allergy, you'll need to use the nasal spray and inhalation solution form of Atrovent. Because it doesn't contain soy lecithin, this form of the drug is safe for patients who are allergic to peanuts.

Route trouble

Danger zone

Many medication errors stem at least in part from problems related to the route of administration. The risk of error increases when a patient has several lines running for different purposes.

Caught in a tangle of lines

Consider this example. A nurse prepared a dose of digoxin elixir for a patient who had a central I.V. line and a jejunostomy tube — and she mistakenly administered the drug into the central I.V. line. Fortunately, the patient had no adverse reaction. To help prevent such mix-ups in route of administration, prepare all oral medications in a syringe that has a tip small enough to fit an abdominal tube but too big to fit a central line.

Bubble trouble

Here's another error that could have been avoided: To clear air bubbles from a 9-year-old patient's insulin drip, a nurse disconnected the tubing and raised the pump rate to 200 ml/hour to flush the bubbles through quickly. She then reconnected the tubing and restarted the drip, but she forgot to reset the rate back to 2 U/hour. The child received 50 units of insulin before the error was detected. To prevent this kind of error, never increase a drip rate to clear bubbles from a line. Instead, remove the tubing from the pump, disconnect it from the patient, and use the flow-control clamp to establish gravity flow.

You carry a great deal of responsibility for making sure that patients get the right drugs in the right concentrations at the right times and by the right routes. By diligently applying the advice offered here, you can minimize your risk of medication errors and maximize the therapeutic effects of your patients' drug regimens.

Container confusion

Even a confusing container can cause a medication error if you aren't careful. For example, it's easy to mistake eyedrops for the developers used for the Hemoccult test. Some patients have sustained permanent eye damage as a result. The best way to avoid this mistake is to keep Hemoccult developers in an appropriate room (such as the utility room). Never keep them in a patient's room.

We all make mistakes. Be professional. Let someone double-check your orders. And do the same for her!

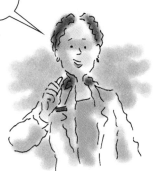

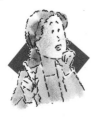

Quick quiz

1. Which type of inpatient medication order remains in effect indefinitely or for a specified period?

    A. Standard
    B. Single
    C. Standing
    D. Stat

Answer: A. A standard order is a prescription that remains in effect indefinitely or for a specified period.

2. The patient is ordered Lasix 40 mg I.V. at 10 p.m. × 1 dose. This is an example of which type of order?

    A. Stat
    B. Single
    C. Standing
    D. Standard

Answer: B. A single order is written when a medication should be given only once.

3. Which type of order poses the highest risk for error?

    A. Verbal
    B. Telephone
    C. Standard
    D. P.R.N.

Answer: B. The risk of error is highest when a prescriber gives an order over the telephone.

4. As the nurse, you aren't the only one at risk for making medication errors. Who is at an even higher risk?

    A. Doctors
    B. Pharmacists
    C. Residents
    D. Patients

Answer: D. Patients are at a higher risk for making medication errors because they lack knowledge about medications.

Scoring

☆☆☆ If you answered all four questions correctly, excellent! Here's an order for you: Bask in your glory stat!

☆☆ If you answered two or three correctly, congratulations are still in order! You delivered a fine performance!

☆ If you answered fewer than two correctly, don't worry! You've got the right attitude and now's the right time to get it right.

Measurement systems and dosage calculations

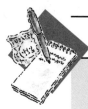

Just the facts

In this chapter, you'll learn:

♦ measurement systems for medication administration

♦ how to perform conversions between measurement systems

♦ how to perform dosage calculations.

A look at conversions and calculations

An increasing number of medications are becoming available in unit-dose formulations, which may decrease the need for you to do dosage calculations — and decrease the risk of calculation-based medication errors as well. However, you still need to be familiar with the measurement systems used for ordering and administering medications, and you need to be able to calculate within measurement systems and convert between systems. This chapter reviews what you need to know to calculate doses and convert measurements accurately.

Measurement systems

In theory at least, a doctor may order a medication using one of four different measurement systems:

• metric
• household
• apothecaries'
• avoirdupois.

Taking measure of the measurement systems

You'll almost always use one of the first two when working with medications. In fact, the metric and household systems are so common that cups used to measure liquid medications usually show both types of calibration marks.

The apothecaries' system is less common, and the avoirdupois system is usually used for ordering and purchasing pharmaceutical products and sometimes for weighing patients.

Metric system

The metric system is the most widely used international system of measurement and the one used by the U.S. Pharmacopoeia. The units of the metric system are:
- gram (g) for measuring weight
- liter (L) for measuring volume
- meter (m) for measuring distance. (See *Metric measures*.)

Weighing in

Many drugs are ordered and administered in milligrams (mg); 1 mg is 1/1,000 of a gram. Body weights are commonly recorded in kilograms (kg), each of which equals 1,000 g.

Filling up

A liter is about equal to a quart in volume, and a milliliter (ml) equals 1/1,000 of a liter. Solutions for I.V. use are commonly ordered and administered by the liter. Many parenteral and some oral drugs are ordered and administered by the milliliter.

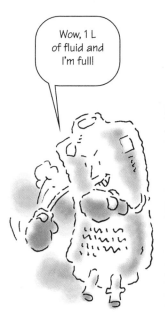

Wow, 1 L of fluid and I'm full!

Let's hear it for the metric system!

The metric system offers many advantages when ordering and administering medications, not least of which is that most people in the world know how to use it. What's more, it provides a reliable way to accurately measure small amounts—a provision crucial for many drug dosages. And it uses Arabic numerals, which most health care professionals prefer. Most drugs are calibrated using the metric system.

Here are some examples of medication orders that use the metric system:
- 1 L of dextrose 5% in water I.V. over 8 hours
- 30 ml milk of magnesia P.O. h.s.
- cefazolin sodium 1 g I.V. piggyback q 6 h
- digoxin 0.125 mg P.O. daily
- maintain 10 kg continuous traction.

Metric measures

This table shows the relationships among some commonly used metric measures. Several less commonly used measures, such as the hectogram, also appear.

Liquids

1 milliliter (ml)	=	1 cubic centimeter (cc)
1 deciliter (dl)	=	100 ml
1,000 ml	=	1 liter (L)
100 centiliters (cl)	=	1 L
10 dl	=	1 L
10 L	=	1 dekaliter (dkl)
100 L	=	1 hectoliter (hl)
1,000 L	=	1 kiloliter (kl)

Solids

1,000 micrograms (mcg)	=	1 mg
1,000 milligrams (mg)	=	1 g
1,000 grams (g)	=	1 kilogram (kg)
100 centigrams (cg)	=	1 g
10 decigrams (dg)	=	1 g
10 g	=	1 dekagram (dkg)
100 g	=	1 hectogram (hg)

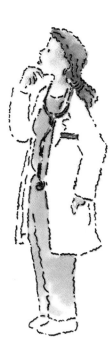

The new standard

In January 1995, the U.S. Pharmacopoeial Convention changed its standards to require that all drug prescriptions state the quantity and strength of the ordered drug in metric units. It also stipulated that, if other units are used to express strength or quantity, only the metric equivalent should be dispensed.

This change is particularly significant for you because, if you receive a medication order that uses the apothecaries' system, you'll need to know how to convert the dosage into the metric system, in which the drug must be dispensed.

Household system

Most people in the United States are more familiar with the household system of weights and measures than they are with the metric system. The household system is based on the:
- ounce (oz) and the pound (lb) for measuring weight
- teaspoon (tsp), tablespoon (tbs), and cup for measuring volume
- inch (″), foot (′), and yard for measuring distance.

Most foods, recipes, over-the-counter drugs, and home remedies in the United States are sold under the household system of measurement.

A problem with precision

The problem with the household system is that it lacks precision, both in the quantities ascribed to each measurement and in the conversions used to switch between measurements. For example, not all teaspoons and tablespoons hold the same amount. The clinical teaspoon and tablespoon have been standardized to 5 ml and 15 ml, respectively. Thus, 3 tsp equals 1 tbs, and 6 tsp equals 1 oz.

Home schooling

In clinical settings, you'll rarely use the household measurement system for preparing or administering drugs. However, the patient may need to use teaspoons or tablespoons to take drugs prescribed for home use. You'll need to help him translate prescribed medications into common measurements. And you'll need to make sure he has medication spoons calibrated to deliver the precise dose.

Here are some examples of medication orders that use the household system:
- 2 tsp Bactrim P.O. b.i.d.
- Riopan 2 tbs P.O. 1 h a.c. and h.s.

Apothecaries' system

Although used occasionally to measure some medications, the apothecaries' system is outdated, imprecise, and being phased out. It's based on the:
- grain (gr) and dram (dr) for measuring weight

• minim (min) for measuring volume. (See *Apothecaries' measures.*)

A grain equals about 60 mg and was originally designed to represent the weight of an average grain of wheat. A dram equals about 60 gr. The apothecaries' pound equals 12 oz. A minim is about the size of a drop of water; 15 or 16 min equal about 1 ml.

Where are the numbers?

The apothecaries' system has two unique features: the use of Roman numerals and the placement of the numeral after the measurement amount. For example, 5 grains would be written "grains v." The apothecaries' system is also the only system of measurement that uses special symbols instead of abbreviations to represent units of measure.

Avoirdupois system

The solid measures or units of weight in the avoirdupois system include the dram (27.344 gr), the ounce (16 drams or 437.5 gr), and the pound, which contains 16 oz or 7,000 gr. This system may be used for ordering and purchasing pharmaceutical products.

Mixed systems

As you've seen, several units of measurement appear in more than one measurement system. For example, the pound appears in the household system, the apothecaries' system, and the avoirdupois system. Typically, it contains 16 oz. However, in the apothecaries' system, it contains 12 oz.

Drop everything — let's discuss drops

Other measurement terms may have rather imprecise meanings as well. The drop, for instance, which appears in the household and apothecaries' systems, is traditionally considered equal to a drop of water. However, the drop is an inexact measure that varies in size depending on the physical characteristics of the liquid being measured and the equipment used to form the drop.

Nonetheless, you'll use the drop as a unit of measure when instilling liquid medication into a patient's ear, nose, or conjunctival sac. You'll also use it when monitoring the flow of I.V. solutions. When held vertically, a standard medication dropper usually is calibrated to deliver 20 drops of liquid per ml. Standard I.V. administration sets usually deliver 10 to 20 drops/ml. Microdrip sets deliver 60 drops/ml.

Apothecaries' measures

This table shows some of the values in the apothecaries' system of drug measurement and their metric equivalents.

Liquids

1 minim	= 0.06 ml
1 fluid dram	= 4 ml
1 fluid ounce	= 30 ml
1 pint	= 500 ml
1 quart	= 1,000 ml

Solids

1/600 grain	= 100 mcg
1/60 grain	= 1 mg
1 grain	= 60 mg
60 grains (1 dram)	= 4 g
1 ounce	= 30 g

Special measures

Some drugs are measured using special terms, such as:

- units
- international units
- milliequivalents.

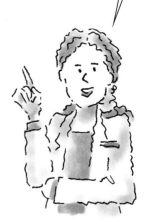

Keep in mind that some drug measurements have special terms, such as units, international units, and milliequivalents.

Units

Several important and widely used drugs, such as insulin, heparin, and some antibiotics, are measured in units (U). As you know, insulin is available in many types; all are measured in units. In fact, the international standard of U-100 insulin means that 1 ml of insulin solution contains 100 U of insulin, regardless of type.

Several antibiotics (in liquid, solid, and powder forms for oral or parenteral use) also are measured in units. Each drug maker provides information about how its drugs are measured. For example, an oral liquid preparation of nystatin contains 100,000 U/ml.

Here are some examples of orders that use units:

- 14 U NPH insulin S.C. this a.m.
- heparin 5,000 U S.C. b.i.d.
- nystatin 200,000 U P.O. q 6 h.

Unit measurements aren't universal

Keep in mind that the unit isn't a standard measure. In other words, you can't assume that 100 U of a drug made by one company will have a level of activity similar to 100 U of an analogous drug made by another company.

International units

International units are used to measure biologicals, such as vitamins, enzymes, and hormones. For example, the activity of calcitonin, a synthetic hormone used in calcium regulation, is expressed in international units. The doctor may order Calcitonin (salmon) 100 international units (IU) daily S.C. for the initial treatment of Paget's disease of bone.

Milliequivalents

Electrolytes may be measured using the milliequivalent (mEq), which is the number of grams of a solute contained in 1 ml of a normal solution. Electrolyte solutions are supplied with instructions about the number of metric units required to provide the prescribed number of milliequivalents.

Here are some examples of orders that use milliequivalents:

- 30 mEq KCl P.O. b.i.d.

• 1 L of dextrose 5% in normal saline solution with 40 mEq KCl to run at 125 ml/hour.

Conversions between systems

Occasionally, you'll need to convert a measurement from one system to another. To perform conversion calculations, you'll need to know the equivalents among the different systems of measurement. (See *Measure for measure*.)

In your comfort zone

You can use several methods to convert a drug measurement from one unit to another. Use the one that feels most comfortable and that you know the best. The conversion methods discussed here — the fraction method and the ratio method — are two of the most commonly used. Remember, you may need to convert from one

---

Measure for measure

This table shows some approximate liquid equivalents among the household, apothecaries', and metric systems.

Household	Apothecaries'	Metric
1 teaspoon (tsp)	1 fluidram (f℈)	5 ml
1 tablespoon (tbs)	½ fluidounce (f℥)	15 ml
2 tbs	1 f℥	30 ml
1 measuring cup	8 f℥	240 ml
1 pint (pt)	16 f℥	473 ml
1 quart (qt)	32 f℥	946 ml (1 L)
1 gallon (gal)	128 f℥	3,785 m

This table shows some approximate solid equivalents between the apothecaries' system and the metric system.

Apothecaries'	Metric
15 grains (gr)	1 gram (g) (1,000 mg)
1 gr	0.06 g (60 mg) or 0.065 g (65 mg)
½ gr	0.03 g (30 mg)
$\frac{1}{100}$ gr	0.6 mg
$\frac{1}{120}$ gr	0.5 mg
$\frac{1}{150}$ gr	0.4 mg

This table lists some approximate solid equivalents among the avoirdupois, apothecaries', and metric systems.

Avoirdupois	Apothecaries'	Metric
1 gr	1 gr	0.065 g
15.4 gr	15 gr	1 g
1 ounce (oz)	480 gr	28.35 g
0.75 pound (lb)	1 lb	373 g
1 lb	1.33 lb	454 g
2.2 lb	2.7 lb	1 kilogram (kg)

measure to another within the same system, or you may need to convert from one system to another.

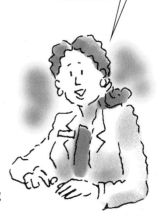

Fraction method

The fraction method for conversions requires an equation made up of two fractions.

First, set up a fraction by placing the ordered dose (the one you need to convert) over x units of the available dose. For example, the doctor orders 300 mg of aspirin, and the bottle is labeled "aspirin gr v per tablet." The mg dose is the ordered dose, and the gr dose is the available dose. Because the amount of the available dose is unknown, it's represented by an x. So the first fraction in the equation is:

$$\frac{300 \text{ mg}}{x \text{ gr}}$$

Next, set up a second fraction that includes standard equivalents between the ordered and available measures. Because 60 mg equals 1 gr, the second fraction is:

$$\frac{60 \text{ mg}}{1 \text{ gr}}$$

The same unit of measure appears in the numerator of both fractions, and the same unit of measure appears in both denominators. The entire equation appears as:

$$\frac{300 \text{ mg}}{x \text{ gr}} = \frac{60 \text{ mg}}{1 \text{ gr}}$$

Finally, solve for x, cross-multiply, and follow these steps:

$$300 \text{ mg} \times 1 \text{ gr} = 60 \text{ mg} \times x \text{ gr}$$
$$300 = 60x$$
$$5 \text{ gr} = x$$

Based on this conversion equation, your patient should receive 5 gr (gr v) of aspirin, which in this case equals 1 aspirin tablet.

Ratio method

When using the ratio method to make conversions, first express the ordered dose and available dose as a ratio. For example, the doctor's order calls for Tylenol elixir 2.5 ml for a pediatric patient.

You want to tell the child's mother how many teaspoons to give at home. As a result, the first ratio appears as 2.5 ml : x tsp. The x represents the unknown teaspoon amount. The second ratio represents the standard equivalents between the ordered and available measures. Because 5 ml equals 1 tsp, the second ratio appears as 5 ml : 1 tsp. Note that the same unit of measure (ml) appears in the first half of each ratio, and the same unit (tsp) appears in the second half.

The equation should appear as:

☝ Set up the following ratio

$$2.5 \text{ ml} : x \text{ tsp} :: 5 \text{ ml} : 1 \text{ tsp}$$

✌ Solve for x by multiplying the means of the ratio (inner portions) and the extremes (outer portions):

$$x \text{ tsp} \times 5 \text{ ml} = 2.5 \text{ ml} \times 1 \text{ tsp}$$
$$x = 0.5 \text{ tsp}$$

Based on this calculation, you'd tell the child's mother to give ½ tsp, which equals the ordered 2.5-ml dose.

Nonparenteral dosage calculations

Computing drug dosages is a two-step process:

☝ First, determine whether the drug is available in the ordered system of measurement. If it's available only in another system of measurement, perform either the fraction method or the ratio method as explained above to convert between the two systems.

✌ Next, calculate the quantity of the available drug form that you'll need to administer.

For example, if the dose to be given is 250 mg, determine the quantity of tablets, powder, or liquid needed to deliver that dose. To do so, you can use the fraction or ratio method again—as described below—or you can use the desired-available method.

Fraction method

When using the fraction method to compute a drug dosage, write an equation that includes two fractions. The first shows the ordered dose over x, where x represents the quantity of the drug form you'll be giving. (See *Delving into dimensional analysis*, page 90.)

Delving into dimensional analysis

Dimensional analysis is an alternative way of solving mathematical problems. It's a basic and easy approach to calculating drug dosages because it eliminates the need to memorize formulas.

Key factors

When using dimensional analysis, a series of ratios called factors are arranged in a fractional equation. Each factor, written as a fraction, consists of two quantities of measurement that are related to each other in a given problem. Dimensional analysis uses the same terms as fractions, specifically the terms numerator and denominator.

Let's give it a try

Here's how it works: A patient is ordered 70 mg of enoxaparin (Lovenox). It's available in vials that contain 30 mg per 0.3 ml. How much should be prepared?

- Begin by identifying the given quantity:

$$70 \text{ mg}$$

- Then isolate what you're looking for:

$$X \text{ ml}$$

- Next, know your conversion factor:

$$30 \text{ mg} = 0.3 \text{ ml}$$

- Now set up your equation:

$$\frac{70 \text{ mg}}{1} \times \frac{0.3 \text{ ml}}{30 \text{ mg}}$$

- Identify and cancel units that appear in both the numerator and denominator

$$\frac{70 \ \cancel{\text{mg}}}{1} \times \frac{0.3 \text{ ml}}{30 \ \cancel{\text{mg}}}$$

- Finally, multiply the numerators and denominators and divide the products:

$$\frac{70 \times 0.3 \text{ ml}}{1 \times 30} = \frac{21 \text{ ml}}{30} = 0.7 \text{ ml}$$

The patient would receive 0.7 ml of Lovenox.

Set up the first fraction. If a doctor orders a 250-mg dose and the drug is available in tablets, the first fraction would be:

$$\frac{250 \text{ mg}}{\text{x tab}}$$

Set up the second fraction. The second fraction shows what's available in the form of the drug you need to give. Usually, this information is available on the drug label. For this example, each tablet contains 125 mg of the drug. The second fraction is:

$$\frac{125 \text{ mg}}{1 \text{ tab}}$$

Remember that the same units of measure must appear in the numerators of each fraction. The denominators should show the same units of measure as well. The entire equation should appear as:

$$\frac{250 \text{ mg}}{\text{x tab}} = \frac{125 \text{ mg}}{1 \text{ tab}}$$

To solve the equation, you cross-multiply to find that x equals 2 tablets.

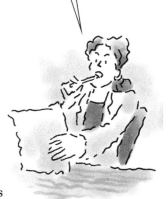

Now let's see. The same units of measure must be present in the numerator and denominator.

Ratio method

To use the ratio method, follow these steps:

Write the amount of the drug to be given and the quantity of the dose (x) as a ratio. Using the example shown above, you would write:

250 mg : x tab

Complete the equation by forming a second ratio from the number of units in each tablet (or whatever form the drug comes in). The manufacturer's label provides this information. Again using the example from above, the entire equation is:

250 mg : x tab :: 125 mg : 1 tab

Solve for x by multiplying the means (inner portions) and extremes (outer portions) of the equation. The patient should receive 2 tablets.

Desired-available method

This method combines the typical two-step process (the conversion of ordered units into available units and the computation of drug dosage) into one step.

You'll use this equation:

$$\begin{array}{c} \text{ordered} \\ \text{units} \end{array} \times \begin{array}{c} \text{conversion} \\ \text{fraction} \end{array} \times \dfrac{\begin{array}{c} \text{quantity of} \\ \text{drug form} \end{array}}{\begin{array}{c} \text{stated quantity} \\ \text{of drug in} \\ \text{each drug form} \end{array}} = \begin{array}{c} \text{quantity} \\ \text{to give} \end{array}$$

For example, the doctor orders 60 mEq of potassium chloride liquid, but the solution you have on hand contains 20 mEq/15 ml. You need to know how many tablespoons to give.

☝ Convert ml to tbs after consulting a table of equivalents. (See the table in *Measure for measure*, page 87.) You'll see that 15 ml equals 1 tbs. Set up the first fraction with the amount desired over the amount you have:

$$\dfrac{60 \text{ mEq}}{20 \text{ mEq}}$$

✌ Set up the second fraction with the unknown amount desired—represented by x—in the appropriate position:

$$\dfrac{\text{x tbs}}{1 \text{ tbs}}$$

🤟 Put these fractions into a proportion:

$$\dfrac{\text{x tbs}}{1 \text{ tbs}} = \dfrac{60 \text{ mEq}}{20 \text{ mEq}}$$

🖖 Now cross-multiply the fractions:

$$\text{x tbs} \times 20 \text{ mEq} = 1\text{tbs} \times 60 \text{ mEq}$$

🖐 Solve for x by dividing each side of the equation by 20 mEq and canceling units that appear in the numerator and denominator:

$$\dfrac{\text{x tbs} \times 20 \text{ } \cancel{\text{mEq}}}{20 \text{ } \cancel{\text{mEq}}} = \dfrac{1\text{tbs} \times 60 \text{ } \cancel{\text{mEq}}}{20 \text{ } \cancel{\text{mEq}}}$$

You'll find that x = 3 tbs, which is the amount of potassium chloride liquid the patient should receive.

Avoiding errors

Although the desired-available method has the advantage of using only one equation, it's a more elaborate equation than either the fraction or ratio methods. If you think that having to memorize a more complex equation will increase your risk of making an error, you're better off sticking with the two-step process.

Make the difference 10% or less

Keep in mind that converting drug measurements from one system to another and then determining the amount of a drug form to give can easily produce inexact doses. You may determine a precise drug amount to be given, such as 0.97 tablet, only to find it impossible to administer that amount.

Follow this general rule to help prevent calculation errors and discrepancies between theoretical and real doses: Allow no more than a 10% variation between the dose ordered and the dose given. According to this rule, if you find that the patient should receive 0.97 tablet, you may safely give the patient a full tablet.

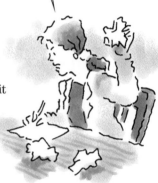

When I make a mistake with the one-step method, I go back to the two-step process.

Parenteral dosage calculations

Methods for computing nonparenteral drug dosages also apply to parenteral dosages. You'll need to know how to reconstitute powders for injection and how to calculate I.V. drip rates, I.V. flow rates, and percentage solutions.

Reconstituting powders for injection

Usually, a pharmacist reconstitutes powdered drugs for parenteral use. Sometimes, however, you'll have to do it by following the directions on the drug label that specify the amount of drug in the vial or ampule, the type and volume of diluent to add to the powder, and the strength and shelf life (expiration date) of the resulting solution. (See *Diluent dilemma*, page 94.)

This takes concentration

To determine the amount of solution to administer after the drug is reconstituted, use the manufacturer's information about the concentration of the solution. For example, if you want to administer 500 mg of a drug, and the concentration of the prepared solution is 1 g (1,000 mg) per 10 ml, you can set up a fraction equation as follows:

$$\frac{500 \text{ mg}}{\text{x ml}} = \frac{1,000}{10 \text{ ml}}$$

Set up a ratio equation as follows:

$$500 \text{ mg} : \text{x ml} :: 1,000 \text{ mg} : 10 \text{ ml}$$

The patient should receive 5 ml of the prepared solution.

Calculating I.V. drip and flow rates

The number of drops (gtt) needed to deliver a specified quantity of I.V. solution varies with the type of administration set you use and the manufacturer. To calculate the needed flow rate, you have to know the calibration of the drip rate for each manufacturer's product. Then you can use an equation to determine the drip rate you need. (See *Calculating an I.V. drip rate.*)

Coming up with the solution

First, set up a fraction showing the volume of solution to be delivered over the number of minutes in which that volume must be infused. For example, if a patient must receive 100 ml of solution over 1 hour, you would use this fraction:

$$\frac{100 \text{ ml}}{60 \text{ min}}$$

Next, multiply the fraction by the drip factor (the number of drops needed to supply 1 ml) to determine the drip rate (the number of drops per minute to be infused).

This equation works for I.V. solutions that infuse over many hours or for small-volume infusions, which are given in less than 1 hour.

Always follow directions

Carefully follow the manufacturer's directions when determining drip factor. Standard administration sets have drip factors of 10, 15, or 20 drops/ml. However, the drip factor varies among different I.V. sets; it appears on the package for the I.V. tubing administration set. A microdrip (minidrip) set has a drip factor of 60 drops/ml.

Diluent dilemma

When you add diluent to a powder, the powder increases the fluid volume. That's why the drug label calls for less diluent than the total volume of the prepared solution. For example, you may have to add 1.7 ml of diluent to a vial of powdered drug to obtain a 2-ml total volume of prepared solution.

Calculating an I.V. drip rate

The doctor's order is 1,000 ml dextrose 5% in half-normal saline solution to infuse over 12 hours. The administration set delivers 15 drops per milliliter. What should the drip rate be?

- Use the equation:

$$\frac{\text{Total no. of ml}}{\text{Total no. of min}} \times \text{drip factor} = \text{drip rate}$$

- Set up the equation using the given data:

$$\frac{1,000 \text{ ml}}{12 \text{ hr} \times 60 \text{ min}} \times 15 \text{ gtt/ml} = \text{X gtt/min}$$

- Multiply the elements in the denominator:

$$\frac{1,000 \text{ ml}}{720 \text{ min}} \times 15 \text{ gtt/ml} = \text{X gtt/min}$$

- Divide the fraction:

$$1.39 \text{ ml/min} \times 15 \text{ gtt/ml} = \text{X gtt/min}$$

The final answer is 20.85 gtt/min, which can be rounded to 21 gtt/min. The drip rate is 21 drops per minute.

A modification

You can modify the equation by first determining the number of milliliters to be infused over 1 hour (the flow rate). Next, divide the flow rate by 60 minutes. Multiply the resulting calculation by the drip factor to determine the number of drops you should give per minute.

You'll also use the flow rate when working with I.V. infusion pumps to set the number of milliliters to be delivered in 1 hour. For some administration sets, you may not need to use an equation at all. (See *Quicker drip-rate calculations*, page 96.)

Calculating percentage solutions

In most clinical settings, a pharmacist or the drug maker prepares solutions of drugs for I.V. infusion. However, you'll need to prepare special percentage solutions for emergencies such as resuscitation attempts after cardiac arrest. What's more, if you work in home care, you may need to prepare large-volume solutions if prepared solutions aren't available to the patient.

Quicker drip-rate calculations

Here's a quicker way to compute an administration rate for an I.V. solution. If you're using a microdrip set, which has a drip rate of 60, you can simply set the flow rate in milliliters (ml) to match the drip rate (because it's 60 drops per minute).

If you were using an equation, you would divide the flow rate by 60 minutes and multiply by the drip factor, which in this case also equals 60. For example, if you need to administer 125 ml of fluid per hour, the equation would be:

$$\frac{125 \text{ ml}}{60 \text{ min}} \times 60 = \text{drip rate (125)}$$

When flow equals rate (things are great)

Because the flow rate and drip factor are the same, mathematically they cancel each other out. So rather than taking time to set up and solve the equation, you can simply use the number assigned to the flow rate as the drip rate. If your administration set delivers 15 drops/ml, divide the flow rate by 4 to get the drip rate. If your administration set has a drip factor of 10, divide the flow rate by 6 to find the drip rate.

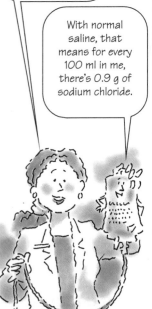

When dealing with solutions, percentages mean grams per 100 ml.

With normal saline, that means for every 100 ml in me, there's 0.9 g of sodium chloride.

Playing the percentages

An example of a percentage solution is 0.9% sodium chloride, which means that every 100 ml of solution contains 0.9 g of sodium chloride. Expressed as a fraction, the figures would appear as:

$$\frac{0.9}{100}$$

The ratio form would appear as 0.9 : 100. A liter of 0.9% sodium chloride solution would contain 9 g of sodium chloride. Expressed as a fraction, the figures for 1 L would be:

$$\frac{9}{1,000}$$

The ratio form would appear as 9 : 1,000.

Solute + solvent = solution

You may prepare percentage solutions by adding solute (solid or liquid forms of drugs) to solvents (also known as diluents). Examples of commonly used solvents are sterile water and 0.9% sodium chloride solution. As a general rule, when preparing solutions, you can consider a solid drug form—such as crystals, powders, or tablets—to be of 100% strength. Liquid forms, also known as stock solutions, may vary in strength.

To calculate the strength of percentage solutions, you can use two formulas for the fraction method, or you can use two formulas for the ratio method. The fraction method includes these formulas:

$$\frac{\text{weaker solution}}{\text{stronger solution}} = \frac{\text{solute}}{\text{solvent}}$$

$$\frac{\text{small \% strength}}{\text{large \% strength}} = \frac{\text{small volume}}{\text{large volume}}$$

The ratio method includes these two formulas:

$$\text{weaker} : \text{stronger} :: \text{solute} : \text{solvent}$$
$$\text{small \% strength} : \text{large \% strength} :: \text{small volume} : \text{large volume}$$

When the difference becomes meaningful

Although a solid combined with a diluent increases the total volume of the prepared solution, sometimes the increase is negligible and may not need to be calculated. If you're adding a large amount of solid or a small amount of diluent, however, you'll probably have to calculate the total volume.

When adding a liquid, subtract the amount of liquid to be added from the total volume desired to find how much diluent you should use. For example, if you need to include 50 ml of a liquid drug in 1 L of solution, add the 50 ml of liquid drug to 950 ml of diluent.

Let's go over that again

Here's another example. Suppose you need to prepare 500 ml of a 0.5% lidocaine solution using dextrose 5% in water (D_5W) as the diluent. You have a 2% lidocaine solution and D_5W on hand. You must now determine how much lidocaine solution to use and how much D_5W to use. Using the ratio method, set up the following equation:

$$0.5\% : 2\% :: x \text{ ml} : 500 \text{ ml}$$

Multiplying the means and the extremes yields $2x = 250$. Dividing by 2 then gives you a final figure of 125 ml of 2% lidocaine solution.

Because you want a total volume of 500 ml and you need to use 125 ml of lidocaine solution, you next need to determine how much D_5W to use as the diluent. To do so, simply subtract 125 from the 500-ml total to obtain your answer: Use 375 ml of D_5W.

Calculating pediatric dosages

If you're caring for a child, you'll need to use different calculations to determine the correct drug dosages. One is based on the child's weight in kilograms; the other uses body surface area.

Body weight

Most drug companies provide guidance about safe dosage ranges for drugs given to children. Typically, drugs are labeled with a safe dosage range in mg/kg of body weight. To determine a safe pediatric dosage range, follow these directions.

Defining the limits

The doctor orders a drug with a suggested dosage range of 10 to 12 mg/kg of body weight/day. The child weighs 12 kg. To find the safe daily dosage range, you need to calculate the lower and upper limits of the range provided by the manufacturer.

First, calculate the dosage based on 10 mg/kg of body weight. Next, calculate the dosage based on 12 mg/kg of body weight. The answers you obtain represent the lower and upper limits of the daily dosage range, expressed in mg/kg of the child's weight. (See *Calculating pediatric dosages.*)

Body surface area

Another acceptable method for calculating safe pediatric dosages uses the child's body surface area (BSA) as a guide. In fact, this method may provide the most accurate calculation because the child's BSA probably parallels his metabolic rate and organ growth and maturation.

No problems with a nomogram

You can determine a child's BSA using what's called a nomogram. Simply find the child's height in the first column and weight in the third column. Place a straight-edge so it connects the two measurements. The point at which the straight-edge intersects the second column shows the child's approximate BSA in square meters.

To calculate the child's approximate drug dose, use the BSA measurement in the following equation:

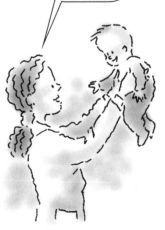

A child's BSA provides a good indication of his metabolic rate as well.

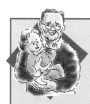

Ages and stages

Calculating pediatric dosages

The doctor orders 150 mg of a drug to be given q 6 h to an 18-kg child. (Remember that 1 kg equals 2.2 lb). The package insert indicates that the safe dosage range for the drug is 30 mg/kg to 35 mg/kg per day, to be given in divided doses. Can you safely administer the ordered dosage?

• Use the ratio method to determine the lower limit of the safe dosage range:

$$30 \text{ mg} : X \text{ mg} :: 1 \text{ kg} : 18 \text{ kg}$$

• Cross-multiply the means and the extremes to find that X = 540 mg, which represents the low dosage. Use the same method to calculate the upper limit of the safe dosage range:

$$35 \text{ mg} : X \text{ mg} :: 1 \text{ kg} : 18 \text{ kg}$$

• Cross multiply the means and the extremes to find that

$$X = 630 \text{ mg, the high dosage.}$$

The safe dosage range for the child is 540 to 630 mg per day. Because the doctor ordered 150 mg to be given every 6 hours, the child would receive four doses per day, or a total daily dose of 150 mg x four doses per day = 600 mg per day. This daily dose falls within the safe range, so the nurse can safely administer 150 mg q 6 hours.

$$\frac{\text{child's BSA}}{1.73 \text{ m}^2 \text{(average adult BSA)}} \times \frac{\text{average}}{\text{adult dose}} = \text{child's dose}$$

Crunching the numbers

Here's an example. You know that your patient weighs 25 lb and is 33″ (84 cm) tall. Using a nomogram, you find that he has a BSA of 0.52 m². You also know that the average adult dose is 100 mg. To determine the appropriate drug dose, set up the equation this way:

$$\frac{0.52}{1.73 \text{ m}^2} \times 100 \text{ mg} = 30.06 \text{mg (child's dose)}$$

Based on your calculation, you know that your patient should receive 30 mg of the drug.

Your knowledge of measurement systems, understanding of conversion procedures, and ability to perform dosage calculations accurately is crucial to delivering appropriate drug dosages.

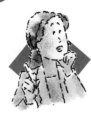

Quick quiz

1. The U.S. Pharmacopoeial Convention require that all drug prescriptions state the strength and quantity of the ordered drug in which units?

A. Apothecaries'
B. Metric
C. Avoirdupois
D. Household

Answer: B. The U.S. Pharmacopoeial Convention mandated that all drug prescriptions contain metric units.

2. A patient is ordered 2 tsp Bactrim P.O. b.i.d. How many ml of the drug should you administer?

A. 15 ml
B. 5 ml
C. 20 ml
D. 10 ml

Answer: D. A teaspoon is equivalent to 5 ml; therefore, 2 tsp is equivalent to 10 ml. You should administer 10 ml of Bactrim.

3. When you reconstitute a powder for injection, the drug label calls for:

A. less diluent than the total volume of prepared solution.
B. the same diluent as the total volume of prepared solution.
C. more diluent than the total volume of prepared solution.
D. your professional judgment in deciding on the amount of diluent to add.

Answer: A. When you add diluent to a powder, the powder increases the fluid volume. Therefore, the drug label calls for less diluent than the total volume of prepared solution.

Scoring

☆☆☆ If you answered all three questions correctly, wow! Using any measurement system, your abilities are off the charts!

☆☆ If you answered fewer than three correctly, review the chapter and see if you can't get the trick of the metric system!

Documenting drug administration

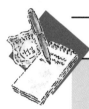

Just the facts

In this chapter you'll learn:

♦ medication documentation basics and how to avoid common errors

♦ how to document administering p.r.n. and single-dose medications

♦ how to document administering narcotics

♦ how to document I.V. therapy

♦ when and how to report adverse drug reactions.

Medication documentation basics

Medication administration is one of the most important practice areas to document completely, accurately, and on time. Besides creating a legal record of your clinical care, documenting drug delivery also helps other caregivers continue your patient's drug regimen safely and accurately.

What, when, how — and what happens

No matter what kind of drug regimen your patient receives, you'll need to document:
- what he receives
- when he receives it
- how he receives it
- what happens as a result.

In most facilities, you'll use a medication administration record (MAR) to compile this information. An *MAR* is a document that serves as the central record for a patient's medication orders and their execution. The MAR is commonly included in a card file (a medication Kardex) or on a separate medication administration sheet. (See *Medication Kardex*, pages 102 and 103.)

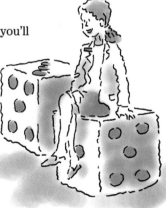

Don't take chances when documenting medication administration — do it completely, accurately, and on time.

Medication Kardex

The medication Kardex contains a permanent record of the patient's medications. It may also display the patient's diagnosis and information about allergies and diet. This partial form shows typical notations.

NURSE'S FULL SIGNATURE, STATUS AND INITIALS		
	INIT.	
Roy Charles, RN	RC	
Theresa Hopkins, RN	TH	

DIAGNOSIS: _Heart failure, Atrial flutter_

ALLERGIES: _ASA_

ROUTINE/DAILY ORDERS/FINGERSTICKS/ INSULIN COVERAGE			DATE: 2/24/02		DATE: 2/25/02	
ORDER DATE	MEDICATIONS DOSE, ROUTE, FREQUENCY	TIME	SITE	INT.	SITE	INT.
2/24/02	digoxin 0.125 mg	0900	℞ s.c.	RC		
RC	I.V. q.d.	HR	68			
2/24/02	furosemide 40 mg	0900	℞ s.c.	RC		
RC	I.V. q12h	2100	℞ s.c.	TH		
2/24/02	enalapril 1.25 mg	0500	℞ s.c.	TH		
RC	I.V. q6h	1100	℞ s.c.	RC		
		1700	℞ s.c.	RC		
		2300	℞ s.c.	TH		

(continued)

Mastering MARs

When using an MAR, follow these guidelines:
• Know and follow your facility's policies and procedures for recording drug orders and administration.

Medication Kardex *(continued)*

	Addressograph		A

INITIAL	SIGNATURE & STATUS	INITIAL	SIGNATURE & STATUS
RC	Roy Charles, RN		
TH	Theresa Hopkins, RN		

YEAR 19 _2002_

ORDER	RENEWAL	DISCONTINUED	DATE	
DATE: 2/24	DATE: /	DATE: /		2/24
MEDICATION: acetaminophen		DOSE 650 mg	TIME GIVEN	0930
DIRECTION: q 6 h PRN mild pain		ROUTE: P.O.	DATA	P.O.
			INIT.	RC

ORDER	RENEWAL	DISCONTINUED	DATE	
DATE: 2/24	DATE: /	DATE: /		2/24
MEDICATION: MSO4		DOSE 2 mg	TIME GIVEN	0930
DIRECTION: 15 minutes prior to changing		ROUTE: IV.	DATA	® S.C.
® bed dressing			INIT.	RC

ORDER	RENEWAL	DISCONTINUED	DATE	
DATE: 2/24	DATE: /	DATE: /		2/24
MEDICATION: milk of magnesia		DOSE 30 ml	TIME GIVEN	2115
DIRECTION: q6 H p.r.n.		ROUTE: P.O.	DATA	P.O.
			INIT.	TH

ORDER	RENEWAL	DISCONTINUED	DATE		
DATE: 2/25	DATE: /	DATE: 2/25		2/25	2/25
MEDICATION: prochlorperazine		DOSE 5 mg	TIME GIVEN	1100	2230
DIRECTION: q 8h p.r.n.		ROUTE: I.M.	DATA	® glut	Ⓛ glut
p.r.n. nausea and vomiting			INIT.	RC	TH

ORDER	RENEWAL	DISCONTINUED	DATE	
DATE: /	DATE: /	DATE: /		
MEDICATION:		DOSE	TIME GIVEN	
DIRECTION:		ROUTE:	DATA	
			INIT.	

ORDER	RENEWAL	DISCONTINUED	DATE	
DATE: /	DATE: /	DATE: /		
MEDICATION:		DOSE	TIME GIVEN	
DIRECTION:		ROUTE:		

• Make sure that all drug orders include the patient's full name, date, time, drug name, dose, administration route or method, and frequency.
• When appropriate, include the specific number of doses given or the stop date. When you administer a stat order, make sure to record the time.
• Note any drug allergies prominently.
• Write legibly.
• Use only standard abbreviations approved by your facility. If you're not sure whether an abbreviation is approved, don't use it. Instead, write out the full word or phrase.
• After giving the first dose of a drug, sign your full name, licensure status, and initials in the appropriate space in the MAR.
• When transcribing a one-time order to be given on another shift, make sure to communicate the order in your report to the next shift, or use a medication alert sticker to flag the order.
• If you can't administer a prescribed drug as scheduled, document the reason. For instance, the patient may be scheduled for a test that requires you to hold his medications.
• Document drug administration immediately after completing it so another nurse doesn't give the drug again. This is especially important if you document medication administration by computer.

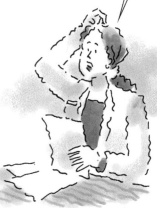

When in doubt, S-P-E-L-L it out.

Documenting p.r.n. medications

For drugs given as necessary (p.r.n.), document what you gave and when and how you gave it. For example, for sublingual nitroglycerine pills a patient required for chest pain, document the number of pills, the date and time you gave them, and the strength of the drug.

Go the extra step

You will also need to include any other clinically relevant information. For example, include additional information about the patient's chest pain (such as radiation to his left arm) and vital signs. Also note his response to the medication. You might write, "Relief of chest pain was obtained after one sublingual nitroglycerine pill."

Documenting single-dose medications

A single-dose medication, such as a supplemental dose or a stat dose, should be documented not only in the patient's MAR, but also in your progress notes.

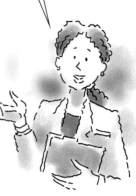

Remember to document a single-dose medication, such as a supplemental dose or a stat dose, not only in the patient's MAR, but also in your progress notes.

Sign on the dotted line

Document who gave the order, why the order was given, and the patient's response to the medication. For example, if you administered a one-time order of I.V. furosemide (Lasix), you could write: "Lasix 40 mg given I.V. per Dr. Singh's order. Patient with SOB, crackles bilaterally, and oxygen (O_2) saturation decreased to 89% on room air." Include your signature, your title, the date, and the time you gave the drug.

Follow up on your previous note with an update on the patient's response to the medication. You might write something like, "Patient responded with urine output of 1,500 ml, decreased SOB, and O_2 saturation increased to 97% on room air." Once again, include your signature, your title, the date, and the time.

> You need to document narcotics according to federal, state, AND facility regulations.

Documenting narcotics

Any time you give a narcotic, you're required to document its administration according to federal, state, and facility regulations. These requirements may differ somewhat depending on what storage system your facility uses.

Big Brother is watching

If your facility uses an automated storage system, you'll use an ID and password to obtain narcotics (and other drugs and floor stocks for nursing units).

You can remove one or more drugs by entering the patient's name, medication, and amount needed on the keypad. Then you must figure the amount of drug remaining in the system and enter it. Each transaction is recorded, and copies are sent to the pharmacy and billing department.

If something goes wrong

If your facility doesn't use an automated storage and dispensing system, you'll need to take a couple of additional steps. Before giving a narcotic, verify the amount of drug in the container and sign out the medication on the appropriate form, usually a narcotic sheet. Someone will need to count the remaining narcotics at the end of each shift.

> If you need to discard a narcotic dose...

> ...be sure to have another nurse present to document it.

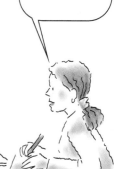

Incidentally

Whether your facility has an automated system or not, you may need to have another nurse observe and document your actions if you have to discard all or part of a narcotic dose. If you discover a discrepancy in the narcotic count, follow your facility's policy for reporting it. Also, file an incident report. An investigation will follow.

Reporting adverse reactions

If you think a medication has caused an adverse reaction in your patient, follow your facility's policy for reporting it internally.

Talking to the feds

You may also need to report the adverse reaction to the Food and Drug Administration (FDA) on an official MedWatch form. Complete a MedWatch form when you suspect that a drug, medical device, nutritional product, or any FDA-regulated product causes:
- a death
- a life-threatening illness
- an initial or prolonged hospitalization
- a disability
- a congenital anomaly
- the need for medical or surgical intervention to prevent a permanent impairment or an injury.

Just the facts, ma'am

When filling out a MedWatch form, remember that you aren't expected to establish a connection between the product and the problem. You don't have to include copious details; simply describe the adverse event or problem that you observed with a drug or product. Send your completed form to the FDA by using the fax number or mailing address on the form.

Don't double up

File a separate MedWatch form for each patient. Attach additional pages, if needed. If appropriate, report product problems to the manufacturer as well as to the FDA. Also, remember to comply with your facility's protocols for reporting adverse events. Your supervisor should keep a copy of your report and the product lot number in case the FDA needs to identify, track, or recall the product.

Also, promptly inform the FDA of product quality problems, such as a defective device, an inaccurate or unreadable product label, packaging or product mix-ups, intrinsic or extrinsic contamination or stability problems, particulates in injectable drugs, or product damage.

Documenting I.V. therapy

At least 8 of 10 hospitalized patients receive some form of I.V. therapy. You may use I.V. therapy to deliver fluids, electrolytes, total parenteral nutrition (TPN), or drugs.

In all cases, document all facets of I.V. therapy carefully and completely, including not only administration but also any complications that arise. You may need to use a special I.V. therapy sheet or nursing flow sheet. (See *Using a flow sheet to document I.V. therapy*, page 108.)

Don't round the corner

Whenever you insert an I.V. line, remember to document the:
- date
- time
- venipuncture site
- equipment used, such as the type and gauge of catheter or needle.

Always chart the exact time you performed a procedure rather than charting on the hour or half hour. (See *Documenting an infusion therapy procedure*, page 109.)

A-one, and a-two...and done

The Infusion Nurses Society (INS) recommends making only two attempts to start an I.V. line. Document the number of attempts you made and the type of assistance you needed to start the line. Follow your facility's policy.

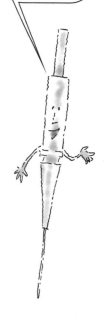

When you insert an I.V., note the date, time, site, and equipment you used.

Documenting I.V. assessment

When documenting an I.V. assessment, review previous assessments and keep them in mind when documenting the latest assessment. Watch for any assessment findings that differ markedly from earlier ones.

Say, for example, the previous nurse wrote, "Slight discomfort at right-hand I.V. site" at the 8 a.m. assessment. At 11 a.m., you inspect the site and note some redness. Because of the change from the earlier assessment, you should suspect phlebitis and consider removing the line, assessing for other complications, or both.

The latest news

Update your records each time you change an insertion site, a venipuncture device, a site dressing, or I.V. tubing. Also, document any reason for changing the I.V. site, such as:
- extravasation

Using a flow sheet to document I.V. therapy

This sample shows some typical features of an I.V. therapy flow sheet. To document, use the flow sheet's key to abbreviations and numbers (not shown).

I.V. THERAPY FLOW SHEET

Diagnosis: ® Mastectomy

Venipuncture limitations: Ⓛ arm only

Permanent access: None

Date and time	2/24/02 1400	2/27/02 1800	
Patient visit	2	1	
Site status	1	1	
Procedure	R	C	
Gauge I.V. device	20	✓	
Catheter type	J	J	
Location	LPF	LPF	
Date of insertion	2/26	2/26	
Routine site rotation	—	—	
Phlebitis	1+	1	
Infiltration	1	0	
Other	1	—	
Number of failed attempts	0	—	
Lock status	—	—	
Flush	—	—	
Tubing: Macrodrip	✓	✓	
Minidrip			
Valleylab			
Filter			
Extension	✓	✓	
Dressing change	✓	—	
Blood sample drawn	—	—	
Subcutaneous access port	—	—	
Patient response	1	1	

Document all facets of I.V. therapy carefully and completely.

Documenting an infusion therapy procedure

Precise, accurate documentation of infusion therapy is critical for effective communication among staff members caring for the patient. This list summarizes the information that should be contained in each notation about initiating, monitoring, and discontinuing an I.V.

Initiating	Monitoring	Discontinuing
• Site chosen • Condition of the insertion site before and after insertion (bruising, burns, and other observations) • Type of cannula used • Length and gauge of the cannula • Time and date of insertion • Number of attempts at cannulation • Name and title of person responsible for insertion • Type of medication administered • Flow rate	• Condition of the insertion site and surrounding area • Flow rate • Type of medication being administered • Intake and output • Description of any complications as well as what was done about them • Name and title of person making the assessment	• Condition of the site and surrounding area • Condition of the cannula upon removal (documented only if a problem occurred) • Reason for discontinuation • Date and time of discontinuation • Name and title of person removing the infusion device

- phlebitis
- occlusion
- patient removal
- facility policy.

On each shift, make sure to document the type, amount, and flow rate of I.V. fluid and the condition of the I.V. site. Make a note each time you flush an I.V. line, and document the fluid used to flush the line.

Take the time to document any complication precisely and in a timely manner. For example, if you note erythema and swelling at an I.V. site, document the amount of redness and swelling at the site, your nursing interventions, to whom the incident was reported, and what treatment, if any, was ordered.

Extra, extra, extravasation!

If extravasation occurs, stop the I.V. infusion. Then assess the approximate amount of fluid infiltrated, provide appropriate nursing intervention, and notify the doctor. Be sure to document all pertinent information. (See *Documentation sampler: I.V. therapy,* page 110.)

If a chemotherapy drug extravasates, follow your facility's procedure. Document the appearance of the I.V. site, the type of treatment given (especially any drug used as an antidote), the kind of dressing applied to the site, and that the doctor was notified. Also,

---

Documentation sampler: I.V. therapy

Effective charting for I.V. therapy means covering key aspects of the therapy in a consistent, easily understandable manner. Here are samples written by a nurse about several different patients receiving various forms of peripheral infusion therapy.

I.V. start

I.V. started in right lower cephalic vein with a 20G 1¼" after two attempts. The site before and after insertion was unremarkable. 0.9% NaCl and 20 mEq KCL infused at 125 ml/hour without difficulty.

0812
1/4/02
M. Black, RN

I.V. site problems

I.V. in left hand infiltrated; approximately 2 cm-size area slightly puffy with no discomfort. I.V. dc'd, and warm pack applied.

1323
2/23/02
M. Black, RN

Patient pulled out I.V. in left forearm. Small hematoma at site. Pressure dressing applied for 10 minutes. Restarted in right basilic vein with 20G, 1" protective catheter; two attempts. Site was benign before and after insertion. Lactated Ringer's infused at 75 ml/hour without difficulty.

1214
4/25/02
M. Black, RN

Routine I.V. site change not done due to limited vein access. No redness, tenderness, or swelling at I.V. site.

1632
6/1/02
M. Black, RN

Patient refusal

Patient refused routine I.V. site change. Patient informed of site rotation policy. Patient states, "Leave it alone. It feels fine."

1129
7/11/02
M. Black, RN

Discharge instructions

Patient instructed to apply warm packs if tenderness at I.V. site persists and to notify doctor if fever develops or I.V. site becomes more sore.

1053
10/31/02
M. Black, RN

---

be sure to make a note every time you flush this kind of I.V. line and the type and amount of fluid used.

Stay hypersensitive to allergic reactions

If your patient has an allergic reaction while receiving I.V. therapy, notify a doctor immediately and complete an incident report.

Document all pertinent information about the reaction, such as the type of reaction, when it was discovered, the extent of the reaction, and that it was reported to the doctor. Also document treatments and the patient's response to them.

Teacher's notes

Finally, record any patient teaching that you offer to the patient and his family, including:
- the purpose of I.V. therapy
- description of the procedure itself
- discussion of any possible complications.

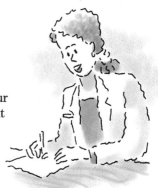

Record any patient teaching you do.

Documenting total parenteral nutrition

If you're administering TPN, you'll need to document the:
- TPN solution and bottle or bag number
- type and location of the central line
- condition of the insertion site
- volume and rate of the infusion.

Label all tubing with the date and time it was hung plus your initials. Assess the patient for adverse reactions, and document your observations and interventions.

Crossing the finish line

When you discontinue a central TPN line, record the date and time it was removed and the type of dressing applied. Also, describe the appearance of the administration site.

Avoiding common errors

Remember how to avoid common errors in documentation. As you become an expert at medication administration — and you become busier than ever — you must never forget how important it is to fully document all aspects of medication administration. Make sure you chart fully, accurately, and legibly.

Do's and don'ts

Along with the "do's" of charting, pay attention to the "don'ts." For instance:
- don't chart ahead of time
- don't chart at arbitrary times rather than charting immediately
- don't chart for someone else, in most cases, because doing so could make you liable for that person's inappropriate or incorrect medication administration
- don't forget to document any patient teaching you provide on the topic of drugs or their administration. Include in your documentation any patient teaching aids you used and any response either the patient or family members had to your teaching.

I know we're close, but I still can't chart for you.

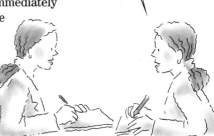

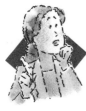

Quick quiz

1. If you aren't sure whether an abbreviation is approved by your facility, you should:
    A.   Still use it if it's common.
    B.   Use it and inform your supervisor.
    C.   Not use it, and write out the full word instead.
    D.   Use it, and explain its meaning at report.

Answer: C. Use only standard abbreviations approved by your facility. If you aren't sure whether an abbreviation is approved, don't use it. Instead, write out the full word or phrase.

2. If you suspect that a drug caused a life-threatening illness in your patient, which form would you use to report it to the FDA?
    A.   MedWatch form
    B.   MAR form
    C.   Internal incident report form
    D.   Facility Adverse Drug Reaction form

Answer: A. To report an adverse reaction to the FDA, complete a MedWatch form. Use this form when you suspect that a drug, medical device, nutritional product, or any FDA-regulated product causes a death, a life-threatening illness, an initial or prolonged hospitalization, a disability, a congenital anomaly, or the need for medical or surgical intervention to prevent impairment or injury.

3. According to the INS, how many attempts should you make to start an I.V. line?
    A.   One
    B.   Two
    C.   Three
    D.   Four

Answer: B. The INS recommends making only two attempts to start an I.V. line. Document the number of attempts you make and the type of assistance you needed to start the line. Be sure to follow your facility's policy.

Scoring

☆☆☆   If you answered all three items correctly, make a note! You're ready to document completely, accurately, and on time!

  ☆☆   If you answered fewer than three items correctly, no need to inform the FDA. Just review the chapter, and you'll be ready to move to the top of the charts.

Part II Drug administration methods and routes

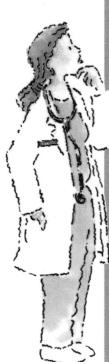

7

Topical administration

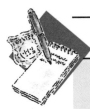

Just the facts

In this chapter, you'll learn:

♦ different methods of topical drug administration

♦ procedures you should follow for safe, effective topical drug therapy

♦ how to administer various types of transdermal medications.

Administering topical drugs

Topical drugs exert their effects after being applied to a patient's skin or the mucous membrane in the patient's mouth or throat.

Topical drugs may take the form of a lotion, cream, ointment, paste, powder, or spray, which you apply to an affected skin area. Or you may use a spray, mouthwash, gargle, or lozenge to treat a problem in the patient's mouth or throat.

Uptown local

Usually, you'll use these topical administration methods to obtain local, rather than systemic, drug effects. The drug moves through the epidermis and into the dermis based in part on the vascularity of the region to which it's applied.

Interstate transport

Certain types of topical drugs are known as transdermal drugs. A *transdermal drug* is a type of topical drug meant to enter the patient's bloodstream and exert a systemic effect after you apply a paste or patch to the patient's skin.

> Topical drugs are usually applied to the skin, but can also treat a problem in the mouth or throat.

Applying lotions, creams, ointments, and pastes

Keep in mind the following differences between lotions, creams, ointments, and pastes:
• A *lotion* contains an insoluble powder suspended in water or an emulsion. When you apply a lotion, it leaves a uniform layer of powder in the film on the patient's skin.
• A *cream* is an oil-in-water emulsion in semisolid form. It lubricates the skin and acts as a barrier.
• An *ointment* is a semisolid substance that, when applied to the skin, helps to retain body heat and provides prolonged contact between the skin and the drug.
• A *paste* is a stiff mixture of powder and ointment. It provides a uniform coat to reduce and repel moisture.

What you need

Prescribed medicated lotion, cream, ointment, or paste ✳ gloves ✳ towels or linen-saver pads ✳ sterile tongue blade ✳ sterile 4″ × 4″ gauze pads

Getting ready

• Verify the order in the patient's chart.
• Identify the patient by checking his armband.
• Explain what you'll be doing, and help the patient into a comfortable position. Expose only the body part on which you'll apply the topical drug.
• Wash your hands and put on gloves.
• Place a linen-saver pad or towel under the affected area.
• As needed, wash and dry the affected skin area to remove crusts, epidermal scales, or residue left after previous topical applications. (See *Removing an ointment.*)
• Change your gloves after you clean debris from the skin or if they become soiled for another reason.

How you do it

For a lotion

• Shake the lotion container well and pour a small amount of lotion into your gloved hand.
• Gently smooth a thin layer of lotion onto the patient's skin in the affected area.

For a cream, ointment, or paste

• Open the medication container and place the lid or cap upside down to keep the inside from becoming contaminated.

Memory jogger

Trans- means "across" or "through"; *dermal* means "related to the skin." A transdermal drug moves THROUGH THE SKIN and into the bloodstream.

Peak technique

Removing an ointment

Because ointments don't dissolve in water, they can be tough to remove from your patient's skin. To remove old ointment, follow these steps.

Solve the problem
First, get a solvent, such as cottonseed oil, and some sterile 4" × 4" gauze pads and gloves. Wash your hands, put on the gloves, and saturate a gauze pad with some of the cottonseed oil as shown.

Next, use the saturated pad to swab the ointment gently from the patient's skin. Rub in the direction of hair growth, and don't wipe too hard or you may irritate the skin. After you've removed the ointment, use another gauze pad to remove excess cottonseed oil. Then remove your gloves and wash your hands.

Home improvement
If the patient will be removing old ointment at home, teach him the procedure and ask for a return demonstration. After removing ointment, record the date and time, solvent used, condition of the patient's skin, and patient teaching you provided.

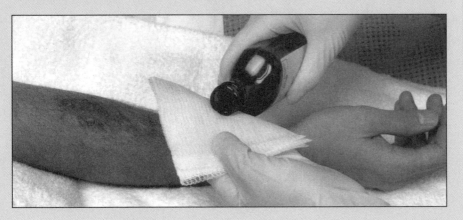

- Remove a tongue blade from its sterile wrapper and cover one end with the medication from the tube or jar.
- Transfer the medication from the tongue blade to your gloved hand.
- Apply the medication to the affected area using long, smooth strokes. Remember to move in the direction of hair growth. (See *Moving in the right direction*, page 118.)
- Remove your gloves and wash your hands.

Peak technique

Moving in the right direction

When applying a topical medication, be sure to move in the direction of hair growth using long, smooth strokes as shown in the illustrations below. Moving in the right direction will avoid forcing the drug into the patient's hair follicles, which can lead to irritation and folliculitis.

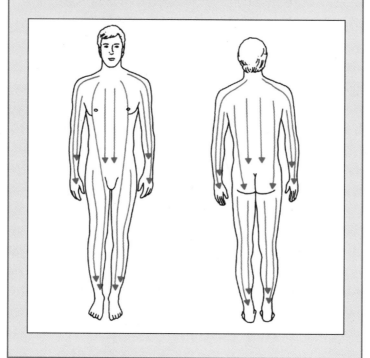

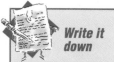

Write it down

Documenting topical drug administration

Be sure to record:
• date and time you applied a topical medication
• medication contained in the topical preparation
• condition of the patient's skin
• effects of the topical medication
• patient teaching you provided.

When you're done
• Afterward, assess the patient's skin for local irritation.

Practice pointers
• Make sure you apply the lotion, cream, ointment, or paste only to affected skin areas. Don't use them on uninvolved areas because you could encourage skin breakdown.
• Never apply an ointment to a patient's eyelids or ear canal unless specifically instructed to do so. The ointment could congeal and occlude the tear duct or ear canal.

What to teach

• Tell the patient to wash his hands before and after applying the topical medication.
• Teach him how to apply the medication properly.
• Be sure to stress that his skin should be clean and dry before he applies the medication.
• Teach him to apply the lotion only to the affected area.
• Be sure to show him how to avoid contaminating the lid or cap of the container.
• Warn the patient to stop using the medication and to call his doctor if he develops skin irritation, ulcers, or signs and symptoms of infection or a worsening skin reaction.

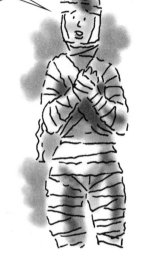

To prevent skin breakdown, expose only affected skin areas to lotions or other drugs.

Administering a powder

A *powder* is an inert chemical that may contain medication. It helps dry the skin and reduces maceration and friction.

What you need

Powder ✳ towels or linen-saver pads ✳ gloves

Getting ready

• Verify the order in the patient's chart.
• Identify the patient by checking his armband.
• Explain what you'll be doing, and help the patient to a comfortable position. Expose only the body part on which you'll apply the powder.
• Wash your hands and put on gloves.
• Place a linen-saver pad or towel under the affected area.

How you do it

• Dry the skin surface. Make sure you spread and dry all skin folds that could collect moisture.
• Shake a small amount of the powder onto your hand and then gently apply a thin layer to the affected skin area.
• Don't let the patient inhale airborne powder. Be sure to shake the powder away from the patient's face.

Practice pointers

• Make sure the patient knows why you're applying the powder.

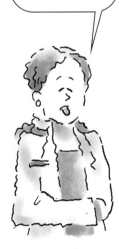

Be sure to shake the powder away from the patient's face — and yours.

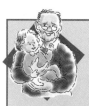

Ages and stages

Topical tips for tots

Remember these tips when administering topical drugs to pediatric patients:
• When applying powder, shake it into your hand, then apply it to the child; doing so avoids creating puffs of powder that you or the child could accidentally inhale.
• Use topical corticosteroids cautiously and sparingly on diaper-covered body areas. A disposable diaper or rubber pants mimics an occlusive dressing, possibly increasing systemic absorption of the drug.

• Remember these tips when administering a topical drug to pediatric patients. (See *Topical tips for tots*.)

What to teach

• Tell the patient to first make sure the skin is dry, including all skin folds.
• Teach him to apply only a thin layer of powder unless the doctor has ordered otherwise.

Administering a topical spray

A *topical spray* allows even application of a thin film of medication.

What you need

Prescribed medicated spray ✻ towels or linen-saver pads ✻ gloves

Getting ready

• Verify the order in the patient's chart.
• Identify the patient by checking his armband.
• Explain what you'll be doing, and help the patient to a comfortable position. Expose only the body part on which you'll apply the topical spray.
• Wash your hands and put on gloves.
• Place a linen-saver pad or towel under the affected area.

How you do it

• Dry the skin surface. Make sure you spread and dry all skin folds that could collect moisture.

Write it down

Documenting medicated powder administration

Be sure to record:
• date and time you applied the powder
• medication it contained
• condition of the patient's skin
• effects of the powder
• patient teaching.

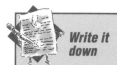

Write it down

Documenting topical spray administration

Be sure to record:
• date and time you administered a spray
• medication it contained
• condition of the patient's skin
• effects of the medication
• patient teaching you provided.

Shake it up

- Shake the container, if indicated, to mix the medication.
- Hold the container 6″ to 12″ (15 to 30.5 cm) from the skin or as specified on the container's label.
- Spray the medication evenly over the treatment area to apply a thin film.

Practice pointers

- To keep the patient from inhaling aerosol, tell him to turn his head and hold his breath when you're about to spray. You may also cover his face lightly with a towel.

I'd like a thin film, please!

What to teach

- Tell the patient to dry his skin before using a spray.
- Show him how to evenly spray a thin layer.
- Warn him not to inhale the aerosol.

Applying medication to the scalp

You may apply a medicated lotion, cream, or shampoo to a patient's scalp.

What you need

Scalp medication or shampoo ✱ towels ✱ linen-saver pads ✱ comb or brush ✱ gloves

Getting ready

- Verify the order in the patient's chart.
- Identify the patient by checking his armband.
- Explain what you'll be doing, and help the patient to a comfortable position.
- Wash your hands and put on gloves.

How you do it

- Wet the patient's hair thoroughly and wring out excess water.
- Shake the shampoo bottle to mix the contents, if appropriate.
- Apply the amount of shampoo specified on the label.

Lather, rinse — and don't repeat

- Work the shampoo into a lather, adding water as necessary. Part the hair and work the shampoo into the patient's scalp, taking care not to use your fingernails.

• Leave the shampoo on the scalp and hair for as long as instructed (usually 5 to 10 minutes). Then rinse the patient's hair thoroughly.

Off the top of his head

• Remove excess water with a towel.
• Comb or brush the hair to remove tangles.
• If you're applying a medicated lotion or cream, use your fingertips, as shown below, to apply medication to the scalp. Start at the point where the hair parts naturally, and spread the medication evenly.

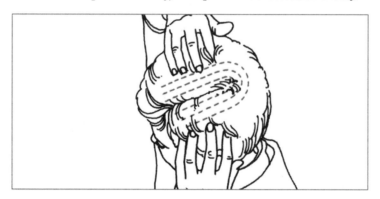

• Continue applying the medication every ½″ (1.3 cm), following the label instructions.
• As appropriate, massage the medication into the scalp using your finger tips, taking care not to use your fingernails.
• Remove your gloves and wash your hands.

Practice pointers

• Take care to apply the medication as directed on the label.
• Keep the medication out of the patient's eyes and mucous membranes.

Head it off

• Make sure you know what to do in case the medication accidentally comes in contact with the patient's eyes or mucous membranes.

What to teach

• Have the patient apply the medication, if possible, especially if he'll be continuing treatment at home.
• Make sure he can spread the medication evenly onto his scalp.
• Remind the patient not to get the medication in his eyes, and to flush them liberally with water if he does.

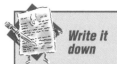

Write it down

Documenting scalp medication administration

Be sure to record:
• date and time you applied a scalp medication
• medication it contained
• condition of the patient's scalp
• effects of the medication
• patient teaching you provided.

Be sure to keep the medication out of the patient's eyes.

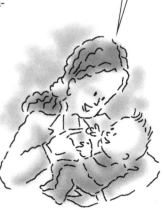

Applying medication to the face

You may apply an ointment, paste, or lotion to a patient's face.

What you need

Soap ✳ water ✳ gloves ✳ cotton-tipped applicators ✳ sterile 4″ × 4″ gauze pads ✳ prescribed medication ✳ towels ✳ wash-cloth

Getting ready

- Verify the order in the patient's chart.
- Identify the patient by checking her armband.
- Wash your hands and put on gloves.
- Wash or have the patient wash her face with mild soap and water to remove any medication residue or exudate.

How you do it

- If you'll be applying the medication to the patient's forehead or chin, or under her eyes, place a small amount of the medication on the tip of a cotton-tipped applicator.
- If you'll be applying the medication to a larger area of the patient's face, place some of it on a 4″ × 4″ gauze pad.

Don't lose face

- Apply the medication as shown. (See *Applying medication to a patient's face*, page 124.)

Practice pointers

- Apply the medication according to the directions on the tube.
- Don't get the medication in the patient's eyes or mucous membranes.

What to teach

- Instruct the patient to wash her hands before and after applying the drug.
- Teach her how to apply the drug properly and only on clean, dry skin.

Face facts

- Stress the importance of applying the medication in the direction of hair growth.
- Tell her to apply the drug only to affected skin areas, and to keep it out of her eyes and mucous membranes.

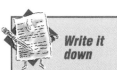

Write it down

Documenting face medication administration

Be sure to record:
- date and time you applied medication to the patient's face
- name of the medication
- condition of the patient's face
- effects of the medication
- patient teaching you provided.

Peak technique

Applying medication to a patient's face

Follow these steps when applying a medicated ointment, paste, or lotion to a patient's face:
• Begin applying the medication on the patient's forehead.
• Spread it down each side of the face to the jaw.
• Be sure to stroke only in one direction, using the pattern shown in the illustration.

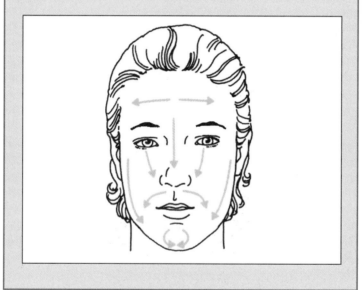

• Be sure to show her how to avoid contaminating the lid or cap of the medication container.

In the face of danger

• Warn the patient to stop using the drug and to call the doctor if she develops skin irritation, ulcers, or signs of infection or a worsening skin reaction.

Administering a throat spray

You may administer an antibiotic, antiseptic, or anesthetic into a patient's throat, commonly by spray.

What you need

Prescribed medication ✳ atomizer or spray pump ✳ tongue blade or spoon ✳ gloves

Getting ready

- Verify the order in the patient's chart.
- Identify the patient by checking his armband.

Up you go

- Explain what you'll be doing, and help the patient to a comfortable, upright position. If the patient can't sit up, ask the doctor if you can substitute another form of medication. Spraying the throat of a supine patient increases the risk of aspiration.
- Wash your hands and put on gloves.

How you do it

- Ask the patient to open his mouth.

Take my advice

- If you're administering an anesthetic, such as benzocaine (Vicks Chloraseptic), follow the advice given below. (See *Administering an anesthetic throat spray.*)
- Tell the patient not to inhale as you spray the medication.
- If you're using a spray pump, hold the nozzle just outside the patient's mouth and direct the spray to the back of his throat. If you're using an atomizer, insert the tip just inside the patient's mouth and direct the spray to the back of his throat.
- Press down the spray button or device quickly and firmly, using enough force to propel the spray to the inflamed throat tissues.
- Caution the patient not to swallow for a few moments so the medication can run down his throat and coat the mucous membranes.
- Monitor the patient for aspiration.

Practice pointers

- To increase the drug's effectiveness, tell the patient not to eat or drink for at least 30 minutes after receiving a throat spray.
- If the patient has received an anesthetic, hold foods and fluids for 60 minutes to reduce the risk of aspiration.

Peak technique

Administering an anesthetic throat spray

Drugs, such as antibiotics, antiseptics, and anesthetics, can all be applied as a spray. When you're administering an anesthetic throat spray, follow these steps:

- Invert a teaspoon or place a tongue blade over the patient's tongue before you spray (doing so keeps the patient's tongue from getting numb and it helps you see the irritated area of his throat).
- Ask the patient to hold the spoon or tongue blade in place.

Be sure to monitor your patient for aspiration after administering a throat spray.

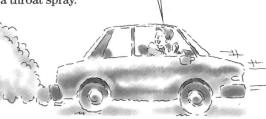

What to teach

• Teach the patient how to administer his own throat medication because he may have to continue treatment at home.

Mirror, mirror on the wall

• Have him try it in front of a mirror, then offer suggestions and correct any errors you observe.

Administering a mouthwash or gargle

You may administer a mouthwash or gargle to address a problem in the patient's mouth or throat.

What you need

Prescribed solution ✳ drinking cup ✳ emesis basin ✳ thermometer

Getting ready

• Verify the order in the patient's chart.
• If necessary, warm the prescribed medication to 100° F (37.8° C) by setting the container in warm water. Check the temperature with a thermometer.
• Identify the patient by checking his armband.
• Explain what you'll be doing, and help the patient to a comfortable, upright position.
• Wash your hands.

How you do it

• If you're using a mouthwash, pour 30 to 120 ml into a drinking cup and tell the patient to swish it around in his mouth, especially over the teeth and gums. Warn him not to swallow it, but to spit it into the emesis basin.

Take a deep breath

• If you're using a gargle, tell him to tilt his head back slightly and take a deep breath. Give him 30 ml of the solution, and tell him to hold it in his mouth.
• Then, tell him to exhale slowly through his mouth to create the gargling effect. Warn him not to swallow the solution (unless it's an anesthetic), but to spit it into the emesis basin when he's finished gargling.

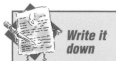

Write it down

Documenting throat spray administration

Be sure to record:
• date and time you administered a throat spray
• medication it contained
• method of administration
• condition of the patient's throat, if pertinent
• effects of the medication
• patient teaching you provided.

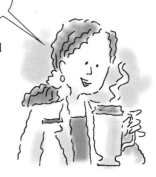

Warm the medication to 100° F (37.8° C) by setting the container in warm water.

Practice pointers

• To increase the drug's effectiveness, tell the patient not to eat or drink for at least 30 minutes after receiving a throat spray.
• If the patient swallows any of the gargling solution, hold foods and fluids for 60 minutes to reduce the risk of aspiration and notify the doctor.

What to teach

• Teach the patient how to administer his own mouth or throat medication because he may have to continue treatment at home.
• Have him try it in front of a mirror, then offer suggestions and correct any errors you observe.

Administering a lozenge

Some mouth and throat medications are delivered by lozenges.

What you need

Prescribed lozenge ✻ gloves

Getting ready

• Verify the order in the patient's chart.
• Identify the patient by checking his armband.
• Explain the purpose of the lozenge, and help the patient to a comfortable, upright position.
• Wash your hands and put on gloves.

How you do it

• Give the patient the lozenge or place it in his mouth.

I'll chew you out

• Tell the patient to keep the lozenge in his mouth until it dissolves. Warn him not to chew or swallow it because doing so will circumvent the intended effect.

Practice pointers

• Some lozenges contain sugar, so if your patient has diabetes or follows a sugar-restricted diet, ask the doctor if this medication is permissible or if a substitute medication should be ordered.
• To increase the drug's effectiveness, tell the patient not to eat or drink for at least 30 minutes after receiving a lozenge.

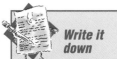

Documenting a mouthwash or gargle administration

Be sure to record:
• date and time you administered a mouthwash or gargle
• medication it contained
• method of administration
• condition of the patient's throat, if pertinent
• effects of the medication
• patient teaching you provided.

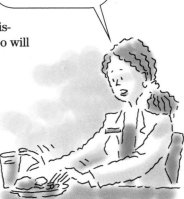

Tell the patient not to eat or drink for at least 30 minutes after taking the lozenge.

What to teach

- Teach the patient how to administer his own lozenge because he may have to continue treatment at home.
- Have him try it in front of a mirror, then offer suggestions and correct any errors you observe.

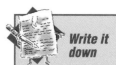

Write it down

Documenting lozenge administration

Be sure to record:
- date and time you administered a lozenge
- medication it contained
- condition of the patient's mouth or throat, if pertinent
- effects of the medication
- patient teaching you provided.

Administering a transdermal drug

Transdermal drugs deliver a constant, controlled amount of medication through the skin and into the bloodstream, thereby achieving a steady, prolonged systemic effect.

Patch him up

To give a transdermal drug, you'll either apply a measured amount of ointment to a selected area of the patient's skin, or you'll apply a transdermal patch that contains medication. (See *Understanding a transdermal patch.*)

The transdermal team

- Nitroglycerin to control angina
- Scopolamine to treat motion sickness
- Estradiol to provide hormone replacement after menopause
- Clonidine to treat hypertension
- Fentanyl to control chronic pain

A matter of time

The appropriate form—ointment or patch—by which to give the drug depends largely on the desired delivery time; typically, a patch delivers the drug for a longer period of time. For example, transdermal nitroglycerin ointment dilates coronary vessels for up to 4 hours, whereas a nitroglycerin patch lasts for up to 24 hours. In patch form, scopolamine lasts up to 72 hours, estradiol up to a week, clonidine up to 24 hours, and fentanyl up to 72 hours.

What you need
Transdermal ointment

Prescribed medicated ointment ✳ application strip or measuring paper ✳ semipermeable dressing or plastic wrap ✳ gloves ✳ washcloth ✳ soap ✳ warm water ✳ towel ✳ adhesive tape

Transdermal patch

Prescribed medicated patch ✳ washcloth ✳ soap ✳ water ✳ towel

Understanding a transdermal patch

A transdermal patch is made up of several layers. The outermost layer is an aluminized polyester barrier that holds the drug in the patch. The next layer is the drug reservoir; it contains the main dose of the drug. The next layer—a membrane—controls release of the drug from the reservoir.

Stick with it

The innermost adhesive layer keeps the patch on the patient's skin and holds a small amount of drug as it moves from the patch into the skin. The dots in the illustration below show the drug moving through the skin and into the bloodstream.

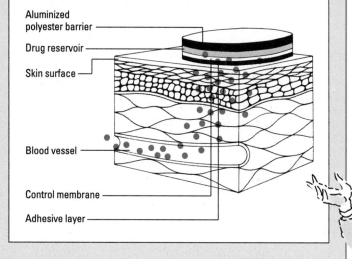

Aluminized polyester barrier

Drug reservoir

Skin surface

Blood vessel

Control membrane

Adhesive layer

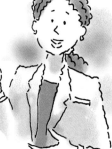

A transdermal patch delivers a constant, controlled amount of medication that achieves a steady, prolonged systemic effect.

Getting ready

- Verify the order in the patient's chart.
- Identify the patient by checking his armband.
- Wash your hands and put on gloves.

How you do it

Applying a transdermal ointment

- Choose the application site—usually a dry, hairless spot on the patient's chest or arm.
- To promote absorption, wash the site with soap and warm water. Dry it thoroughly.

• If the patient has a previously applied medication strip at another site, remove it and wash this area to clear away any drug residue.

Splitting hairs

• If you must use an area that's hairy, clip excess hair rather than shaving it; shaving causes irritation, which may be exacerbated by the drug.

Hands off

• Squeeze the prescribed amount of ointment on the application strip or measuring paper as shown below. Don't let the drug touch your skin.

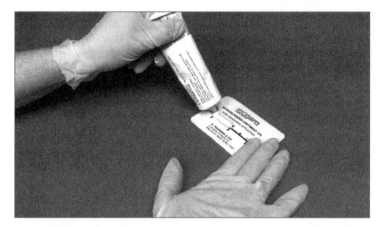

• Apply the strip, drug side down, directly to the patient's skin.
• Maneuver the strip slightly to spread a thin layer of the ointment over a 3″ (7.5 cm) area, but don't rub the ointment into the skin.
• Secure the application strip to the patient's skin by covering it with a semipermeable dressing as shown below.

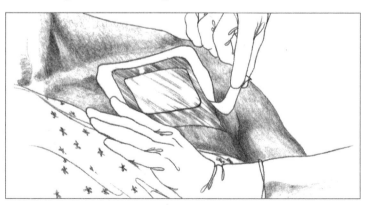

Skin tight

• Press firmly with the palm of one hand to ensure that the dressing adheres well, especially around the edges.
• Label the strip with the date, time, and your initials.
• Remove your gloves and wash your hands.

Applying a transdermal patch

• Remove the old patch. (See *Discarding a patch.*)
• Choose a dry, hairless application site. Be sure to rotate application sites. Don't attempt to apply the patch to an area with alterations in skin integrity.
• If necessary, clip any hair from the site, but don't shave the area. The most commonly used sites are the upper arm, chest, and back and behind the ear.
• Clean the application site with soap and warm water. Dry it thoroughly.
• Open the drug package and remove the patch.
• Without touching the adhesive surface, remove the clear plastic backing as shown.
• Apply the patch to the application site, again without touching the adhesive.

Practice pointers

• Apply any transdermal drug at the prescribed intervals to ensure a continuous effect.
• Don't apply the drug if the patient has skin allergies or has experienced skin reactions to the drug.

Saved by his own skin

• Avoid areas of broken or irritated skin; the drug could increase the irritation.
• Don't apply a transdermal drug to scarred or callused skin because either one may impair absorption.
• If you need to defibrillate a patient who has a transdermal patch in place, follow the advice given below. (See *A shocking experience*, page 132.)

What to teach

• Review any drug-specific precautions the patient needs to know. For example, make sure he knows to thoroughly remove an old application of nitroglycerin ointment before applying a new dose.
• Make sure the patient knows how to choose an appropriate application site, and be sure to tell him to avoid scarred or callused areas, bony prominences, and hairy surfaces.

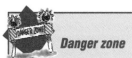

Danger zone

Discarding a patch

Because there's still a substantial amount of drug remaining in a used patch, fold the patch in half, with the adhesive layer inside, before disposing it. This will avoid possible harm to children or animals.

When administering a transdermal patch, remember to rotate application sites.

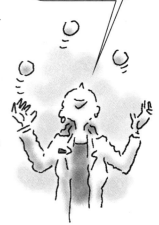

Danger zone

A shocking experience

Don't place a defibrillator paddle on a transdermal patch. The aluminum on the patch can cause electrical arcing during defibrillation, resulting in smoke, thermal burns and, possibly, ineffective electrical cardioversion. If a patient's patch is on a standard paddle site, remove the patch before applying the paddle.

• Warn him not to get any transdermal ointment on his hands, and to wash them thoroughly after applying a transdermal drug.

Dry as a bone

• Make him aware that he needs to keep the area around the application site as dry as possible.
• If the patient will be applying scopolamine, tell him not to drive or operate machinery until he knows how the drug is affecting him.
• If the patient will be using clonidine patches, tell him to check with his primary health care provider before using any nonprescription cough preparations: Over-the-counter preparations may counteract the effects of the drug.
• Warn the patient about the possible adverse reactions that can occur with transdermal drug delivery, such as skin irritation, itching, and rashes.

Here's the facts, Jack

Also, be sure to alert the patient to any adverse reactions to the particular drug being delivered. For example:
• Nitroglycerin may cause headaches and, in elderly patients, postural hypotension.
• Scopolamine most commonly causes a dry mouth and drowsiness.
• Transdermal estradiol may increase the risk of endometrial cancer, thromboembolic disease, and birth defects.
• Clonidine may cause severe rebound hypertension, especially if withdrawn suddenly.

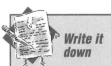

Write it down

Documenting transdermal drug administration

Be sure to record:
• date and time of a transdermal application
• medication used
• location of the ointment or patch on the patient's body
• effects of the medication
• patient teaching you provided.

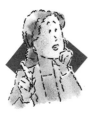

Quick quiz

1. Which of the following topical drug preparations is a semisolid substance that, when applied to the skin, helps to retain body heat and provides prolonged contact between the skin and the drug?
  A. Lotion
  B. Cream
  C. Paste
  D. Ointment

Answer: D. Ointment is a semisolid topical drug that offers prolonged contact between the skin and the applied medication. Its consistency also helps to retain body heat.

2. Which of the following best describes a medicated paste?
  A. An inert chemical that helps dry the skin and reduces maceration and friction.
  B. A stiff mixture of powder and ointment that provides a uniform coat to reduce and repel moisture.
  C. An oil-in-water emulsion in semisolid form that lubricates the skin and acts as a barrier.
  D. An insoluble powder suspended in water or an emulsion that leaves a uniform layer of powder in the film on the patient's skin.

Answer: B. Medicated paste is a topical drug derived from a mixture of a powder and an ointment. It can be applied in a uniform layer to reduce and repel moisture.

3. When applying many topical drugs to the skin, it's important to do which of the following?
  A. Use small, circular strokes.
  B. Force the drug into the patient's hair follicles.
  C. Move in the direction of hair growth.
  D. Apply the drug to the affected and unaffected skin areas.

Answer: C. When applying many topical drugs to the skin, it's important to move in the direction of hair growth to avoid forcing the drug into the patient's hair follicles, which can lead to irritation and folliculitis.

4. If the doctor wants nitroglycerin to dilate the coronary vessels for up to 24 hours, which of the following topical forms would you expect to use for your patient?
  A. Patch
  B. Ointment

C.   Paste
D.   Spray

Answer: A. A nitroglycerin patch lasts up to 24 hours.

Scoring

☆☆☆   If you answered all four questions correctly, congrats! You can help spread the word about topical administration!

☆☆   If you answered three questions correctly, great! You're good to gargle!

☆   If you answered fewer than three questions correctly, there's no need to cry. Just remember to keep medicated shampoos out of your eyes!

8

Ophthalmic, otic, and nasal administration

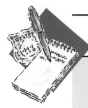

Just the facts

In this chapter, you'll learn:

♦ how to administer drugs into a patient's eye

♦ how to administer drugs into a patient's ear

♦ how to administer drugs into a patient's nose

♦ how to follow procedures for safe, effective therapy.

Administering ophthalmic drugs

Typically, you'll give ophthalmic drugs (diagnostic and therapeutic) as either drops or ointment. To administer some types of drugs, you'll insert a medicated disk into your patient's eye.

Sometimes, you'll need to apply a patch over a patient's eye after you instill an ophthalmic drug.

Instilling eyedrops

Eyedrops can be used for several diagnostic and therapeutic purposes, including:
• dilating the pupil
• staining the cornea to detect abrasions or scars
• anesthetizing the eye
• lubricating the eye
• protecting the vision of a neonate
• treating certain eye disorders, such as infections or glaucoma.

What you need

Prescribed drops ✳ sterile cotton balls ✳ gloves ✳ warm water or normal saline solution ✳ sterile gauze pads ✳ optional: eye dressing

Getting ready

- Verify the order in the patient's chart.
- Read the label to make sure the drug is intended for ophthalmic use.

Seeing is believing

- Check the expiration date on the eyedrop container and inspect the drops for cloudiness, discoloration, and precipitates. If the solution appears abnormal in any way, don't use it.
- Keep in mind that some ophthalmic drugs are in suspension form and normally appear cloudy. When in doubt, check with a pharmacist.

Not the same eye-dea

- Take extra care when verifying an order for eye-drops because different drugs or dosages may be ordered for each eye.
- Identify the patient by checking the armband.
- Explain the procedure to the patient.
- Wash your hands and put on gloves.

Check eyedrops for cloudiness and other abnormalities.

How you do it

- If the patient has an eye dressing in place, remove it by gently pulling it down and away from the patient's forehead.

Careful clean up

- If she has discharge around her eye, moisten sterile cotton balls or sterile gauze pads with warm water or normal saline solution.
- Wipe the eye gently to clean away debris, moving from the inner canthus to the outer canthus as shown below. Use a fresh sterile cotton ball or sterile gauze pad for each stroke.

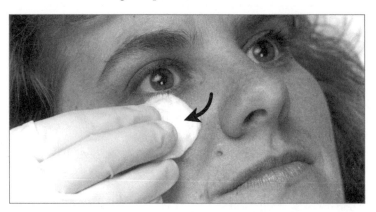

• If the patient has crusted secretions around her eye, moisten a sterile gauze pad with warm water or normal saline solution. Then have the patient close her eye, and place the moist pad over her closed eye for 1 or 2 minutes.
• Remove the pad and reapply new moist sterile gauze pads, as needed, until the secretions become soft enough that you can remove them without injuring the tender ocular tissues.

Full tilt

• Ask the patient to tilt her head back, following the advice below. (See *Instilling eyedrops*.)
• Remove the dropper cap from the bottle (unless the bottle has a built-in dropper) and draw the eyedrops into the dropper, taking care not to contaminate the dropper.
• Ask the patient to look up and away. This moves the cornea away from the lower lid and minimizes the risk of touching the cornea with the dropper if the patient blinks.

Here's a tip

• Steady the hand holding the dropper or eyedrop bottle by resting it against the patient's forehead. Use your other hand to gently pull down the patient's lower eyelid as shown below.

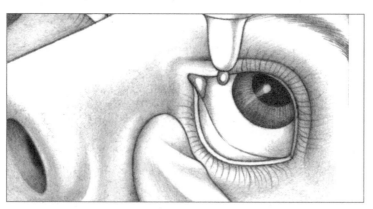

• Instill the prescribed number of drops into the conjunctival sac, not onto the patient's eyeball. Then release the patient's eyelid and have her blink to distribute the drops throughout her eye.

Practice pointers

• If you're opening the drug container for the first time, write the date on the label. Once the container has been opened, the drug should be used within 2 weeks or discarded.
• To prevent contamination, never use the same eyedrop container for more than one patient.

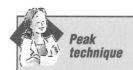

Peak technique

Instilling eyedrops

Have your patient tilt his head back and toward the side of the affected eye to ensure that the drops will flow away from the tear duct at the inner canthus. If you'll be placing drops in his left eye, ask your patient to tilt to the left, to the right if you'll be placing drops in his right eye.

By tilting his head, the patient will reduce the chance that the drops will drain into the tear duct and cause systemic effects.

Memory jogger

When instilling eyedrops, remember UP, UP, AND AWAY — have the patient look up and away from you.

Worth the wait

• If the patient needs more than one type of eye medication, wait at least 5 minutes between administering different doses.
• You can help to minimize systemic reactions to eyedrops by following the advice below. (See *Minimizing systemic reactions to eyedrops.*)

What to teach

• Explain why the doctor prescribed the eyedrops.
• When teaching an older patient, follow the advice below. (See *Managing eyedrop non-sense.*)
• Stress the importance of proper handwashing technique.
• Teach her to make sure she has the right medication, the correct number of drops, and the correct eye.

Warm hands, warm drops

• Tell her that she can warm the drops to room temperature by holding the bottle between her hands for about 2 minutes.
• Teach her that if she's using more than one kind of drop, to wait 5 minutes between them.
• Teach her to protect the container from light and heat.
• Teach her the potential adverse effects of the medication, and when she should notify the doctor.

For your eyes only

• Stress the importance of never placing any medication in her eyes unless the label reads "For Ophthalmic Use" or "For Use in Eyes."
• Teach your patient what to do if the solution is discolored. (See *Checking eye medication.*)
• Provide the patient with written instructions so she can review the proper administration steps after she gets home.

Administering ophthalmic ointment

An ointment formulation helps to keep an ophthalmic drug in contact with the treatment area for as long as possible—an especially useful trait for pediatric patients.

Usually, you'll use an antibiotic ointment to treat eye infections.

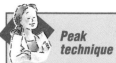

Peak technique

Minimizing systemic reactions to eyedrops

To minimize systemic reactions to eyedrops (tachycardia, palpitations, flushing, dry skin, ataxia, and confusion), have the patient press a finger over his tear duct at the inner canthus as you instill the drops. This compresses the nasolacrimal tear ducts, preventing the drops from draining out.

Write it down

Documenting ophthalmic drug administration

Be sure to record:
• eye treated
• date and time
• prescribed drug and dose
• patient's response to the procedure (Note the appearance of his eye before and after.)
• patient or family teaching you provided.

What you need

Prescribed ointment * sterile cotton balls * gloves * warm water or normal saline solution * sterile gauze pads * facial tissues * optional: eye dressing

Getting ready

• Verify the order in the patient's chart.
• Read the label to make sure the drug is intended for ophthalmic use.

Eye-eye, captain

• Double-check the medication order when administering ophthalmic ointment because different drugs or dosages may be ordered for each eye.
• Identify the patient by checking his armband.
• Explain the procedure to the patient.
• Wash your hands and put on gloves.

How you do it

• If the patient has an eye dressing in place, remove it by gently pulling it down and away from his forehead.
• If he has discharge around his eye, moisten sterile cotton balls or sterile gauze pads with warm water or normal saline solution.
• Gently wipe the eye to clean away debris, moving from the inner canthus to the outer canthus. Use a fresh sterile cotton ball or sterile gauze pad for each stroke.
• If the patient has crusted secretions around his eye, moisten a sterile gauze pad with warm water or normal saline solution. Have the patient close his eye, then place the moist pad over it for 1 or 2 minutes.
• Remove the pad and reapply new moist sterile gauze pads, as needed, until the secretions are soft enough to be removed without injuring the tissue.

Conquering crust

• If the tip of the ointment tube has crusted, wipe it with a sterile gauze pad to remove the crust.
• Ask the patient to look up and away. This moves the cornea away from the lower lid and minimizes the risk of touching the cornea with the tip of the ointment tube if the patient blinks.
• Steady the hand holding the ointment tube against the patient's forehead. Use your other hand to gently pull down his lower eyelid.

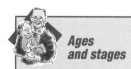

Ages and stages

Managing eyedrop non-sense

If your patient is an older adult, he may have trouble sensing whether a drop has gone into his eye. If so, suggest that he chill his eyedrops before using them. Most people find it easier to feel a drop entering the eye when the drop is cold.

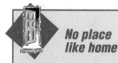

No place like home

Checking eye medication

If your patient can see through the eyedrop container, teach him to hold it up to the light and look at it. If the liquid is discolored or if contains sediment, tell him not to use it. Instead, have him take the container back to the pharmacy and have it checked.

Avoiding eye contact

• Squeeze a small ribbon of ointment along the edge of the conjunctival sac from the inner to the outer canthus as shown below. Don't let the tip of the tube touch the patient's eye. (If it does, discard the tube.)

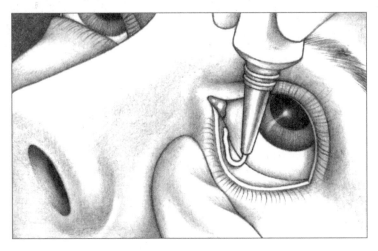

• Cut off the ribbon of ointment by turning the tube. Then release the patient's eyelid and have the patient roll his eyes behind closed lids to help distribute the drug.
• Use a clean tissue to remove any excess ointment that leaks from the patient's eye. Use a fresh tissue for each eye to prevent cross-contamination.
• Finally, apply a new eye dressing, if indicated.

Practice pointers

• If you're opening the drug container for the first time, write the date on the label. Once the container has been opened, the drug should be used within 2 weeks or discarded.

An ounce of prevention is worth a pound of cure

• To prevent contamination, never use the same drug container for more than one patient.
• Systemic reactions are unlikely with ophthalmic ointments because they don't empty quickly into the lacrimal duct, as eyedrops do.

What to teach

• Explain why the doctor prescribed the ointment, and review the proper steps for using the ointment at home.

• Tell the patient to wash his hands before and after applying eye ointment. Be sure to warn him not to contaminate the lid of the ointment tube or touch the tip of the tube to his eye or to the skin around his eye.

• Tell the patient to apply ointment from the inner to the outer corner of his eye. Let him know that his vision may be blurry for several minutes after he puts the ointment in his eye.

Applying an eye patch

Sometimes after you give an ophthalmic drug, you may need to apply a patch over the patient's eye. A patch can:

• protect the eye after injury or surgery
• prevent damage to an anesthetized eye
• promote healing
• absorb secretions
• prevent the patient from touching or rubbing the eye.

Added pressure

A special kind of patch, called a *pressure patch*, is thicker than a conventional patch and requires a doctor's order and supervision. A pressure patch can promote healing of a corneal abrasion; it can also compress edema or control hemorrhage.

What you need

Several sterile eye pads ✳ gloves ✳ tape ✳ protective eye shield

Getting ready

• Verify the order in the patient's chart.
• Wash your hands and put on gloves.
• Identify the patient by checking his armband.

How you do it

• Explain the procedure to the patient, and ask him to close both eyes.
• Grasp the center of a sterile eye pad and place it over the patient's closed eye, so the pad covers the orbit. The pad keeps the patient's eyelid from opening.

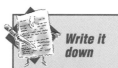

Write it down

Documenting ophthalmic ointment administration

Be sure to record:
• eye treated
• date and time
• prescribed drug
• dose administered
• patient's response to the procedure
• appearance of the patient's eye before and after instillation
• patient or family teaching you provided.

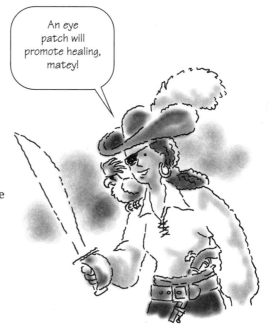

An eye patch will promote healing, matey!

• Secure the pad with parallel strips of tape that extend from the patient's forehead to his cheekbone as shown below. Attach each strip first to the patient's forehead, then to his cheek.

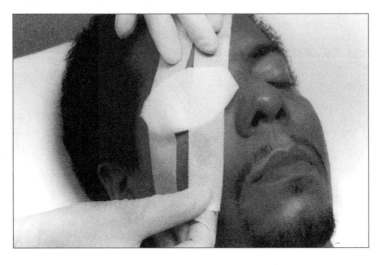

Documenting eye patch application

Be sure to record:
• eye patched
• date and time the patch was placed
• condition of the eye before it was patched
• how the patient tolerated the procedure
• patient or family teaching you provided.

A real eyesore

• If you need to hold the patch in place without tape (if the patient has a facial burn, for instance), use a head dressing to secure the patch.
• To maximize protection of an injured eye, place a plastic shield on top of the eye pad, then apply tape over the shield.

Practice pointers

• When it's time to discontinue the eye patch, carefully remove the tape from the patient's face to avoid damaging the delicate tissues around his eye.

What to teach

• Teach the patient or a family member how to apply an eye patch, if necessary.
• Be sure to tell him to wash his hands before and after applying or removing a patch.
• Instruct the patient to notify a doctor if he develops increased drainage, redness, or swelling.

Inserting a medicated disk

A *medicated ocular disk* is a small, flexible, oval wafer that contains a layer of drug sandwiched between two soft outer layers.

A floppy disk

When it's inserted into a patient's eye, the disk can stay in place for up to 1 week. It floats between the eyelid and the sclera, releasing the drug into the ocular fluid even while the patient sleeps.

What you need

Medicated disk ✳ cotton-tipped applicator ✳ sterile gloves

Getting ready

- Verify the order in the patient's chart.
- Identify the patient by checking his armband.
- Describe the procedure to the patient and explain the purpose of the drug.
- Wash your hands and put on gloves.

How you do it

- Open the disk packet and place it in the palm of your nondominant hand.
- Press a fingertip of your dominant hand against the oval disk. It should stick to your finger. Lift it from its packet.
- After you discard the disk packet, use the fingers of your nondominant hand to gently pull the patient's lower eyelid away from her eye. Place the disk horizontally in the conjunctival sac as shown below.

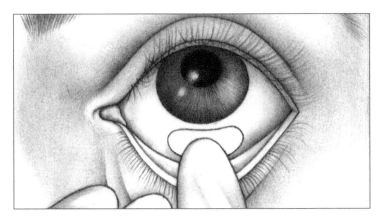

A natural fit

- The disk will naturally adhere to the patient's eye.
- Pull the patient's lower eyelid out, up, and over the disk. Tell him to blink several times. If you can still see the disk, pull the lower lid out, up, and over the disk again.

• Tell the patient that once the disk is in place, he can adjust its position by gently pressing his finger against his closed eyelid. However, caution him not to rub his eye or move the disk across his cornea.

Out of sight

• If the disk falls out, wash your hands, put on gloves, rinse the disk in cool water, and reinsert it. If it looks bent, replace it.

Slipped disk

• If the disk repeatedly slips out of position, reinsert it under the upper eyelid. To do so, use a cotton-tipped applicator to gently lift and evert the patient's upper lid as shown below. Have him look down while you insert the disk horizontally under the upper lid.

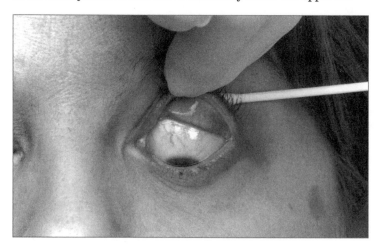

Practice pointers

• The best time to insert a medicated ocular disk is just before bedtime to avoid the blurry vision that may follow insertion.

Powder precautions

• If possible, use unpowdered gloves to insert the disk. If you can't use unpowdered gloves, rinse your gloved hands well before you handle the disk. Rinsing washes away any powder on the gloves, thus preventing it from irritating the patient's eye.
• At the end of the prescribed time, remove the disk as ordered. (See *Removing an ocular disk.*)

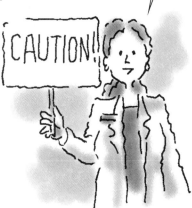

Tell the patient to avoid rubbing his eye or moving the disk across his cornea.

CAUTION!

Peak technique

Removing an ocular disk

You can remove a medicated ocular disk with either one finger or two.

One-finger method
To use one finger, put on gloves and evert the patient's lower eyelid to expose the disk. Use the index finger of your other hand to slide the disk onto the lower lid and out of the patient's eye.

Two-finger method
To use two fingers, evert the patient's lower eyelid to expose the disk. Then use the thumb and forefinger of your other hand to pinch the disk and remove it from the eye.

Yet another way
If the disk is under the patient's upper eyelid, use your finger to make long, circular strokes on the closed eyelid until you see the disk in the corner of the patient's eye. Then place your finger directly on it, move it to the lower sclera, and remove it normally.

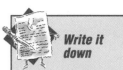

Write it down

Documenting medicated disk administration

Be sure to record:
• eye treated
• date and time the medicated disk was placed
• condition of the patient's eye
• how the patient tolerated the procedure
• patient or family teaching you provided.

An eye for an eye

• If both eyes are being treated with medicated disks, replace both disks at the same time so both eyes receive the drug at the same rate.
• Don't use a medicated ocular disk if the patient has conjunctivitis, keratitis, retinal detachment, or any condition in which pupillary constriction should be avoided.

What to teach

• If the patient wears contact lenses, tell him that he can continue to wear them with the medicated disk in place.

Adverse reactions, my eye!

• Explain that ocular disks can cause adverse reactions, such as:
– a feeling that something is in the eye
– a watery or red eye
– increased mucous discharge
– itchy or red eyelids
– possible blurred vision, headaches, stinging, and swelling.
    These effects usually subside within the first 6 weeks of use.

Administering otic drugs

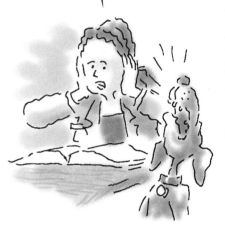

I don't think eardrops will solve this problem!

Otic drugs may be instilled to:
- treat infections and inflammation
- soften cerumen for later removal
- produce local anesthesia
- aid removal of a foreign object trapped in the ear.

Instilling eardrops

You probably won't administer otic drugs to a patient with a perforated eardrum (although it may be permitted with certain medications and with sterile technique).

Not just hearsay

Certain otic drugs may be prohibited in other conditions as well, such as hydrocortisone, if the patient has a viral or fungal infection.

What you need

Prescribed drops ✳ penlight ✳ facial tissues (or cotton-tipped applicators) ✳ cotton balls ✳ emesis basin (for warm water)

Getting ready

- Verify the order in the patient's chart.
- To avoid adverse reactions caused by the instillation of cold eardrops (such as vertigo, nausea, and pain), warm the drops to body temperature by placing the container in a basin of warm water.

Now hear this

- Don't make the drops too hot; if necessary; test their temperature by placing a drop on your wrist.
- Identify the patient by checking his armband.
- Wash your hands.

Within earshot

- Explain the procedure to the patient.

How you do it

- Then have him lie on his side with his affected ear facing up.
- Straighten the patient's ear canal. (See *Positioning a patient for eardrops.*)

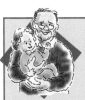

Ages and stages

Positioning a patient for eardrops

Before you instill eardrops, have the patient lie on his side. Then straighten the patient's ear canal to help the drops reach the eardrum. In an adult, gently pull the auricle *up* and *back;* in an infant or young child, gently pull *down* and *back* as shown.

Adult

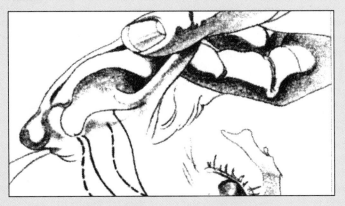

Child

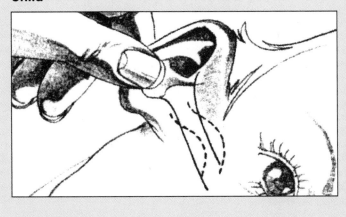

Memory jogger

To straighten your patient's ear canal, remember for an adult or grown-*UP,* gently pull the auricle *UP* and back; for an infant or young child, get *DOWN* to their level and gently pull the auricle *DOWN* and back.

Light the way

• Using a penlight, examine the ear canal for drainage. If you find any, clean the canal with a tissue or cotton-tipped applicator because drainage can reduce the effectiveness of the drug.

• Straighten the patient's ear canal once again and instill the ordered number of drops. To avoid patient discomfort, aim the dropper so the drops fall against the side of the ear canal, not on the eardrum.

Disappearing act

• Hold the ear canal in position until you see the drug disappear down the canal. Then release the ear.
• Tell the patient to stay on his side for 5 to 10 minutes to allow the drug to travel down the ear canal.
• If ordered, tuck a cotton ball loosely into the opening of the ear canal. Don't push it too far into the ear, however, because you'll keep secretions from draining and increase pressure on the eardrum.
• Clean and dry the outer ear.
• Help the patient into a comfortable position
• Remove your gloves, and wash your hands.

Practice pointers

• Some conditions make the normally sensitive ear canal quite tender, so be especially gentle when instilling eardrops.
• Take special care not to injure the eardrum. Never insert any object, even a cotton-tipped applicator, so far into the ear canal that you can't see its tip.
• If the patient has vertigo, keep the side rails of his bed up and assist him as necessary. Also, move slowly to avoid aggravating his vertigo.

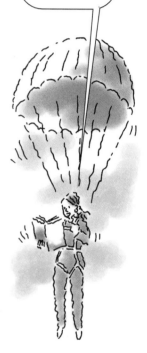

Make sure drops land on the side of the ear canal, not on the eardrum.

Ages and stages

Otic tips for tots

When teaching parents how to administer ear drops to their child, make sure you include the following helpful information:
• Warm the drops for their child's comfort by holding the bottle in their hands for about 2 minutes.
• Gently pull the earlobe down and back to straighten the child's ear canal.
• If necessary, place a cotton ball moistened with the medication at the entrance to the ear canal; remove the cotton after 1 hour. Avoid using dry cotton because it may absorb the medication.

What to teach

- Remind the patient never to insert any object into his ear.
- Review the importance of washing his hands thoroughly.
- Make sure he knows how many drops to give and into which ear.
- Teach him not to use the medication and to call his pharmacist or doctor if the liquid looks discolored or contains sediment.
- When teaching parents how to give eardrops to their child, include the following helpful hints. (See *Otic tips for tots*.)

Not just in one ear and out the other

- Provide written guidelines to parents who will be administering eardrops to a child at home.

Administering nasal drugs

For the most part, nasal drugs produce local effects.

Instilling nose drops

You'll use drops to treat a specific nasal area and sprays and aerosols to diffuse the drug through the nasal passages.

The nose knows

The most commonly administered nasal drugs include:
- vasoconstrictors, which coat and shrink swollen mucous membranes
- local anesthetics, which promote patient comfort during such procedures as bronchoscopy
- corticosteroids, which reduce inflammation caused by allergies or nasal polyps.

What you need

Prescribed medication ✳ gloves

Getting ready

- Verify the order in the patient's chart.
- Identify the patient by checking his armband.

Right on the nose

- Explain the procedure to the patient and position him as needed to make sure the drops reach the intended site. (*See Positioning a patient for nose drops*, page 150.)

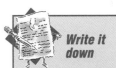

Peak technique

Positioning a patient for nose drops

To reach the ethmoidal and sphenoidal sinuses, have the patient lie on her back with her neck hyperextended and her head tilted back over the edge of the bed. Support her head with one hand to prevent neck strain.

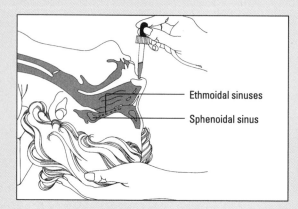

Ethmoidal sinuses

Sphenoidal sinus

To reach the maxillary and frontal sinuses, have the patient lie on her back with her head toward the affected side and hanging slightly over the edge of the bed. Ask her to rotate her head laterally after hyperextension, and support her head with one hand to prevent neck strain.

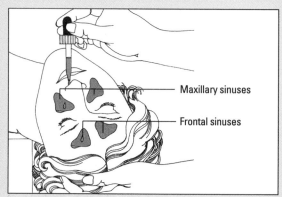

Maxillary sinuses

Frontal sinuses

To administer drops to relieve ordinary nasal congestion, help the patient to a reclining or supine position with her head tilted slightly toward the affected side. Aim the dropper upward, toward the patient's eye, rather than downward, toward her ear.

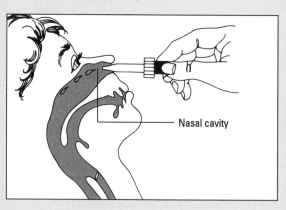

Nasal cavity

Be sure to position the patient properly before instilling nose drops.

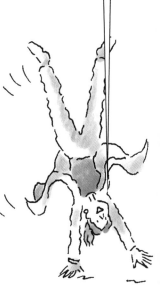

- When administering nose drops to an infant, support the infant on your lap. (See *Positioning an infant for nose drops.*)
- Wash your hands and put on gloves.

How you do it

- Uncap the bottle of nose drops and squeeze the bulb at the top of the dropper to withdraw the drug.

A tip to remember

- Push up gently on the tip of the patient's nose to open his nostrils completely.
- Place the dropper about ⅓″ (1 cm) inside his nostril. Angle the tip of the dropper slightly toward the inner corner of the patient's eye. Squeeze the dropper bulb to dispense the correct number of drops into each nostril.

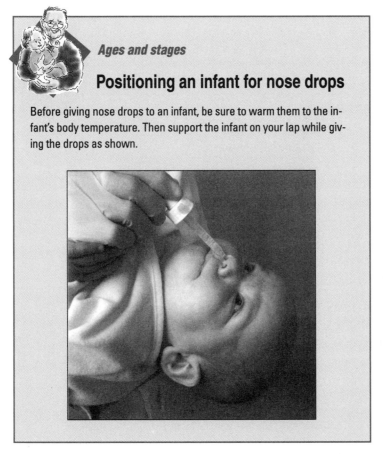

Ages and stages

Positioning an infant for nose drops

Before giving nose drops to an infant, be sure to warm them to the infant's body temperature. Then support the infant on your lap while giving the drops as shown.

• After you've instilled the prescribed number of drops, instruct the patient to keep his head tilted back for about 5 minutes. Encourage him to expectorate any medication that runs into his throat.

Practice pointers

• Stay with the patient after administering nose drops. Urge him to breathe through his mouth. If he coughs, help him to sit up. For several minutes, observe him closely for possible respiratory problems.

What to teach

• Explain the need for proper positioning when nose drops are given
• Tell him to breathe through his mouth during instillation.

Be nose-y

• Make sure the patient can administer the nose drops successfully or that someone at home can help him.
• Instruct the patient to report any changes or adverse reactions caused by the drops or by his nasal condition.

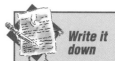

Write it down

Documenting nasal drop administration

Bee sure to record:
• name and amount of medication administered
• date and time of administration
• nostril used
• patient's tolerance for the instillation
• patient teaching you provided.

Administering nasal spray

A *nasal spray* breaks a drug into small particles and distributes it evenly over the mucous membranes.

What you need

Prescribed drug (in an atomizer) ✳ gloves

Getting ready

• Verify the order in the patient's chart.
• Identify the patient by checking his armband.
• Have the patient sit straight with his head upright.
• Wash your hands and put on gloves.

How you do it

• Occlude one of his nostrils with your index finger.
• Place the tip of the atomizer about ½″ (1.5 cm) inside the patient's open nostril. Position the tip straight up his nose toward the inner corner of his eye.

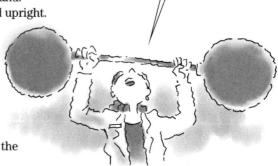

Avoid excessive force when squeezing the atomizer — if spray reaches the sinuses, it can cause a headache.

Taking a nose-dive

- Depending on the drug you're administering, you'll need to have the patient either hold his breath or inhale. Then squeeze the atomizer once, quickly and firmly, just enough for the drug to coat the inside of his nose. Excessive force may propel the spray into his sinuses and cause a headache.
- Repeat the procedure in the other nostril as ordered.

Practice pointers

- Make sure you've placed the tip of the nozzle appropriately — just inside the nostril — to ensure proper delivery of the drug.

What to teach

- If the patient will administer the drug to himself at home, explain the procedure and then have the patient perform it while you supervise.

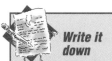

Write it down

Documenting nasal spray administration

Be sure to record:
- name and amount of the drug administered
- date and time you administered it
- nostril or nostrils you used
- patient's tolerance for the nasal spray
- patient teaching you provided.

Administering a nasal aerosol drug

An *aerosol nasal spray* has even finer particles than an atomizer spray, and is especially suited for treating nasal polyps and inflamed areas. A special preparation called dexamethasone turbinaire, given as an aerosol nasal spray, is commonly effective in treating nasal allergies that don't respond to conventional antihistamine-decongestive treatment.

What you need

Prescribed medication (in an aerosol spray) ✳ facial tissues ✳ gloves ✳ plastic bag

Getting ready

- Verify the order in the patient's chart.
- Identify the patient by checking his armband.
- Explain the procedure to the patient.
- Wash your hands.

Some assembly required

- Demonstrate how to assemble the spray device by placing the stem of the medication cartridge into the plastic nasal adapter.

How you do it

• Have the patient blow his nose gently to remove excess mucus. As he does so, shake the cartridge well and remove the protective cap from the adapter tip.
• Put on gloves. Then place the aerosol applicator tip inside the patient's nostril.

Waiting to exhale

• Depending on the drug you're administering, you'll need to have the patient either hold his breath or inhale. As he does, firmly press once on the cartridge, then release it.
• Have the patient continue to hold his breath or inhale for several seconds afterward.
• Remove the adapter tip from the patient's nostril and ask him to exhale.
• If ordered, repeat the procedure.
• Tell the patient not to blow his nose for at least 2 minutes after the procedure.
• Rinse the equipment, replace the protective cap, and store the spray device in a plastic bag to keep it clean.

Practice pointers

• If you're inserting a refill cartridge, you must first remove the plastic cap from the stem.
• Remember to wear gloves, especially if the patient has heavy nasal discharge.

What to teach

• If the patient will be using the aerosol spray at home, have him give you a return demonstration of the procedure so you can assess his technique.

Sit back and relax

• Tell the patient to keep his head tilted back for several minutes after he gives himself the drug to encourage it to stay in place.
• Tell the patient to report any increased nasal irritation, bleeding, nasal congestion, headaches, or dizziness.

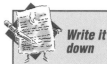

Write it down

Documenting nasal aerosol administration

Be sure to record:
• name and amount of medication you administered
• date and time of administration
• nostril or nostrils you used
• patient's tolerance for the aerosol spray
• patient teaching you provided.

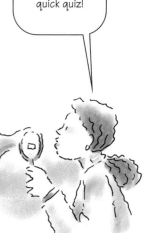

I'll take a break while you take the quick quiz!

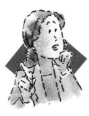

Quick quiz

1. When instilling eyedrops, instruct your patient to do which of the following?
    A.   Look down and away.
    B.   Look up and away.
    C.   Look straight ahead.
    D.   Look up and directly at the dropper.

Answer: B. When instilling eyedrops, ask your patient to look up and away. This moves the cornea away from the lower lid and minimizes the risk of touching the cornea with the dropper.

2. Which of the following is a contraindication to using a medicated ocular disk in your patient?
    A.   Mucous discharge from his eye
    B.   A watery or red eye
    C.   Itchy or red eyelids
    D.   Keratitis

Answer: D. Don't use a medicated ocular disk if the patient has keratitis, conjunctivitis, retinal detachment, or any condition in which pupillary constriction should be avoided.

3. To instill eardrops in your adult patient, you would straighten the ear canal by gently pulling the auricle
    A.   Up and back.
    B.   Down and back.
    C.   Down and out.
    D.   Up and down.

Answer: A. In an adult, gently pull the auricle up and back to straighten the ear canal to help the drops reach the eardrum.

4. Which of the following is better suited for administering a medication to treat nasal polyps and inflamed areas in your patient?
    A.   Atomizer spray
    B.   Aerosol spray
    C.   Nose drops
    D.   Nasal solution

Answer: B. An aerosol spray, which has even finer particles than an atomizer spray, is especially suited for treating nasal polyps and inflamed areas of the nose.

Scoring

☆☆☆ If you answered all four questions correctly, awesome! Your knowledge is a real eye-opener!

☆☆ If you answered three questions correctly, happy day! Get ready for an earful of accolades!

☆ If you answered fewer than three questions correctly, don't take *nose* for an answer. Just read the chapter once more, and you'll surely smell success.

Respiratory administration

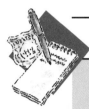

Just the facts

In this chapter, you'll learn:

♦ how to use a metered-dose inhaler

♦ how to use a holding chamber

♦ how to use a dry powder inhaler

♦ how to deliver nebulizer therapy

♦ how to give a medication through an endotracheal tube.

Administering respiratory devices

Several devices and procedures can be used to produce a fine, drug-carrying mist that a patient can inhale deep into his lungs.

Quick route to the capillaries

Once there, the drug moves almost immediately into the lining of the patient's bronchi or alveoli and then into the adjacent capillaries. Drugs are administered in this way because the inhaled route is the most effective method to get the medicine where it's supposed to go, that is, directly to the airways. In addition, the total dose is low and there's little chance for systemic effect.

A breath of fresh air

To deliver drugs to the respiratory tract, you'll typically use some type of handheld inhaler (sometimes with special attachments known as holding chambers called spacers) or a nebulizer. In an emergency, if the patient doesn't have an I.V. line in place, certain liquid drugs can be delivered directly into the respiratory tract through an endotracheal (ET) tube.

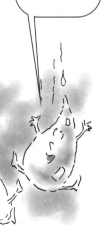

Inhalers and nebulizers produce a fine mist...

...which the patient inhales into his lungs.

Using a metered-dose inhaler

Many inhalant drugs, such as bronchodilators (help to open the bronchial airways of the lungs) and corticosteroids (used as effective anti-inflammatory agents), are available in small canisters, which are then inserted into a metered-dose inhaler, also known as a *puffer*. A *metered-dose inhaler* is a device that can be used to trigger the release of measured doses of aerosol drug from a canister. The patient can then inhale the fine mist deep into his lungs.

What you need

Metered-dose inhaler ✳ prescribed drug ✳ normal saline solution

Getting ready

- Verify the order in the patient's chart.
- Identify the patient by checking his armband.
- Place the patient in a comfortable sitting position.

How you do it

- Shake the inhaler canister well.
- Remove the cap from the canister, turn the canister upside down, and insert the stem of the canister into the small hole in the flattened portion of the mouthpiece as shown below.

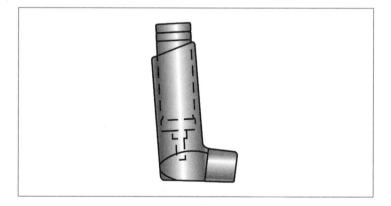

- Ask the patient to exhale, then hold the inhaler about 1″ (2.5 cm) in front of his open mouth (two to three finger widths from his mouth).
- Tell the patient to inhale slowly through his mouth and to continue inhaling until his lungs feel full.

Once is enough

- As he begins to inhale, compress the drug canister into the plastic housing of the inhaler to release a metered dose of the drug. Do this only once.

Whistle while you work

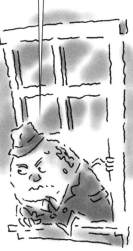

Wanna keep out oral fungal infections? Tell your patient to rinse and gargle after taking the medication.

- Tell the patient to hold his breath for ten seconds or as long as he can. Then instruct him to exhale slowly through pursed lips, as though whistling. Doing so produces back pressure that helps to keep his bronchioles open, thus increasing absorption and diffusion of the drug.
- Have the patient rinse his mouth and gargle with normal saline solution or water to remove the drug from his mouth and the back of his throat. This step helps to prevent oral fungal infections. Warn him not to swallow after gargling, but rather to spit out the liquid.

Practice pointers

- If the patient can't coordinate well enough to inhale the drug as soon as you discharge it, you may need to put a spacer device or holding chamber on the inhaler.
- Some inhaled bronchodilators may cause restlessness, palpitations, nervousness, and hypersensitivity reactions, such as rash, urticaria, or bronchospasm.
- If you're administering a bronchodilator to a patient with heart disease, follow the advice given below. (See *Cardiac cautions.*)

Hoarse sense

- If the patient takes an inhaled corticosteroid, watch for evidence of hoarseness or fungal infection in his mouth or throat.

Danger zone

Cardiac cautions

If you need to administer bronchodilators to a patient with heart disease, proceed with caution. These drugs may cause cardiac arrhythmias, hypotension, hypertension, or anginal symptoms.

Emergency advice
If paradoxical bronchospasm does occur, stop the drug, support the patient's respiratory status, and call a doctor immediately.

• When giving inhaled drugs to pediatric patients, remember these tips. (See *Giving inhaled drugs to pediatric patients.*)

What to teach

• Teach the patient the drug's dose, purpose, and potential adverse effects.
• Teach the patient how to use the inhaler so he can continue his drug therapy at home, if necessary.
• Warn him against using the inhaler more often than the doctor prescribed; doing so can cause the drug to lose its effectiveness.

Note the dose

• Tell the patient to record the date and time of each dose and his response to it. This record will help him keep track of the number of doses left in his drug canister. It's important for the patient to know the total number of doses in each canister. (See *How full is the canister?*) Some canisters come with built-in dose counters.
• Tell the patient to rinse his mouth after using his inhaler to prevent oral fungal infection.
• Instruct the patient to call his doctor if his shortness of breath worsens, the drug becomes less effective, or he develops palpitations, nervousness, or hypersensitivity reactions such as a rash.
• If the patient takes both a bronchodilator and a corticosteroid by inhaler, tell him to inhale the bronchodilator 5 minutes before the corticosteroid. That way, his bronchial tubes will be as open as possible when he takes the corticosteroid.

Not so fast

• Have the patient wait at least 1 minute between doses of a single inhaled drug.

Identification, please!

• If the patient takes an inhaled corticosteroid, urge him to carry medical identification announcing that he may need supplemental corticosteroids during stress or a severe asthma attack.

Using a holding chamber

A *holding chamber,* also called a *spacer,* is a device that attaches to the mouthpiece of an inhaler and is used to make sure a patient gets the entire dose of a drug each time he uses an inhaler.

Holding it all in

Commonly used holding chambers include the InspirEase and the AeroChamber. An *InspirEase system* is a type of holding chamber

Ages and stages

Giving inhaled drugs to pediatric patients

When giving inhaled drugs to pediatric patients, remember these tips:
• If you need to give an inhaled drug to an infant or young child, have a parent or assistant hold the child to gain his cooperation.
• Give the drug through an aerosol nebulizer or spacer so the child doesn't have to hold his breath to retain the drug.
• For an older child, consider using a metered-dose inhaler, but only after you explain its use and you're satisfied that he understands the device and can use it properly. Don't use this type of inhaler if you doubt the patient's ability to get an appropriate dose into his lungs, rather than into his mouth and throat.

No place like home

How full is the canister?

It's important that your patient check his metered-dose inhaler daily, in order to know when it's time to replace it.

Recent studies have shown no correlation between how the inhaler floats and how much medicine remains in the inhaler—some even malfunction after being submerged.

To help your patient keep track of how often he needs to change his inhaler, teach him to use an inhalant canister calendar by following these steps:
• Have the patient check the number of puffs contained in his inhaler, which is printed on the side of the canister (keeping in mind that the number of puffs varies in each inhaler).
• After he uses the number of puffs contained in the inhaler, he must discard it, even if it continues to spray because he won't be getting the amount of medication he needs.

Determining puffs
• If he uses an inhaler every day for prevention, he can determine how long his inhaler will last by dividing the total amount of puffs in the inhaler by the total puffs he uses every day. For example, if the inhaler has 200 puffs and he's prescribed a total of 8 puffs per day, the canister will last 25 days (200 puffs ÷ 8 puffs/day = 25 days).
• As a reminder, he should mark the date of when his medication will run out on his inhaler canister calendar and on the canister itself.

Keeping track
• If he uses his inhaler more often than prescribed, he must remember that his medication will run out sooner. It's important that he replace his inhaler by refilling his prescription before it runs out.
• If he uses his inhaler only when he needs to, he must keep track of how many times he puffs the inhaler.

Counting down
• If necessary he can obtain a device that counts down the number of puffs each time he uses the inhaler. He can purchase such a device from his local pharmacist.

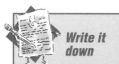

Write it down

Documenting respiratory device administration

Be sure to record:
• date and time
• drug administered and dose
• patient's response to inhaler treatment
• patient's vital signs
• breath sounds before and after treatment
• amount, color, and consistency of sputum produced
• complications; and nursing actions taken
• teaching aids given to the patient.

that has a bag that collapses when the patient inhales and inflates when the patient exhales. An *AeroChamber system* uses a small cylinder called a *valved chamber* to trap medication. It may also include a mask that helps the patient inhale the medication more easily.

What you need

Metered-dose inhaler * holding chamber * prescribed medication * normal saline solution

Getting ready

- Verify the order in the patient's chart.
- Identify the patient by checking his armband.
- Position the patient in a comfortable sitting position.

How you do it

- Shake the inhaler canister well.
- Remove the cap from the canister, turn the canister upside down, and insert the stem into the small hole in the flattened portion of the mouthpiece of the inhaler.
- Place the end of the mouthpiece into the opening in the holding device and twist the device to lock it in place.

Just puff it

- Hold the inhaler in front of the patient's mouth. Ask him to exhale and then to place his lips firmly around the mouthpiece of the holding chamber.
- Compress the canister into the inhaler once to discharge a puff of medication.

Don't get left holding the bag

- Tell the patient to inhale slowly and deeply. If the holding chamber has a bag, it should collapse completely.
- If the patient inhales too quickly, the device will make a whistling sound. Remind him to inhale slowly and deeply.

Waiting to exhale

- Have the patient keep his lips around the mouthpiece of the holding chamber, hold his breath for 5 to 10 seconds, and then exhale slowly into the holding chamber. Then ask him to inhale and exhale once more.
- If the doctor has ordered two puffs of the drug, wait 1 to 2 minutes and then repeat the entire procedure.
- Have the patient rinse his mouth and gargle with normal saline solution or water to remove the drug from his mouth and the back of his throat. This step helps to prevent oral fungal infections. Warn him not to swallow after gargling, but rather to spit out the liquid.

Holding water

- Disconnect the holding chamber from the inhaler; wash the holding chamber in warm, soapy water; rinse it thoroughly; and let it air dry.

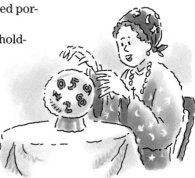

With a holding chamber, I foresee a way to make sure the patient gets the entire dose he needs.

Practice pointers

• Some inhaled drugs may cause restlessness, palpitations, nervousness, and hypersensitivity reactions, such as rash, urticaria, or bronchospasm.
• Remember to administer bronchodilators cautiously to patients with heart disease.
• If the patient takes an inhaled corticosteroid, watch for evidence of hoarseness or fungal infection in his mouth or throat.

What to teach

• Teach the patient how to properly use the inhaler and holding chamber so he can continue his drug therapy at home, if necessary.
• Tell the patient to record the date and time of each dose and his response to it. This record will help him keep track of the number of doses left in his drug canister and the degree to which the drug is helping him.

Too much of a good thing

• Warn him against using the inhaler more often than the doctor prescribed; doing so can cause the drug to lose its effectiveness and may increase the risk of adverse effects.
• Tell the patient to rinse his mouth and gargle with normal saline solution or water after using his inhaler to remove the drug from his mouth and throat. This step helps to prevent oral fungal infections. Be sure to warn him not to swallow after gargling, but rather to spit out the liquid.

Not a rash reaction

• Instruct the patient to call his doctor if his shortness of breath worsens, the drug becomes less effective, or he develops palpitations, nervousness, or hypersensitivity reactions such as a rash.
• If the patient takes both a bronchodilator and a corticosteroid by inhaler, tell him to inhale the bronchodilator 5 minutes before he inhales the prescribed corticosteroid. That way, his bronchial tubes will be as open as possible when he takes the corticosteroid.
• If the doctor ordered two puffs of the drug, instruct him to wait 1 to 2 minutes and repeat the entire procedure.
• If the patient takes an inhaled corticosteroid, urge him to carry medical identification announcing that he may need supplemental corticosteroids during stress or a severe asthma attack.

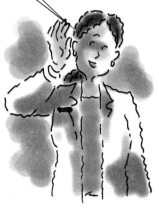

Be sure to document breath sounds before and after treatment.

Write it down

Documenting holding chamber administration

Be sure to record:
• date and time
• drug administered and dose
• patient's response to inhaler treatment
• patient's vital signs
• breath sounds before and after treatment
• amount, color, and consistency of sputum produced
• complications and nursing actions taken
• teaching aids provided to the patient.

Using a dry powder inhaler

Several drugs are available in dry powder form for inhalation, such as salmeterol (Serevent Diskus), albuterol (Ventolin Rotacaps), fluticasone (Flovent Rotadisk), and budesonide (Pulmicort Turbuhaler). Each comes in a product-specific inhalation device. These dry powder inhalers are easier for some patients to use because they don't require coordinating a hand movement with taking a breath unlike other inhalers.

Take a powder

For instance, the Pulmicort Turbuhaler administers budesonide, a corticosteroid used to prevent asthma attacks through its anti-inflammatory effects.

What you need

Administration device ✳ prescribed drug (if it isn't already in the device) ✳ normal saline solution or water

Getting ready

- Verify the order in the patient's chart.
- Identify the patient by checking his armband.
- Position the patient in a comfortable sitting position.

How you do it

- To administer the drug, follow the directions supplied with the device you're using. (The guidelines provided here describe how to use the Pulmicort Turbuhaler.)

Do the twist

- If you're using a new canister, prime the Pulmicort Turbuhaler. First, remove the cover.
- Next, hold the canister upright, with the mouthpiece up and the brown grip down. Twist the brown grip fully to the right and back again to the left. Repeat these steps until you hear a click.
- Don't shake the inhaler after priming it.
- Have the patient turn away from the inhaler and exhale. Make sure he doesn't blow or exhale into the device.

My lips are sealed

- Hold the inhaler in an upright position, and tell the patient to close his lips around the mouthpiece.
- Tell the patient to inhale deeply and forcefully, an action that discharges the drug.
- Afterward, replace the cap on the device and twist it shut.

• Have the patient rinse his mouth or gargle with normal saline solution or water to remove the drug from his mouth and throat. This step helps to prevent oral fungal infections. Warn him not to swallow after gargling, but rather to spit out the liquid.

Practice pointers

• Don't shake a dry powder inhaler to determine whether it's empty. A drying agent inside the device may make noise and mislead you into thinking that more drug is available when it isn't.
• Some dry powder inhalers have a dose-counting indicator that shows when the canister is getting low.
• Some inhaled drugs may cause restlessness, palpitations, nervousness, and hypersensitivity reactions, such as rash, urticaria, or bronchospasm.

Heartfelt advice

• Remember to administer bronchodilators cautiously to patients with heart disease.
• If the patient takes an inhaled corticosteroid, watch for evidence of hoarseness or fungal infection in his mouth or throat.

What to teach

• Teach the patient how to use the prescribed dry powder inhaler so he can continue drug therapy at home, if necessary.
• Warn the patient not to exhale or breathe into the device and not to use a spacer or holding chamber on it.

How dry I am

• Tell the patient not to wash the device and to always keep it dry. Be sure to warn him against immersing it in water to find out how full it is.
• Warn the patient to store the device in a dry place without humidity (not the bathroom) at room temperature.
• Warn the patient not to use the inhaler more than prescribed; doing so can cause the drug to lose its effectiveness, or it may cause uncomfortable adverse effects.
• Warn the patient that unlike other inhaled medications, he may not taste, smell, or feel the dry powder. This may differ from what he's used to. Reassure him that as long as he follows the directions, he'll get the full dose of his medication.

Keep the calendar

• Tell the patient to record the date and time of each dose and his response to it.
• Tell the patient to rinse his mouth and gargle with normal saline solution or water after using his inhaler to remove the drug from

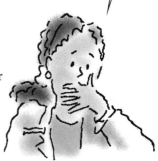

Remember not to shake a dry powder inhaler to determine whether it's empty. A drying agent inside the device may make noise and mislead you.

his mouth and throat. This helps to prevent oral fungal infections. Warn him not to swallow the liquid, but rather to spit it out.
• Instruct the patient to call his doctor if his shortness of breath worsens, the drug becomes less effective, or he develops palpitations, nervousness, or a hypersensitivity reaction such as a rash.
• If the patient takes both a bronchodilator and a corticosteroid by inhaler, tell him to inhale the bronchodilator first, followed by the corticosteroid, and wait 5 minutes between drugs. That way, his bronchial tubes will be as open as possible when he takes the corticosteroid.

Worth the wait

• If the doctor prescribed two puffs of the drug, instruct him to wait 1 to 2 minutes and then repeat the entire procedure.
• If the patient takes an inhaled corticosteroid, urge him to carry medical identification announcing that he may need supplementary corticosteroids during stress or a severe asthma attack.

Delivering nebulizer therapy

A *nebulizer* is a device that uses compressed gas to convert liquid drugs into a fine aerosol for inhalation. It's commonly used to administer such drugs as:
• bronchodilators (drugs that help open the bronchial airways of the lungs)
• antibiotics (drugs that treat respiratory infections)
• mucolytics (drugs that destroy or dissolve mucus).

If your patient is breathing on his own, he'll most likely use a small-volume, handheld nebulizer. If he's being mechanically ventilated, you'll use an in-line nebulizer to deliver his drug treatment. (See *Comparing nebulizers.*)

What you need

Pressurized gas source ✳ a flowmeter or medical air compressor ✳ oxygen tubing ✳ prescribed drug ✳ nebulizer (with a mouthpiece, if you're using a small-volume device) ✳ normal saline solution or sterile water

Getting ready

• Verify the order in the patient's chart.
• Identify the patient by checking his armband.
• Explain the procedure to the patient to ensure his cooperation. Mention that the nebulizer normally makes clicking and sighing noises.

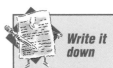

Write it down

Documenting dry powder inhaler administration

Be sure to record:
• date and time
• drug administered and dose
• patient's response to inhaler treatment
• patient's vital signs
• breath sounds before and after treatment
• amount, color, and consistency of sputum produced
• complications and nursing actions taken.
• teaching aids provided to the patient.

Gear up!

Comparing nebulizers

Nebulizer	Characteristics
Ultrasonic 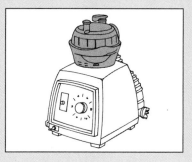	• Uses high-frequency sound waves to create an aerosol mist ***Advantages*** • Provides 100% humidity • About 20% of its particles reach the lower airways • Loosens secretions ***Disadvantages*** • May cause bronchospasm in patients with asthma • Increases risk of overhydration (in infants)
Large volume (Venturi jet) 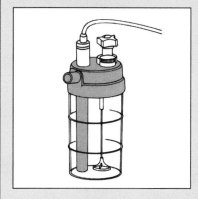	• Supplies cool or heated moisture to a patient whose upper airway has been bypassed by endotracheal intubation or a tracheostomy, or who has recently been extubated ***Advantages*** • Provides 100% humidity with cool or heated devices • Provides oxygen and aerosol therapy • Can be used for long-term therapy ***Disadvantages*** • Increases risk of bacterial growth (in reusable units) • Causes collection of condensate in large-bore tubing • May cause mucosal irritation from breathing hot, dry air (if water level isn't maintained correctly in reservoir) • Increases risk of overhydration from mist (in infants)

(continued)

Comparing nebulizers (continued)

Nebulizer	Characteristics
Small volume (mini-nebulizer, Maxi-mist) 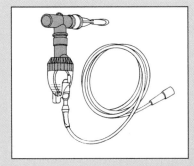	• Uses a handheld device to deliver aerosolized medication **Advantages** • Allows patient to inhale and exhale on his own • Can cause less air trapping than drug administered by intermittent positive-pressure breathing • May be used with compressed air, oxygen, or compressor pump • Allows for portability and disposability **Disadvantages** • Increases time of procedure if patient needs your assistance • Distributes medication unevenly, if patient doesn't breathe properly

Don't hold your breath

* Take the patient's vital signs and listen to his breath sounds.
* Have the patient sit erect in a chair, if possible, to promote lung expansion and aerosol dispersion. Otherwise, help the patient into the semi-Fowler position.
* Wash your hands.

How you do it

Using a small-volume nebulizer

* Obtain the prescribed medication, place it in the nebulizer cup, and add the prescribed amount of normal saline solution or sterile water. Attach the mouthpiece or mask.
* Attach the nebulizer to the flowmeter or air compressor. Then adjust the flow to 6 to 8 L/minute. (Air compressors are internally set at 8 L/minute.)
* Encourage the patient to take slow, even breaths until the drug is gone.
* Stay with the patient during the treatment, which lasts about 15 minutes. Take his vital signs to detect any adverse reactions to the drug.

Have your patient sit erect in a chair, whenever possible, to promote lung expansion and aerosol dispersion.

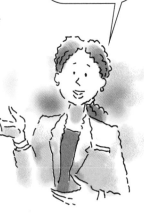

Cough it up

- Encourage the patient to cough and expectorate as needed. Suction him, if necessary.
- Have the patient rinse his mouth and gargle with normal saline solution or water to remove the drug from his mouth and throat. This step helps to prevent oral fungal infection. Tell him not to swallow after gargling, but rather to spit out the liquid.
- Change the nebulizer cup and oxygen tubing according to your facility's policy to prevent bacterial contamination.
- Auscultate breath sounds to evaluate effectiveness of treatment. Do this at the completion of the treatment and again in 15 minutes.

Using an in-line nebulizer

- Make sure the nebulizer is located on the inspiratory side of the ventilatory circuit, as close as possible to the patient's ET tube.
- Obtain the medication and prescribed diluent (if any), remove the nebulizer cup, quickly inject the medication, and then replace the cup. Turn on the nebulizer at the appropriate place on the ventilator.
- Stay with the patient during the treatment, which lasts about 15 minutes. Take his vital signs to detect any adverse reactions to the drug.
- Encourage the patient to cough and expectorate as needed. Suction him, if necessary.

> You're going to take slow, even breaths until the drug is gone.

Listen carefully

- Auscultate the patient's lungs to evaluate the effectiveness of therapy.

Practice pointers

- If the patient is receiving oxygen therapy at a high flow rate via nasal prongs, the nebulizer treatment may be powered with oxygen instead of compressed air.
- Drugs delivered by nebulizer can cause such adverse reactions as tachycardia, hypertension, palpitations, tremors, or hypersensitivity reactions, including rash and urticaria.
- Contaminated equipment can cause a nosocomial infection.

What to teach

- If the patient will be using a small-volume nebulizer at home, teach him how to use the device correctly.

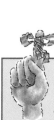

Memory jogger

When using an *IN-LINE* nebulizer, remember to connect it to the *IN-SPIRATORY* side of the ventilatory circuit.

• Make sure arrangements have been made with a supplier of durable medical equipment to set up the nebulizer in the patient's home.

No longer nebulous

• Warn the patient against using the nebulizer more often than the doctor prescribed; doing so can cause the drug to lose its effectiveness, or it may cause uncomfortable adverse effects.
• Tell the patient to record the date and time of each treatment and his response to it.

A fungus among us

• Advise him to rinse his mouth after using the nebulizer to prevent oral fungal infection, and be sure to warn him not to swallow after gargling but to spit out the liquid.
• Instruct the patient to call his doctor if his shortness of breath worsens, the drug becomes less effective, or he develops palpitations, nervousness, or a hypersensitivity reaction, such as a rash.
• If the patient takes more than one nebulized drug, tell him to wait at least 5 minutes between treatments.
• If the patient takes both a bronchodilator and a corticosteroid by inhaler, tell him to inhale the bronchodilator first, followed by the corticosteroid. That way, his bronchial tubes will be as open as possible when he takes the corticosteroid.

Giving medication through an endotracheal tube

If your patient faces a life-threatening emergency and doesn't have an I.V. line in place, you can administer certain liquid drugs directly into his respiratory tree through an *ET tube*, a tube used to provide an airway through the trachea.

Cuff 'em

An inflatable cuff usually surrounds the tube and is inflated after placement. The cuff helps prevent aspiration of foreign material into the bronchus.
Drugs that can be given safely through an ET tube include:
• atropine, an anticholinergic frequently used to increase a patient's heart rate
• lidocaine, an antiarrhythmic used to treat dangerous ventricular arrhythmias
• epinephrine, an endogenous catecholamine used to restore cardiac rhythm.

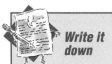

Write it down

Documenting nebulizer therapy

Be sure to record:
• date, time, and duration of therapy
• type and amount of drug administered
• patient's response to the nebulizer treatment
• fraction of inspired oxygen or oxygen flow
• patient's vital signs before and after treatment
• breath sounds before and after treatment
• patient's response to the treatment
• amount, color, and consistency of sputum produced
• complications and nursing actions taken
• teaching aids provided to the patient.

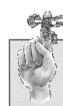

Memory jogger

To help you remember which drug should be inhaled FIRST, remember your ABCs — A Bronchodilator comes before a Corticosteroid!

A brief affair

You'll use this route only until I.V. access becomes available. ET administration allows resuscitation to continue uninterrupted, and it avoids the risks of intracardiac administration, which include coronary artery laceration, cardiac tamponade, and pneumothorax.

Express delivery

Drugs delivered by ET tube take effect more rapidly than those given by intramuscular injection because the bronchial tubes provide a large surface area for drug absorption. Pulmonary circulation propels blood to the left side of the heart, ensuring rapid, central drug dissemination.

Waiting at the depot

Keep in mind, however, that drugs delivered through an ET tube typically have a longer duration of action than they do after I.V. administration. That's because of the depot effect. The *depot effect* refers to sustained absorption, which takes place in the alveoli. Therefore, expect to adjust repeat doses and continuous infusions to prevent adverse reactions.

What you need

Gloves * protective eye wear * stethoscope * self-inflating ventilation bag * prescribed drug * syringe with a needle * sterile water or sterile normal saline solution (for injection as ordered)

Getting ready

• Verify the verbal order with the prescribing doctor.
• Take all necessary equipment to the patient's bedside.
• Identify the patient by checking his armband.
• If possible, explain the procedure to the patient.

How you do it

• If you haven't already done so, calculate the drug dose.
• A drug dose given through an ET tube should be 2 to 2½ times the recommended I.V. dose.
• Dilute the drug with 10 ml of sterile water or sterile normal saline solution for injection as directed.
• Place the patient in a supine position, so his head is even with or slightly higher than his trunk.
• Wash your hands and put on gloves and eye wear.

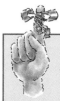

Memory jogger

To remember drugs that can be given safely through an ET tube, use the mnemonic **ale** (Atropine, Lidocaine, Epinephrine).

Hearing is believing

• Auscultate the patient's lungs with a stethoscope while you manually ventilate her with a self-inflating ventilation bag to verify correct placement of the ET tube.
• After confirming correct placement of the tube, give three to five breaths with the self-inflating ventilation bag. Then remove the bag from the ET tube.
• Remove the needle from the syringe and insert the tip of the syringe into the ET tube as shown below. Rapidly instill the drug into the tube.

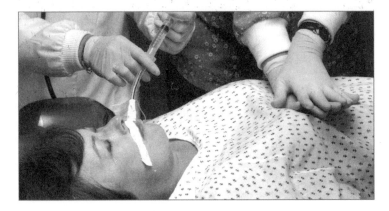

Thumbs up

• Place your gloved thumb briefly over the tube to minimize drug reflux.
• Reattach the resuscitation bag to the ET tube and give the patient five or six brisk breaths. This will propel the drug into her lungs, give her additional oxygen, and clear the ET tube.

Practice pointers

• To prevent dosing errors, which could be fatal for your patient, use extreme caution when giving drugs through an ET tube. Always double-check that you have the right drug and the right amount before instilling it into the ET tube.

What to teach

• If the patient is conscious, calmly tell her what you're doing and explain the need for the drug.

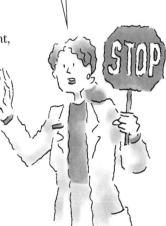

Because dosing errors involving an ET tube can be fatal, be sure to double-check: right drug, right amount.

Not just in one ear and out the other

• Even if the patient can't respond to you, she may still be able to hear you. Remember that talking calmly to your patient and keeping her informed about her care may help to ease some of her anxiety, maintain her dignity, and convey respect for her.

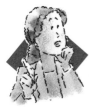

Write it down

Documenting ET drug administration

Be sure to record:
• date and time you administered a drug through an endotracheal (ET) tube
• reason for administration through the ET tube
• drug you administered
• dose you gave
• patient's response
• need to repeat the dose as ordered.

Quick quiz

1. Which device is used to trigger the release of measured doses of an aerosol drug from a canister?
   A.   Holding chamber
   B.   Metered-dose inhaler
   C.   Nebulizer
   D.   Dry powder inhaler

Answer: B. A metered-dose inhaler is a device, which can be used to trigger the release of measured doses of an aerosol drug from a canister.

2. Which of the following types of nebulizers can cause possible bronchospasm in a patient with asthma?
   A.   Ultrasonic
   B.   Large volume
   C.   Small volume
   D.   Mini-nebulizer

Answer: A. An ultrasonic nebulizer, which uses high-frequency sound waves to create an aerosol mist, may cause bronchospasm in patients with asthma.

3. Which of the following drugs can be given safely through an ET tube?
   A.   Morphine
   B.   Atropine
   C.   Procainamide
   D.   Corticosteroids

Answer: B. Atropine, an anticholinergic frequently used to increase a patient's heart rate in an emergency situation, can be given safely through an ET tube when there's no I.V. access available.

4. A drug dose given through an ET tube should be:
A.   One to 1.5 times the recommended I.V. dose.
B.   The same as the I.V. dose.
C.   Three to 3.5 times the recommended I.V. dose.
D.   Two to 2.5 times the recommended I.V. dose.

Answer: D. A drug dose given through an ET tube should be 2 to 2½ times the recommended I.V. dose.

Scoring

☆☆☆   If you answered all four questions correctly, that's inspirational! You've certainly inhaled this chapter!

☆☆   If you answered three questions correctly, not bad! There's nothing nebulous about your response!

☆   If you answered fewer than three questions correctly, take a deep breath. Then give this chapter a quick review, and give it one more try.

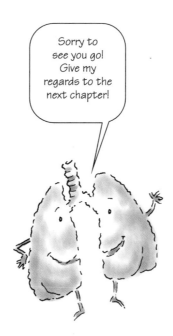

Sorry to see you go! Give my regards to the next chapter!

10

Buccal, sublingual, and translingual administration

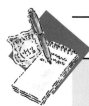

Just the facts

In this chapter, you'll learn:
♦ how to give a buccal drug
♦ how to give a sublingual drug
♦ how to give a translingual drug.

Administering transmucosal drugs

Transmucosal administration refers to giving a drug across the mucous membrane of a patient's mouth. This type of drug administration allows you to produce systemic drug actions while avoiding the damaging effects of gastric juices and liver metabolism.

Rapid transit

Furthermore, unlike traditional oral administration, transmucosal administration offers almost immediate drug effects. The oral mucosa has a thin epithelium and abundant blood vessels, both of which promote rapid absorption of the drug into the patient's bloodstream.

Speedy delivery!

Drugs delivered across the oral mucous membrane may appear in the patient's blood within 1 minute and reach peak blood levels in 10 to 15 minutes—considerably faster than drugs delivered by the traditional oral route. (See *Placing drugs in the oral mucosa,* page 176.)

Transmucosal drugs offer nearly immediate effects—reaching peak blood levels in 10 to 15 minutes.

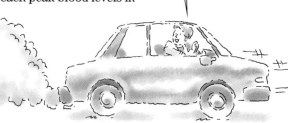

Peak technique

Placing drugs in the oral mucosa

Buccal and sublingual administration routes allow some drugs, such as nitroglycerin and methyl-testosterone, to enter the bloodstream rapidly without being degraded in the GI tract.

What to do

To give a drug buccally, insert it between the patient's cheek and teeth (as shown below left). Ask him to close his mouth and hold the tablet against his cheek until the tablet is absorbed.

To give a drug sublingually, place it under the patient's tongue (as shown below right), and ask him to leave it there until it's dissolved.

Problem solving

Some buccal medications may irritate the mucosa. Alternate sides of the mouth for repeat doses to prevent continuous irritation of the same site. Sublingual medications—such as nitroglycerin—may cause a tingling sensation under the tongue. If the patient finds this annoying, try placing the drug in the buccal pouch instead.

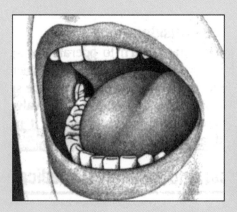

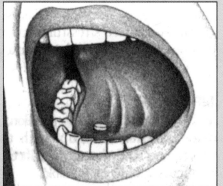

Three choices

You can give drugs across a patient's oral mucous membrane using three administration methods:

 buccal (against the cheek)

 sublingual (under the tongue)

 translingual (on the tongue's surface).

Buccal administration

Buccal administration involves placing a tablet in a patient's mouth so the drug enters the bloodstream via the mucous membrane inside the patient's cheek.

The buc stops here

One benefit of buccal administration is that, if the patient develops excessive or adverse reactions, you can remove what's left of the tablet from his mouth. You may also use the buccal route instead of the sublingual route if a sublingual drug causes too much unpleasant tingling under the patient's tongue.

What you need

Prescribed drug * medication cup * gloves

Getting ready

- Verify the order in the patient's chart.
- Identify the patient by checking his armband.
- Wash your hands and put on gloves.
- Remove the tablet from the patient's drug container and place it in a medication cup.
- Check the patient's medication record to determine on which side of his mouth the drug was last given.

How you do it

- Ask the patient to open his mouth.
- Inspect his mouth for irritation and ulceration.
- Open the tablet package after inspecting the mouth.
- Place the tablet between the patient's cheek and teeth.
- Place it on the side that wasn't used for the previous dose.

To have and to hold

- Ask the patient to close his mouth and to hold the tablet between his cheek and teeth until it dissolves.

Practice pointers

- Make sure the patient doesn't mistakenly swallow a tablet intended for delivery by the buccal route. Swallowing a buccal drug can decrease its effectiveness.

Take turns

- Remember to alternate sides of the patient's mouth when giving more than one dose of a buccal drug.

• Administer buccal drugs after you've given the patient all of his oral drugs.

Rosy-cheeked?

• Inspect the patient's oral mucosa regularly for irritation caused by repeated buccal administration.
• Some buccal drugs take up to 1 hour to be absorbed across the oral mucosa.
• Assess the patient after 30 minutes to determine any effect.

What to teach

• If your patient smokes, tell him not to do so until after his buccal drug has dissolved because the vasoconstrictive effects of nicotine will slow the drug's absorption.

Not too hard to swallow

• Be sure to tell the patient not to eat or drink when he has a buccal tablet in his mouth (especially one that takes a long time to be absorbed) because doing so raises the risk that he'll swallow the tablet.

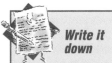

Write it down

Documenting buccal administration

Be sure to record:
• drug administered
• location used
• dose given
• date and time
• patient's reaction
• irritation or ulceration in the patient's mouth
• repeated doses given.

Sublingual administration

In *sublingual administration,* the drug is absorbed across the mucous membrane under the patient's tongue.

Heartfelt relief

Rapid absorption and peak drug effects have made this a popular route for antianginal drugs (agents used to treat anginal symptoms, including chest discomfort, shortness of breath, or cough) such as isosorbide dinitrate (Isordil Tembids). Patients use these sublingual tablets to relieve angina and to prevent it in stressful or other high-risk situations.

What you need

Ordered drug ✳ medication cup ✳ gloves

Getting ready

• Verify the order in the patient's chart.
• Identify the patient by checking the armband.
• Wash your hands and put on gloves.

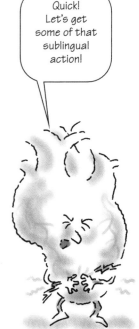

Quick! Let's get some of that sublingual action!

How you do it

- Remove the tablet from the patient's drug container and place it in a medication cup.
- Check the patient's medication record to determine on which side of his mouth the drug was last given.
- Ask the patient to open his mouth and lift his tongue.
- Inspect the patient's mouth for irritation or ulceration.
- Open the tablet package after inspecting the mouth.

Tongue and groove

- Place the tablet under his tongue. Place it on the side that wasn't used for the previous dose.

Put on hold

- Ask the patient to close his mouth and to hold the tablet in place until it dissolves.

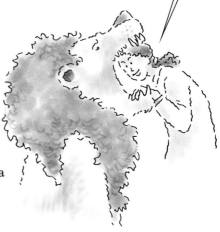

Remember to inspect the patient's mouth for irritation or ulceration before administering the drug.

Practice pointers

- Make sure the patient doesn't mistakenly swallow a tablet intended for delivery by the sublingual route. Swallowing the drug can decrease its effectiveness.

Slip-sliding away

- If your patient has trouble opening his mouth or raising his tongue, place one end of a straw under his tongue and drop the tablet into the other end. The tablet will slide down the straw and into the sublingual space.

Avoid a tongue-lashing

- Remember to alternate sides of the patient's mouth when giving more than one dose of a sublingual drug.
- Administer sublingual drugs after you've given the patient all of his oral drugs.
- Inspect the patient's oral mucosa before each dose of medication for irritation caused by repeated sublingual administration.

What to teach

- Make sure the patient understands that a sublingual drug goes under his tongue and that he shouldn't chew or swallow it.

No smoking, please

- If your patient smokes, tell him not to do so until after his sublingual drug has dissolved because the vasoconstrictive effects of nicotine will slow the drug's absorption.

No place like home

That tingling feeling

If your patient will be taking sublingual nitroglycerine at home, teach him to wet the tablet with saliva before putting it under his tongue. Doing so speeds absorption.

Sign of success

Also, teach your patient to expect a tingling sensation when he places the tablet under his tongue. If he feels no tingling, the drug may not be working; he should discard it and seek medical assistance. Conversely, if the tingling bothers him, tell him he can move the tablet to the buccal pouch between his teeth and cheek.

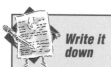

Write it down

Documenting sublingual administration

Be sure to record:
• drug administered
• location used
• dose given
• date and time
• patient's reaction
• irritation or ulceration in the patient's mouth
• repeated doses given.

• If your patient takes nitroglycerin tablets at home, include the helpful hints below in your teaching. (See *That tingling feeling*.)
• Tell the patient not to eat or drink when he has a sublingual tablet in his mouth because doing so raises the risk that he'll swallow the tablet.

Translingual administration

In *translingual administration*, a drug is applied to the top surface of the patient's tongue, usually as a mist or spray. This route offers rapid drug absorption and can be used to deliver nitroglycerin (Nitrolingual).

What you need

Ordered drug ✳ gloves

Getting ready

• Verify the order in the patient's chart.
• Identify the patient by checking his armband.
• Wash your hands and put on gloves.

How you do it

• Remove the spray canister from the patient's medication drawer.
• Ask the patient to open his mouth.
• Inspect the patient's mouth for irritation or ulceration.

Don't breathe a word

• Tell the patient not to inhale while you spray the drug onto his tongue.
• Hold the spray canister in a vertical position, with the valve head at the top and the spray opening within 1″ (2.5 cm) of the patient's mouth.
• Spray the dose onto the patient's tongue by firmly depressing the valve head button.

Practice pointers

• Some translingual drugs may be sprayed under the patient's tongue instead of on top of the tongue.
• Make sure the patient doesn't inhale the spray.

What to teach

• Encourage the patient to become familiar with the location of the spray opening in the canister's valve head, especially if the patient will be using the spray at night. Show him how to use the finger rest on top of the valve to identify the direction of the spray opening.
• Be sure to warn the patient not to rinse his mouth after administering the drug because doing so will decrease its effectiveness.

Early warning

• Tell him to record the number of sprays administered so he'll know when the canister is nearly empty and can replace it before the drug runs out.

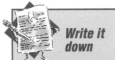

Write it down

Documenting translingual administration

Be sure to record:
• drug administered
• location used
• dose or number of sprays given
• date and time
• patient's reaction
• irritation or ulceration noted in the patient's mouth
• repeated doses given.

> Some translingual drugs may be sprayed under the patient's tongue instead of on top.

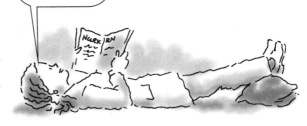

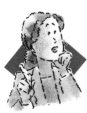

Quick quiz

1. Which of the following administration techniques is designed to move the drug across the mucous membrane inside the patient's cheek?
  A. Buccal administration
  B. Sublingual administration
  C. Translingual administration
  D. Oral administration

Answer: A. Buccal administration is a type of transmucosal drug administration that involves placing a tablet in a patient's mouth so the drug will move into the bloodstream across the mucous membrane inside the patient's cheek.

2.   Which of the following best describes transmucosal drug administration?
    A.   Peak drug levels are usually reached in 45 to 60 minutes.
    B.   Almost immediate drug effects are offered.
    C.   Considerably slower delivery occurs compared with drugs delivered by the traditional oral route.
    D.   Initial drug effects obtained 20 minutes after administration.

Answer: B. Unlike traditional oral administration, transmucosal administration offers almost immediate drug effects. Drugs delivered across the oral mucous membrane may appear in the patient's blood within 1 minute and reach peak blood levels in 10 to 15 minutes — considerably faster than drugs delivered by the traditional oral route.

3.   Swallowing a buccal drug will most likely:
    A.   equal the effectiveness of a sublingual drug.
    B.   increase its effectiveness.
    C.   not change its effectiveness.
    D.   decrease its effectiveness.

Answer: D. Mistakenly swallowing a tablet intended for delivery by the buccal route can decrease its effectiveness.

4.   Sublingual drugs should be administered:
    A.   after all oral drugs are given.
    B.   before all oral drugs are given.
    C.   at the same time as oral drugs.
    D.   alternating sublingual and oral drugs.

Answer: A. Sublingual drugs should be administered after you've given the patient all of his oral drugs.

Scoring

☆☆☆   If you answered all four questions correctly, marvelous! You've mastered transmucosal administration!

☆☆   If you answered three questions correctly, super! You're certain about sublingual drugs (and buccal and translingual, too!).

☆   If you answered fewer than three questions correctly, hold your tongue! Remember that unlike transmucosal drugs, this chapter may take a while to absorb.

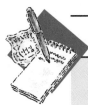

Oral and gastric administration

Just the facts

In this chapter, you'll learn:

♦ how to give a tablet or capsule by the oral route

♦ how to administer a liquid drug by the oral route

♦ how to give drugs through a nasogastric tube

♦ how to give drugs through a gastrostomy tube

♦ how to give drugs through a jejunostomy tube.

Administering oral drugs

Oral drug administration offers the safest, most convenient, and least costly way to administer a host of drugs. Usually, you'll give tablets, capsules, or liquid drugs (such as an elixir, syrup, or suspension) by the oral route. However, oral drugs are also available as powders, granules, and oils.

Giving a tablet or capsule

You may need to mix some drug forms in juice or applesauce before delivery to make them more palatable.

What you need

Prescribed drug ✳ medication cup ✳ glass of water or other liquid

Tablet talk

If you need to crush a tablet, get a mortar and pestle. If you need to split a scored tablet, get a paper towel or cutting device as well. (See *Crushing a tablet*, page 184, and *Splitting a scored tablet*, page 185.)

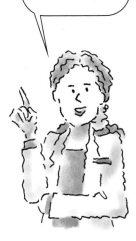

The oral route is the safest, most convenient, and least costly way to administer a host of drugs.

Peak technique

Crushing a tablet

To crush a tablet, follow these steps:
• Wash your hands.
• Remove the unit-dose tablet from the patient's medication drawer or pour the tablet from its container.
• Make sure the mortar and pestle are clean and contain no remnants of a previously crushed tablet.
• Place the tablet in the mortar and crush it completely with the pestle as shown.
• To save time and keep the mortar and pestle clean, crush a unit-dose tablet in its unopened wrapper. Then make sure you empty the wrapper completely.
• Place the crushed tablet into the fluid or food in which you'll administer it, and mix it thoroughly.

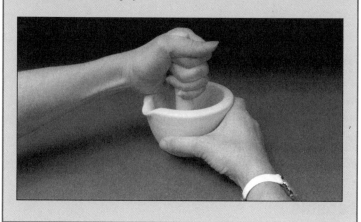

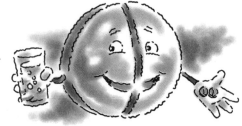

You may need to crush or split me, but that's okay, as long as I'm helping the patient.

Getting ready
• Verify the order for a tablet or capsule in the patient's chart.
• Wash your hands.

How you do it
• If you're giving a unit-dose tablet or capsule, re-move it from the patient's medication drawer. Then place the unwrapped medication into the cup.

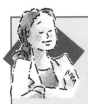

Peak technique

Splitting a scored tablet

To split a scored tablet, follow these steps:
- Wash your hands.
- To split a scored tablet using your fingers, start by placing the tablet in a paper towel.
- Notice the location of the score mark.
- Use both hands to grip the tablet on either side of the score mark, then push down on the edges to break the tablet along the score line.
- To split a tablet using a cutting device, place the tablet into the device so the score mark lines up with the blade.
- Close the lid of the cutting device to force the blade through the tablet as shown.
- Place the correct dose in a medication cup.
- Administer the prescribed dose with sufficient liquid for the patient to swallow it comfortably.

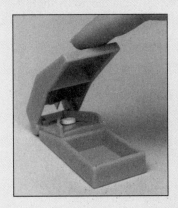 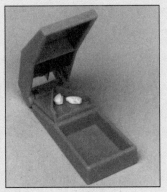

Keeping tabs

- If you need to pour the drug from its container, open the container and pour the required number of tablets or capsules into the lid of the container. Then put them in the medication cup.
- Assess your patient's ability to swallow before giving him an oral drug. Impaired swallowing can lead to aspiration.
- Identify the patient by checking his armband.
- Help the patient to a sitting position.

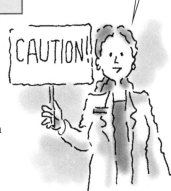

Impaired swallowing can lead to aspiration.

CAUTION!

One at a time please

• Offer the tablets or capsules one at a time. Have the patient place it in his mouth and then take enough liquid to swallow it comfortably.
• If the drug is chewable, make sure the patient chews it thoroughly before swallowing it.

Practice pointers

• Assess the patient's ability to swallow before administering tablets or capsules to prevent choking or aspiration.

Look for the designer label

• Don't give tablets or capsules from a poorly labeled or an unlabeled bottle.
• Never give a tablet or capsule that has been poured by someone else.

No returns, no surprises

• Never return an opened or unwrapped drug to the patient's medication drawer. Instead, properly dispose of it and notify the pharmacy.

Gotta get a witness

• Remember that another nurse will need to witness and co-sign your disposal of a narcotic.
• If the patient questions you about the drug you're giving or the amount you're giving, double-check his medication record. If the drug and dose are correct, reassure and inform the patient about his drug and any changes in dosage.

What to teach

• Caution the patient not to chew tablets that aren't supposed to be chewed, especially enteric-coated ones.
• Teach him about the drug you're administering, including its name, purpose, and possible adverse effects.
• If the patient will be taking the tablets or capsules independently at home, make sure he thoroughly understands and plans to follow the regimen.
• Be sure to tell him to report anything that could be an adverse effect of the drug.

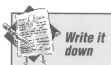
Write it down

Documenting tablet or capsule administration

Be sure to record:
• drug given
• dose given
• date and time of administration
• signing out of the drug on the patient's medication record
• patient's ability to swallow the drug you administered (if the patient has had problems swallowing oral drugs)
• patient's vital signs if you give a drug that could affect them
• adverse effects that arise
• patient's refusal and notification of a doctor as needed (if a patient refuses a tablet or capsule)
• omission or withholding of a drug for any reason.

Administering a liquid drug

For an infant, a child, or any patient who has trouble swallowing pills, you may give a liquid drug. (If the patient has a nasogastric

(NG), gastrostomy, or jejunostomy tube, you may give the drug through the tube rather than orally.)

What you need

Prescribed drug ✳ measuring cup ✳ damp paper towel

Getting ready

- Verify the order in the patient's chart.
- Wash your hands.
- Take the bottle from the patient's medication drawer or from the shelf.

How you do it

- Shake the bottle well, and then uncap it. Place the cap upside down on a clean surface to avoid contaminating the inside surface.

Graduate to the next level

- While holding a graduated medicine cup at eye level, pour the drug into the cup until the bottom of the meniscus reaches the correct dose mark. (See *Measuring liquid drugs*, page 188.)

Give lip service

- Clean liquid drug from the lip and then the side of the bottle with a damp paper towel, if necessary, and replace the cap.
- Identify the patient by checking the armband prior to administering the drug.
- To administer a liquid drug to an infant, follow the steps below. (See *Administering a liquid drug to an infant*, page 189.)

Practice pointers

- Don't give medication from a poorly labeled or an unlabeled container.
- Never give a medication that has been poured by someone else.
- Assess your patient's ability to swallow before administering a liquid drug.
- If the patient or a parent questions you about the drug you're giving or the amount you're giving, double-check the patient's medication record. If the drug and dose are correct, reassure and inform the patient or parent about the drug and any changes in dosage.

Peak technique

Measuring liquid drugs

To measure a liquid drug accurately, hold the graduated medication cup at eye level. Use your thumb to mark the correct level on the cup.

Hold the bottle so the liquid flows from the side opposite the label; this way, the liquid won't stain or obscure the label if it runs down the bottle.

Pour the liquid into the cup until the bottom of the meniscus reaches the correct dose amount. Then set the cup down and read the bottom of the meniscus again — still at eye level — to double-check your accuracy. If you've poured too much, discard the excess rather than pouring it back into the bottle.

Remove any drips from the lip of the bottle using a damp paper towel. Then clean the outside of the bottle, if necessary.

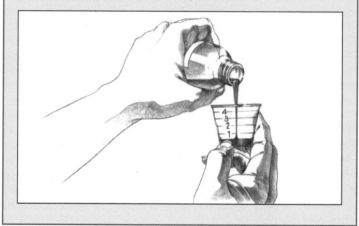

Sip tips

- To avoid damaging or staining the patient's teeth, give acidic drugs or iron preparations through a straw.
- Liquid drugs that have an unpleasant taste are usually more palatable when taken through a straw because the liquid contacts fewer taste buds.
- Remember the following helpful hints when administering oral medications to pediatric patients. (See *Administering oral medications to pediatric patients,* page 190.)

Ages and stages

Administering a liquid drug to an infant

To administer a liquid drug to an infant, be sure to follow these steps.

- Wash your hands.
- Place a bib or towel under the infant's chin.
- Withdraw the correct amount of liquid drug from the medication bottle by squeezing the bulb on the dropper.
- If the dropper is calibrated, hold it in a vertical position at eye level to check the dose amount.
- If the dropper holds too much drug, squeeze some into a sink or trash container. Don't return excess drug to the bottle.
- Identify the infant by checking the armband.
- Hold the infant securely in the crook of your arm and raise his head to about a 45-degree angle.
- Place the dropper at the corner of the infant's mouth so the drug will run into the pocket between his cheek and gum as shown. This action keeps him from spitting out the drug and also reduces the risk of aspiration.
- If the dropper isn't calibrated, hold it vertically over the corner of the infant's open mouth and instill the prescribed number of drops.
- You may also place the drug in a nipple and allow the infant to suck the contents. Lift the

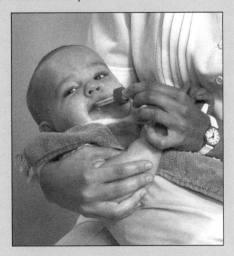

infant's head and give the drug slowly to prevent aspiration. Be sure never to mix a medication in a bottle because if the infant doesn't drink all of the contents of the bottle, he may not receive the full drug dosage.
- If the dropper touches the infant's mouth, wash it thoroughly before returning it to the bottle. Then close the bottle securely.

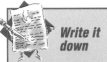

Write it down

Documenting liquid drug administration

Be sure to record:
- drug given
- dose given
- date and time of administration
- signing out of the drug on the patient's medication record
- patient's vital signs if you give a drug that could affect them
- adverse reactions that arise
- ability to swallow the liquid drug you administered (if the patient's record shows that he's had problems swallowing oral drugs)
- refusal and notification of a doctor as needed (if the patient or parent refuses a liquid drug)
- omission or withholding of a drug for any reason.

What to teach

- Teach the patient or parent about the drug, including its purpose and possible adverse reactions.
- If the patient or parent will be administering the drug at home, review the regimen, administration procedures, and any adverse reactions that should prompt a call to the doctor.

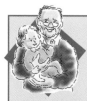

Ages and stages

Administering oral medications to pediatric patients

The oral route of drug administration is the preferred route in children because it's more comfortable and usually safer and easier to use. When administering oral medications to pediatric patients, use the following guidelines:

• Techniques that aid in successful liquid medication administration to young children include administering the medication into the corner pocket of the patient's cheek to prevent the medication from running back out.

• If the patient is a toddler, don't mix a drug with food or call it "candy," even if it has a pleasant taste. Have the child drink a liquid drug from a calibrated medication cup, rather than from a spoon, because it's easier and more accurate. Rinsing the device with water before pouring the drug into it keeps the drug from sticking and delivers a more accurate dose. If the drug is available only in tablet form, crush it and mix it with a compatible syrup after consultation with a pharmacist. Check with the pharmacist first to make sure it's safe to crush the tablet.

• If the patient is an older child, who can swallow a tablet or a capsule by himself, have him place the pill on the back of his tongue and swallow it with water or fruit juice. Remember, milk or milk products may interfere with drug absorption.

Administering a gastric drug

If your patient has an NG or gastrostomy tube, you can deliver drugs directly to the gastric mucosa through the tube. If he has a jejunostomy tube, you can deliver drugs to the intestinal lumen.

Going down the tubes

An *NG tube* extends from the patient's nose into the stomach. Your patient may have an NG tube in place if he has trouble swallowing or he has an altered level of consciousness. In either case, it may be necessary to administer his oral drugs through the tube rather than through the oral route.

Just passsing through

All drugs delivered through an NG tube must be in liquid form so they can pass easily through the tube. If your patient's drug comes in tablet form, you'll need to crush it and dissolve it in water. If the drug comes in capsule form, you'll need to empty the contents of the capsule into water.

Consult with the pharmacist in your facility prior to crushing a pill or emptying the contents of a capsule to verify that this is acceptable practice based on the drug and its intended action.

Crossing over

Unlike an NG tube, a *gastrostomy tube* crosses the abdominal wall to enter the stomach. It may be surgically inserted, or it may be placed during an endoscopic, a laparoscopic, or a radiologic procedure.

A gastrostomy tube reduces the risk of aspiration, and it's more comfortable for the patient than an NG tube. You'll use the tube to deliver feeding solutions and drugs directly into the patient's stomach.

Floating along

A *jejunostomy tube* may be inserted directly into the jejunum across the abdominal wall, or it may be inserted through the nose and allowed to float through the stomach, through the pylorus and into the small intestine. You'll use it to administer feeding solutions and drugs.

Also, patients with a GI obstruction or a high risk of aspiration (as from an altered level of consciousness or the effects of a stroke) may need long-term nutritional therapy. Usually, it's delivered through a jejunostomy tube.

To pass me through an NG tube, you can crush me.

But first, you must ask me if it's acceptable practice in your facility.

Or, you can empty me.

What you need

Prescribed medication * towel or linen-saver pad * stethoscope * gloves * facial tissues * container of water * 50- or 60-ml piston-type, catheter-tipped syringe

Got a crush on you

If you'll be giving a crushed tablet, get a mortar and pestle for crushing it and a liquid in which to dissolve the drug just before instilling it.

Getting ready

• Verify the order in the patient's chart.
• Prepare the drug for delivery by crushing a tablet and mixing it in water or opening a capsule and mixing the contents in water, after consultation with a pharmacist.

- Identify the patient by checking his armband.
- Wash your hands and put on gloves.
- Help the patient into semi-Fowler's position.

What to teach

- Explain the purpose of the NG tube, gastrostomy tube, or jejunostomy tube to the patient.
- Stress the importance of remaining upright after drug administration to avoid aspiration.
- Instruct the patient about possible adverse reactions to the prescribed drug, and tell him which adverse reactions should be reported immediately to the doctor.
- If the patient will be receiving drugs through a gastrostomy tube at home, teach him or a caregiver how to administer them safely and accurately. Send the patient home with written instructions.

> **Memory jogger**
>
> To help you remember which direction to move the syringe when you want to slow down the flow through the tube, remember LOWER IS SLOWER or SLOW DOWN.

Giving drugs through an NG tube

To give drugs through an NG tube, follow these steps.

How you do it

- To protect the patient from spills, place a towel or linen-saver pad across his upper torso.
- Next, remove the clamp from the NG tube and check the position of the tube. (See *Checking the position of a NG tube.*)
- After you've confirmed that the tube is in the proper position, remove the syringe from the end of the tube.
- Draw water into the syringe and use it to irrigate the tube with about 30 ml of water. Then remove the syringe from the tube and remove the piston from the syringe.
- Insert the catheter tip into the distal end of the NG tube, making sure it fits snugly.
- With the syringe attached to the opening of the tube, hold the syringe upright and slightly above the level of the patient's nose.
- Slowly pour the drug into the syringe, using it as a funnel.

Slow flow

- Allow the drug to flow slowly through the tube. If it flows too quickly, lower the syringe. If it flows too slowly, raise the syringe slightly.
- As the syringe empties, add more of the drug. To prevent air from entering the patient's stomach, don't let the syringe drain completely before you add more drug to it.
- After you've given the full dose, pour 30 to 50 ml of water into the syringe.

> To prevent air from entering the patient's stomach, don't let the syringe drain completely before you add more drug to it.

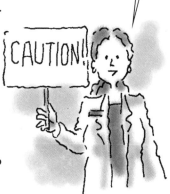

CAUTION!

Peak technique

Checking the position of an NG tube

Before administering a drug through your patient's nasogastric (NG) tube, you'll need to confirm proper placement of the tube by following these steps:
• Insert a catheter-tipped syringe into the distal end of the tube and place the diaphragm of your stethoscope over the patient's stomach as shown.
• Then use the syringe to insert about 10 ml of air into the tube as you listen through the stethoscope. If the tube is in the patient's stomach, you'll hear a loud gurgle when you inject the air.

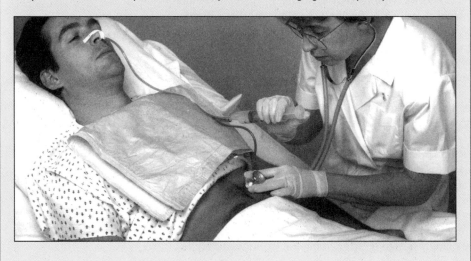

Getting carried away

• Let the water flow through the tube to rinse it and to carry all of the drug into the patient's stomach.
• Next, clamp the tube and remove the syringe.
• If the tube is attached to suction, clamp it for 30 to 60 minutes after you give a drug, if the patient will tolerate it and the patient's doctor agrees and writes an order.

No backsies

• Have the patient remain in semi-Fowler's position or in a side-lying position for at least 30 minutes after administration to prevent esophageal reflux (backward or return flow of stomach contents into the esophagus).
• Clean and store the equipment, or dispose of it as appropriate.

Practice pointers

• Remember that all drugs instilled through the tube must be in liquid form. Check with a pharmacist if you aren't sure whether a tablet can be safely crushed or a capsule safely opened.
• Never crush an enteric-coated or a sustained-release drug.

Full follow-through

• Because capsules tend not to dissolve completely, always follow them with water to flush the tube and prevent occlusion.
• Dilute liquid drugs with about 30 ml of water to decrease their osmolality.
• If you need to give more than one drug through an NG tube, give each one separately, flushing the tube with 10 to 15 ml of water between doses to avoid drug interactions.
• Irrigate the tube with 30 ml of irrigant before and after drug instillation.

Free to vent

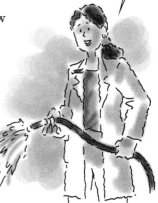

Irrigate the tube with 30 ml of irrigant before and after giving the drug.

• If the patient has a large-bore silastic NG tube, such as the Argyle Salem sump tube, watch for fluid reflux in the vent lumen. Reflux means that pressure in the patient's stomach exceeds atmospheric pressure, possibly because the primary lumen is clogged or the suction system was set up incorrectly. Don't clamp the vent tube in an attempt to stop the reflux.
• Some drugs, such as phenytoin (Dilantin), are altered by the presence of feeding solutions in the patient's stomach. Check with a doctor to see whether you should stop the patient's tube feeding for 1 or 2 hours before or after giving the prescribed drug.

Giving drugs through a gastrostomy tube

To give drugs through a gastrostomy tube, follow the steps below.

How you do it

• Gently lift the dressing around the insertion site and assess the skin around the site for irritation caused by gastric secretions.

Putting it on hold

• If the patient is receiving continuous feedings, touch the pump's HOLD button to interrupt the feedings. Then clamp the gastrostomy tube and disconnect the tubing that leads to the pump.
• Remove the piston from the catheter-tipped syringe, and insert the catheter into the gastrostomy tube.

Royal flush

• Instill 30 ml of water into the syringe to flush the feeding solution through the tube and into the patient's stomach. This allows you to check the tube's patency and to clear the tube before you give a drug through it.

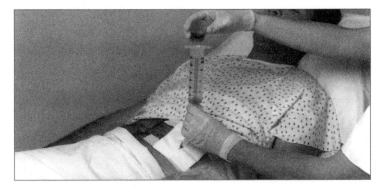

• Slowly pour up to 30 ml of the drug at a time into the syringe, using it as a funnel as shown above.
• Allow the drug to flow slowly through the tube. If it flows too quickly, lower the syringe. If it flows too slowly, raise the syringe slightly.
• As the syringe empties, add more of the drug. To keep air from entering the patient's stomach, don't let the syringe drain completely before adding more drug to it.
• After giving the full dose, place about 30 ml of water into the syringe to rinse the tube and carry all of the drug into the patient's stomach.
• Remove the syringe from the tube. Then tighten the clamp or replug the opening of the tube.

Change for the better

• Change the dressing that covers the insertion site, if necessary, as well as the dressing or plug at the distal tip of the tube.
• Keep the patient in the semi-Fowler position for at least 30 minutes after giving a drug through the tube to prevent esophageal reflux.

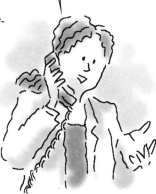

That's right, 30 minutes in semi-Fowler's position after giving the drug.

Practice pointers

• Determine the amount of residual fluid in the patient's stomach, especially when tube feedings are infusing. A high residual fluid level may indicate decreased motility; if this occurs, drugs may not be absorbed completely.
• Give the full dose of the prescribed drug through the gastrostomy tube before you restart any tube feedings as ordered.

Alterations not included

- The actions of some drugs are altered by the presence of feeding solutions in the patient's intestine. Check with a doctor to see whether you should stop the patient's tube feeding for 1 or 2 hours before or after giving the prescribed drug.
- When flushing a gastrostomy tube, use about 30 ml of water if the patient is an adult or about a 15 ml if the patient is a child.

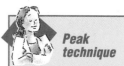

Giving drugs through a jejunostomy tube

To give drugs through a jejunostomy tube, follow the steps below.

How you do it

- Remove the dressing that covers the tube, if necessary, as well as the dressing or plug at the distal tip of the tube. Clamp or pinch the tubing before you remove the plug.
- If the patient is receiving continuous feedings, touch the pump's HOLD button to interrupt the feeding. Then disconnect the tubing that leads to the pump from the jejunostomy tube.

Psssst, don't forget the piston

- Remove the piston from the catheter-tipped syringe, and then insert the tip of the catheter into the jejunostomy tube.
- Instill 30 ml of water into the syringe to flush the feeding solution through the tube and into the patient's jejunum. This allows you to check the patency of the tube before you give a drug through it.
- Slowly pour up to 30 ml of the drug at a time into the syringe, using it as a funnel.
- Allow the drug to flow slowly through the tube. If it flows too quickly, lower the syringe. If it flows too slowly, raise the syringe slightly.
- As the syringe empties, add more of the drug. To keep air from entering the patient's jejunum, don't let the syringe drain completely before you add more of the drug to it.

Out with the rinse water

- After giving the full dose, place about 30 ml of water into the syringe to rinse the tube and carry all of the drug into the patient's jejunum.
- Carefully remove the syringe from the tube, and be sure to tighten the clamp or replug the opening of the tube.
- Change the dressing that covers the insertion site, if necessary, as well as the dressing or plug at the distal tip of the tube.
- Keep the patient in semi-Fowler's position for at least 30 minutes, or as tolerated.

Peak technique

Flush with success

Over the years, nurses have used an assortment of fluids to open clogged feeding tubes, from carbonated soda to cranberry juice. However, the acidic nature of some of these fluids may actually worsen the problem. Studies — and clinical experience — show that water is still the best solution for a clogged tube.

To help avoid the problem altogether, flush the tube with 30 ml of water before and after giving a drug through it; give intermittent feedings, if possible; and check residual levels every 4 to 6 hours.

Practice pointers

• Assessing the amount of residual fluid in the patient's jejunum may be difficult because of the rapid absorption that takes place in the small intestine. If you do withdraw residual fluid from a jejunostomy tube, notify a doctor. It may mean that the patient isn't tolerating the tube feedings and may have decreased motility. As a result, drugs may not be absorbing completely.

Clogged pipes

• Because small-bore feeding tubes are more likely to occlude than larger bore tubes, thus preventing instillation of drugs and feeding solutions, make sure you flush the tube before and after giving a drug. (See *Flush with success.*)
• The actions of some drugs are altered by the presence of feeding solutions in the patient's intestine. Check with a doctor to see whether you should stop the patient's tube feeding for 1 or 2 hours before or after giving the prescribed drug.
• Give the full dose of the prescribed drug through the jejunostomy tube before you restart any tube feedings as ordered.

Taking a shortcut

• Because a jejunostomy tube doesn't empty into the stomach, absorption of the drug you instill doesn't take place in the patient's stomach and duodenum. Consequently, some drugs (such as antacids and antidiarrheals) shouldn't be administered through this kind of tube.

Write it down

Documenting gastric administration

Be sure to record:
• drug given
• amount of drug given
• date and time of the instillation
• condition of the patient's skin around the tube insertion site
• patient's tolerance of the procedure
• placement of the patient's nasogastric tube before you administered a drug through it
• amount of fluid instilled on the patient's intake and output sheet.

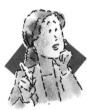

Quick quiz

1. When administering tablets or capsules by the oral route, you would:

    A.   assess the patient's ability to swallow before administering the drug.

    B.   give a drug that had been poured by someone else to save time.

    C.   return any unused opened or unwrapped drug to the patient's medication drawer to avoid unnecessary waste.

    D.   give a drug from a poorly labeled or an unlabeled bottle.

Answer: A. Before administering tablets or capsules by the oral route, assess the patient's ability to swallow to prevent aspiration.

2. If a patient questions you about the drug you're giving or the amount you're giving, you should:

    A.   remain with the patient until he takes the drug.

    B.   discard the drug.

    C.   double-check the patient's medication record.

    D.   inform the patient that he shouldn't question the doctor's order.

Answer: C. If the patient questions you about the drug you're giving or the amount you're giving, double-check his medication record. If the drug and dose are correct, reassure and inform the patient about his drug and any changes in dosage.

3. Which of the following tubes should be positioned in the second portion of the small bowel?

    A.   NG tube

    B.   Gastrostomy tube

    C.   Salem sump tube

    D.   Jejunostomy tube

Answer: D. A jejunostomy tube may be inserted directly into the jejunum across the abdominal wall, or it may be inserted through the nose and allowed to float through the stomach, through the pylorus, and into the small intestine.

4. Which of the following solutions is the best to use to open your patient's clogged feeding tube?

    A.   Carbonated soda

    B.   Cranberry juice

    C.   Water

    D.   Any acidic solution

Answer: C. Studies and clinical experience have shown that water is still the best solution for a clogged tube.

Scoring

★★★ If you answered all four questions correctly, out of sight! You're on track with oral administration.

★★ If you answered three questions correctly, thumbs up! You've got the thread of tube administration.

★ If you answered fewer than three questions correctly, don't get choked up. There's a lot to remember about correct tube technique, so give it another shot.

Rectal and vaginal administration

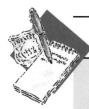

Just the facts

In this chapter, you'll learn:

♦ the local and systemic effects of administering drugs into the rectum or vagina
♦ how to administer a drug rectally
♦ how to administer a drug vaginally.

Administering rectal medication

You may administer a drug rectally to a patient who is unconscious, vomiting, or unable to swallow or take anything by mouth. The most commonly used forms of rectal medication include:
- suppositories
- ointments
- medicated enemas.

Rectally administered drugs can produce either local or systemic effects.

Dodging digestive enzymes

Because rectal administration bypasses the upper GI tract, drugs given by this method aren't destroyed by digestive enzymes in the stomach or small intestine. Also, these drugs don't irritate the upper GI tract, as some oral drugs can.

Bypassing the first pass effect

Rectal drugs bypass the portal system, thus avoiding biotransformation in the liver. *Biotransformation* or drug metabolism refers to the body's ability to change a drug from its dosage form to a more water-soluble form that can be excreted. Once in the liver, drugs are metabolized by enzymes.

Rectal drugs do have some disadvantages, however. The administration procedure may cause discomfort or embarrassment to the patient. Also, the drug may be incompletely absorbed, especially if the patient can't retain it or if his rectum contains feces. As a result, the patient may need a higher dose than if he had taken the same drug in oral form.

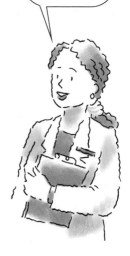

Don't forget that the drugs you give rectally can have far-reaching, or systemic, effects.

Administering rectal suppositories

A *suppository* is a firm, bullet-shaped object made from a substance that melts at body temperature (such as cocoa butter). As the suppository melts, it releases the drug into the patient's rectum, where it can be absorbed across the rectal mucosa. Most suppositories are about 1½″ (3.5 cm) long—smaller for infants and children.

Rectal suppositories commonly contain drugs that reduce fever, induce relaxation, stimulate peristalsis and defecation, or relieve pain, vomiting, and local irritation.

What you need

Prescribed drug ✻ several 4″ × 4″ gauze pads ✻ gloves ✻ linen-saver pad ✻ water-soluble lubricant ✻ bedpan, if necessary

Getting ready

- Verify the order on the patient's chart.
- Identify the patient by checking his armband.
- Provide privacy.

How you do it

- Place the patient on his left side in Sims' position (semi-prone with the right knee and thigh drawn up and the left arm along the patient's back). Cover him with the bedcovers, exposing only his buttocks.
- Place a linen-saver pad under his buttocks to protect the bedding.
- Wash your hands and put on gloves.
- Remove the suppository from its wrapper, and apply a water-soluble lubricant to it.
- Using your nondominant hand, lift the patient's upper buttock to expose his anus.

Take a deep breath and relax

- Tell the patient to take several deep breaths through his mouth to relax the anal sphincter and reduce anxiety and discomfort during insertion.

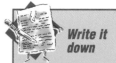

Write it down

Documenting rectal suppository administration

Be sure to record:
- drug given
- dose given
- date and time of administration
- patient's response.

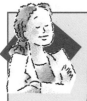

Peak technique

Inserting a rectal suppository in an adult

Use your index finger to direct the suppository along the rectal wall toward the patient's umbilicus, as shown below, so the membrane can absorb the drug. Continue to advance it about 3″ (7.5 cm), or about the length of your finger, until it passes the internal anal sphincter.

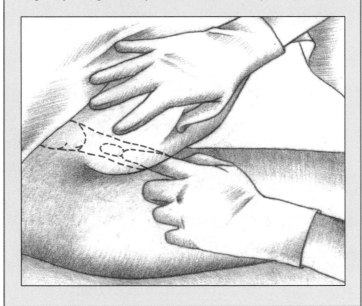

Ages and stages

Using rectal suppositories in pediatric patients

Rectal administration via suppository may be a good alternative when the oral route can't be used, but remember that it's a less reliable method in children than in adults. Remember to insert the suppository only up to the first knuckle joint of your finger. If your patient is an infant, use your little finger to insert the drug.

Tapered end first

• Using your dominant hand, insert the tapered end of the suppository into the patient's rectum. (See *Inserting a rectal suppository in an adult.*)

• If your patient is a child, you'll want to follow these guidelines. (See *Using rectal suppositories in pediatric patients.*)

• Ensure the patient's comfort. Encourage him to lie quietly and, if applicable, to retain the suppository for an appropriate time. A suppository given to relieve constipation should be retained as long as possible (at least 20 minutes) for it to be effective. If necessary, press on the patient's anus with a gauze pad until the urge to defecate passes.

Danger zone

Contraindications for rectal suppositories

You'll want to avoid rectal suppositories in these situations:
• Because inserting a rectal suppository typically stimulates the vagus nerve, rectal drug administration is contraindicated in patients who have cardiac arrhythmias or who have had a myocardial infarction.
• Don't give a rectal drug (or a laxative) to a patient with undiagnosed abdominal pain. If the pain stems from appendicitis, the peristalsis caused by rectal administration could rupture the appendix.
• Because rectal suppositories increase the risk of local trauma, rectal drug administration should be avoided in patients who have recently had colon, rectal, or prostate surgery.

• If the patient can't retain the suppository and pressing on his anus with a gauze pad doesn't relieve his urge to defecate, place the patient on a bedpan.

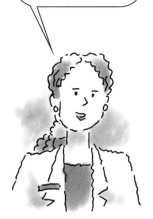

To reduce anxiety and discomfort, have your patient take several deep breaths during insertion of a rectal suppository.

Practice pointers

• Store rectal suppositories in the refrigerator, as indicated, to keep them firm and to maintain the drug's effectiveness.
• Before administering any rectal medication, inspect the patient's anus. If the tissues are inflamed or if hemorrhoids are present, withhold the suppository and notify a doctor. The drug could aggravate the condition.
• To minimize the risk of local trauma, you may need to avoid this route if the patient has had recent rectal, colon, or prostate surgery.
• Rectal suppositories are contraindicated in certain patients. (See *Contraindications for rectal suppositories*.)

What to teach

• Teach the patient about the purpose of the rectal medication.
• Stress to the patient the necessity of retaining the suppository as long as possible to promote the drug's effectiveness.

Applying anal ointment

An ointment is a semi-solid medication that's used to produce local effects.

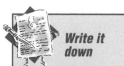

You may apply an ointment to the patient's anus to treat an infection or inflammation. Medicated ointments are also used as lubricants to help protect the skin.

What you need

Prescribed anal ointment ✳ gloves ✳ several 4″ × 4″ gauze pads

Dress for success

After applying an ointment, you may need to apply a dressing as well to keep the ointment from staining the patient's clothes or bed linens.

Getting ready

• Verify the order on the patient's chart.
• Identify the patient by checking his armband.
• Provide privacy.

Side order

• Help the patient onto his side with his knees flexed to allow access to his anus.
• Wash your hands and put on gloves.

How you do it

• Next, lift the patient's upper buttock and inspect his anus.

Main squeeze

• Squeeze a small amount of ointment onto your gloved finger.
• Lift the patient's upper buttock again, and spread the ointment over the anal area, using your finger or a gauze pad.
• Place a folded 4″ × 4″ gauze pad between the patient's buttocks to absorb excess ointment.

Practice pointers

• Before administering an anal ointment, inspect the patient's anus.
• Store ointments as indicated on the tube.

What to teach

• Teach the patient about the purpose of the anal ointment.
• If the patient will be continuing the treatment at home, teach him how to apply the ointment safely and correctly.

Write it down

Documenting anal ointment application

Be sure to record:
• drug given
• dose given
• date and time of administration
• appearance of the patient's anus before you applied the ointment.

Absorb excess ointment by placing a folded 4″ × 4″ gauze pad between your patient's buttocks.

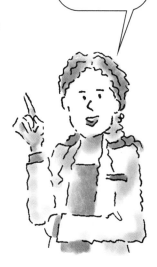

Administering rectal ointment

Some ointments are administered inside the rectum. These internal ointments are used to:
- decrease inflammation
- treat rectal infection
- relieve pain
- treat hemorrhoids.

On the fast tract

Internal ointments are absorbed more quickly than external ointments because of the properties of the mucosal lining.

What you need

Prescribed rectal ointment (with tube and applicator) ✳ water-soluble lubricant ✳ several 4″ × 4″ gauze pads ✳ gloves

Getting ready

- Verify the order on the patient's chart.
- Identify the patient by checking his armband.
- Provide privacy.
- Wash your hands and put on gloves.

How you do it

- Remove the cap from the ointment tube, and attach the applicator to the tube.

Water-soluble lubricants only

- Coat the applicator with water-soluble lubricant. For internal administration, expect to use about 1″ (2.5 cm) of ointment. To judge the pressure needed to extract this amount, squeeze a small amount from the tube before you attach the applicator.
- With your nondominant hand, lift the patient's upper buttock to expose the anus.
- Ask the patient to breathe deeply through his mouth to relax the anal sphincter and reduce anxiety or discomfort during insertion.
- Gently insert the applicator, directing it toward the umbilicus, as shown at top of next page.
- Slowly squeeze the tube to eject the ointment.
- Withdraw the applicator, and place a folded 4″ × 4″ gauze pad between the patient's buttocks to absorb excess ointment.
- Remove the applicator from the tube, and recap the tube. Clean the applicator with soap and water.

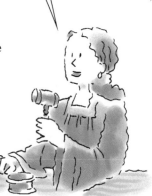

Here's good judgment. Squeeze some ointment from the tube before you attach the applicator to determine the pressure needed to extract it.

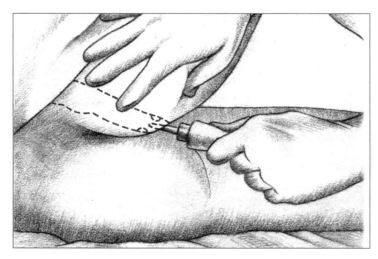

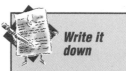
Practice pointers

• Before administering a rectal medication, inspect the patient's anus.
• Store the ointment as indicated on the tube.

What to teach

• Teach the patient the purpose of the rectal ointment.
• If the patient will be continuing the treatment at home, teach him how to administer the rectal ointment safely and correctly.

Giving medicated enemas

When you give an enema, you instill fluid into a patient's rectum for a variable amount of time. If you're preparing the patient for a diagnostic or surgical procedure, or if you're giving the enema to relieve constipation, you may administer a cleansing enema.

Cleaning crew

A *cleansing enema* is a type of enema that involves instilling unmedicated fluid into a patient's rectum to simply clean the patient's rectum and colon. The patient expels the irrigant almost completely within about 15 minutes.

Pay attention. The topic is retention.

Enemas can also be used to deliver such drugs as lactulose, which acidifies the colon contents and lowers blood ammonia levels. To deliver a drug, you'll probably give a retention enema. A *retention enema* is a type of enema that requires the patient to retain the fluid in his rectum and colon for 30 to 60 minutes, if possible, before expelling it. A retention enema can also be used as an emollient to soothe irritated colon tissues.

Enema enemies

Enemas stimulate peristalsis by distending the colon and stimulating nerves in the rectal walls. Consequently, you shouldn't give an enema to a patient who has had:
- recent colon or rectal surgery
- a myocardial infarction
- undiagnosed abdominal pain (which could be caused by appendicitis).

Giving an enema to a patient with appendicitis can irritate the inflamed area of the appendix and precipitate perforation.

Most important, give an enema cautiously to any patient who has cardiac arrhythmias.

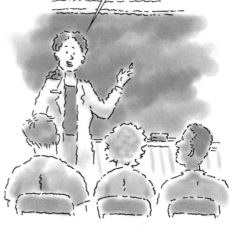

Retention enemas are typically used to deliver drugs. Can you retain that?

What you need

Prescribed solution (usually in a premixed, commercially prepared container) ✳ disposable enema kit ✳ gloves ✳ 4″ × 4″ gauze pads ✳ bedpan ✳ toilet paper ✳ emesis basin ✳ linen-saver pad ✳ water-soluble lubricant (see *Choosing enema supplies*)

Grab bag

If you need to prepare the solution for a patient's enema or you need a large volume of fluid, you'll use an enema bag to perform the procedure instead of commercially prepared solution and a disposable enema kit. You may need an I.V. pole from which to hang the enema bag and a bath thermometer to test the temperature of the solution.

Getting ready

- Verify the order on the patient's chart.
- Identify the patient by checking his armband.
- Explain the procedure to the patient.
- To minimize peristalsis, have the patient empty his bladder and rectum before you begin.

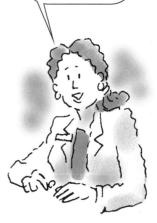

Before administering the enema have the patient empty his bladder and rectum.

Explain the need to retain

- Explain to the patient that, after you instill the enema solution, he'll need to retain it in his rectum for a prescribed length of time until the drug is absorbed.
- Have the patient wear a gown, and provide privacy.

Gear up!

Choosing enema supplies

When choosing supplies for an enema, you should consider the drug prescribed as well as the patient's age, size, and condition. Remember that physical size is always more important than age. For example, if your patient is a small 9-year-old, you'll want to use the smallest tube possible for his age-group.

Remember to use smaller tubing and a smaller volume of fluid when giving a retention enema, so you'll create less pressure in the patient's rectum and make it easier for him to retain the fluid.

Retention enema
Follow these general guidelines when selecting supplies for your patient's retention enema:
• For an adult, select a #14 to #20 French rectal tube. Plan to insert the tube 3″ to 4″ (7.5 to 10 cm) and to use 150 to 200 ml of fluid.
• For a child over age 6, select a #12 to #14 French rectal tube. Plan to insert it 2″ to 3″ (5 to 7.5 cm) and to use 75 to 150 ml of fluid.

Nonretention enema
Follow these general guidelines when selecting supplies for your patient's nonretention enema:
• For an adult, select a #22 to #30 French rectal tube. Plan to insert the tube 3″ to 4″ (7.5 to 10 cm) and to use 750 to 1,000 ml of fluid.
• For a child older than age 6, select a #14 to #18 French rectal tube. Plan to insert it 2″ to 3″ (5 to 7.5 cm) and to use 300 to 500 ml of fluid.
• For a child ages 2 to 6, select a #12 to #14 French rectal tube. Plan to insert it 1½″ to 2″ (4 to 5 cm) and to use 250 to 350 ml of fluid.
• For a child under age 2, select a #12 French rectal tube. Plan to insert it 1″ to 1½″ (2.5 to 4 cm) and to use 150 to 250 ml of fluid.

How you do it
• Help the patient onto his left side in Sims' position. If he's uncomfortable in that position, reposition him onto his right side or, if necessary, onto his back. Place a linen-saver pad under him to protect the bedding.

For disposable enemas
• Put on gloves, and remove the cap from the rectal tube.
• Check the amount of lubricant that's already on the tube. If needed, squeeze water-soluble lubricant onto a 4″ × 4″ gauze pad and dip the tip of the rectal tube into the lubricant.
• Gently squeeze the enema container to expel air.
• With your nondominant hand, lift the patient's upper buttock to expose his anus.

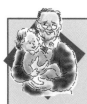

Ages and stages

Administering enemas to children

For a child age 11 or older, advance the rectal tube about 4″ (10 cm). For children ages 4 to 10, advance the tube about 3″ (7.5 cm). For children ages 2 to 4, advance the tube about 2″ (5 cm). For infants, advance the tube about 1″ (2.5 cm).

Flow rate

Regulate the flow rate by lowering or raising the bag according to the patient's retention ability and level of comfort. Don't raise it higher than 12″ (30.5 cm) for a child, or 6″ to 8″ (15 to 20 cm) for an infant.

Waiting to inhale

- Tell the patient to take a deep breath. As he inhales, insert the rectal tube into his rectum, pointing the tube toward his umbilicus.
- If the patient is an adult, advance the tube about 4″ (10 cm). Child patients require different guidelines. (See *Administering enemas to children*.)

Squeeze until empty

- Squeeze the solution container until it's empty. Then remove the rectal tube and discard the used enema container, the packaging it came in, and your gloves.

For enema bags

- Prepare the prescribed solution and warm it to 105° F (40.6° C). Test the temperature using a bath thermometer, or pour a small amount of solution over your wrist.
- Put on gloves, close the clamp on the enema tubing, and fill the enema bag with the solution.
- Hang the enema bag on an I.V. pole, and adjust the bag so it's slightly above bed level.

Tip of the day

- Remove the protective cap from the end of the enema tubing. The tip of the tubing should be prelubricated. If it isn't, lubricate it with a small amount of water-soluble lubricant.
- Unclamp the tubing, and flush solution through it; then reclamp the tubing.

> You can't predict the temperature of the solution — use a bath thermometer or pour a small amount of solution over your wrist to test it.

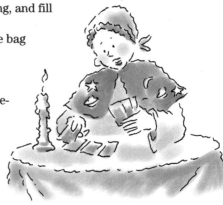

• With your nondominant hand, lift the patient's upper buttock. While holding the tube in your other hand, touch the patient's anal sphincter with the tip of the tube to stimulate contraction. Then insert the tube into the patient's anus.
• As the sphincter relaxes, tell the patient to breathe deeply through his mouth as you gently advance the tube.

Hold on

• Release the clamp on the tubing. Make sure you continue holding the tube in the patient's rectum because bowel contractions and pressure from the anal sphincter can expel the tube.
• Regulate the flow rate by lowering or raising the bag according to the patient's retention ability and level of comfort. Don't raise it higher than 18″ (45.7 cm) for an adult.

Blocked!

• If the flow stops, the tubing may be blocked with feces or wedged against the rectal wall. Gently turn the tubing to free it without stimulating defecation.
• If the tubing becomes clogged, withdraw it, flush it with solution, and then reinsert it.
• To avoid inserting air into the patient's rectum, clamp the tubing to stop the flow just before the enema bag empties.
• Remove the tubing, and dispose of the setup.

A matter of time

• Tell the patient to retain the solution for the prescribed time. If necessary, hold a 4″ × 4″ gauze pad against the anus until the patient's urge to defecate passes.
• If the patient is apprehensive, place him on a bedpan and have him hold toilet tissue or a rolled washcloth against his anus.
• Dispose of your gloves, and place the call button within easy reach. Tell the patient to call for help if he wants to get out of bed, especially if he feels weak or faint.

Practice pointers

• Before giving a retention enema, check the patient's elimination pattern. A constipated patient may need a cleansing enema to keep feces from interfering with drug absorption. A patient with a fecal impaction may need to have the drug delivered by another route.
• Keep in mind that a patient with diarrhea may not be able to retain the enema solution for the prescribed time.
• Before administering a rectal medication, inspect the patient's anus.

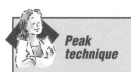

Peak technique

Tips for a weak anal sphincter

If your patient has a weak anal sphincter, try using a baby-bottle nipple to hold the catheter of the enema tubing in place. Enlarge the hole at the nipple's tip. Pass the catheter inside the nipple and out through the tip. The nipple should act as a seal to help the patient retain the enema.

• If the patient has a weak anal sphincter, follow the advice given in *Tips for a weak anal sphincter,* page 209.

What to teach

• Teach the patient about the purpose of the enema.
• Stress to the patient the importance of retaining it as long as possible.
• Advise the patient to report any increase in cramping or pain.
• If the patient will be giving himself an enema at home, provide him with written instructions, if necessary.

Administering vaginal drugs

Vaginal drugs are available in many forms, including:
• suppositories
• creams
• gels
• ointments
• solutions.
    These medicated preparations can be inserted to treat infection — particularly *Trichomonas vaginalis* and candidiasis — or inflammation, or to prevent conception. Vaginal administration is most effective when the patient can remain lying down afterward to retain the medication.

Giving a vaginal drug

Most vaginal drugs come packaged in or with an applicator that you or the patient can use to insert the drug into the anterior and posterior fornices. When in contact with the vaginal mucosa, suppositories melt, diffusing medication as effectively as creams, gels, and ointments.

What you need

Prescribed vaginal drug (with an applicator, if necessary) ✳ gloves ✳ water-soluble lubricant ✳ small sanitary pad ✳ absorbent towel ✳ linen-saver pad ✳ small drape ✳ cotton balls ✳ 4″ × 4″ gauze pad ✳ paper towel ✳ soap and water, if necessary

Getting ready

• Verify the order on the patient's chart.
• If possible, plan to give the drug at bedtime, when the patient is recumbent.

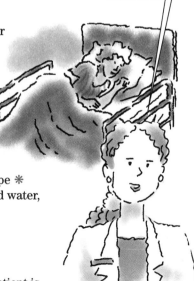

With vaginal administration, have your patient lie down.

- Identify the patient by checking her armband.
- Explain the procedure to the patient, and provide privacy.
- Ask the patient to empty her bladder.

Self-administration is an option

- Ask her whether she would rather insert the medication herself. If so, provide appropriate instructions.

How you do it

- If the patient decides not to self-administer, help her into the lithotomy position.
- Place a linen-saver pad under her buttocks and a small drape over her legs. Expose only her perineum.
- Wash your hands and put on gloves.
- Squeeze a small portion of water-soluble lubricant onto a 4″ × 4″ gauze pad.

Package deal

- Unwrap the suppository, and coat it with the lubricant. If the medication is a small suppository in a prepackaged applicator, lubricate the tip of the suppository with water-soluble lubricant. If the medication is a foam or gel, fill the applicator as prescribed, and lubricate the tip of the applicator with the water-soluble lubricant.
- Next, separate the patient's labia.

Examination before administration

- Examine the patient's perineum. If you find that it's excoriated, withhold the medication and notify a doctor. The patient may need a different type of medication.
- If you see any discharge, wash the area.
- To do this, soak several cotton balls in warm, soapy water.
- Then, while holding the labia open with one hand, wipe once down the left side of the patient's perineum with a cotton ball.
- Discard the cotton ball, pick up another one, and use the new cotton ball to wipe once down the right side of the perineum.
- Discard the cotton ball, pick up another one, and use it to wipe once down the middle of the patient's perineum.

Rounded tip first

- With the patient's labia still separated, insert the rounded tip of a suppository into her vagina, advancing it about 3″ to 4″ (7.5 to 10 cm) along the posterior wall of the vagina, or as far as it will go.
- If you're using an applicator, insert it into the patient's vagina. (See *How to administer a vaginal drug using an applicator,* page 212.)

Peak technique

How to administer a vaginal drug using an applicator

If you're using an applicator to administer a vaginal drug to your patient, follow these steps:
• Use your dominant hand to insert it about 2″ (5 cm) into the patient's vagina. Direct the applicator down initially, toward the patient's spine, and then back up toward the cervix, as shown below.
• Press the plunger until you empty all of the medication from the applicator.
• Remove the applicator, and place it on a paper towel to prevent the spread of microorganisms.
• Discard the applicator, or wash it with soap and warm water before storing it, as appropriate.

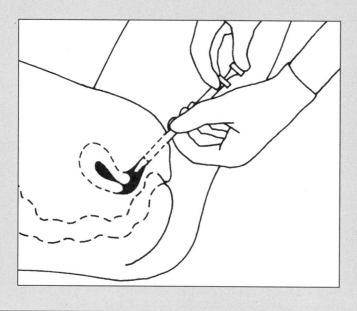

Time to lie down

• Tell the patient to lie down for about 5 to 10 minutes with her knees flexed to help promote absorption and allow the medication to flow into the posterior fornix. If you inserted a suppository, tell her to remain recumbent for at least 30 minutes to allow time for it to melt.
• Place a small sanitary pad in the patient's underwear to keep her clothes or bedding from becoming soiled.

Documenting vaginal drug administration

Be sure to record:
• drug given
• method by which you gave it
• date and time of administration
• color and consistency of any vaginal discharge
• adverse effects the patient experienced
• patient's tolerance of the procedure
• whether the patient prefers to insert vaginal medications independently or with nursing assistance.

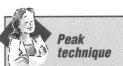

Peak technique

Vaginal administration of 5-FU

Avoid getting the vaginal drug 5-FU on the patient's genital area. Apply petroleum jelly to the vulva and perineal area prior to inserting 5-FU. Then follow its insertion with a tampon.

• When giving vaginal 5-fluorouracil (5-FU), a chemotherapeutic agent, you'll need to take special precautions. (See *Vaginal administration of 5-FU.*)

Practice pointers

• Refrigerate vaginal gels, foams, and suppositories that melt at room temperature.

What to teach

• If the patient will be inserting vaginal medication on her own, show her how to do it correctly and provide her with written instructions.
• Tell the patient not to insert a tampon after using a vaginal medication, unless specifically instructed to do so, because the tampon will absorb the drug and make it less effective.
• Instruct the patient to continue administering vaginal medications as prescribed, even when she has her menstrual period.

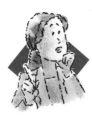

Quick quiz

1. Which of the following is correct concerning rectal drug administration?
   A. Rectal drugs are destroyed by digestive enzymes in the stomach and small intestine.
   B. Rectal drugs undergo biotransformation in the liver.

    C.   Rectal drugs avoid irritating the upper GI tract, as some oral drugs can.

    D.   Rectal drugs are always completely absorbed.

Answer: C. Rectal drugs avoid irritating the upper GI tract, as some oral drugs can.

2.   A patient should retain a retention enema for what period of time?

    A.   10 to 20 minutes

    B.   20 to 30 minutes

    C.   60 to 90 minutes

    D.   30 to 60 minutes

Answer: D. A retention enema requires the patient to retain the fluid in the rectum and colon for 30 to 60 minutes before expelling it.

3.   When choosing supplies for a nonretention enema, what size rectal tube would you select for a child under age 2?

    A.   #12 French

    B.   #14 French

    C.   #18 French

    D.   #26 French

Answer: A. For a child under age 2, select a #12 French rectal tube.

4.   When using an applicator to administer a vaginal drug, how should you initially direct the applicator?

    A.   Toward the patient's spine

    B.   Toward the patient's umbilicus

    C.   Toward the patient's cervix

    D.   Toward the patient's sternum

Answer: A. When using an applicator to administer a vaginal drug, direct the applicator down initially, toward the patient's spine, and then back up, toward the cervix.

Scoring

☆☆☆ If you answered all four questions correctly, excellent! Once again you've navigated the right routes to success!

☆☆ If you answered two or three correctly, great! You absorbed the material well!

☆ If you answered fewer than two correctly, it looks as if you had a little trouble retaining some of the information. Review the chapter, and you'll get the right effect!

13

Intradermal, subcutaneous, and intramuscular administration

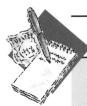

Just the facts

In this chapter, you'll learn:

♦ the principles of administering drugs through injection

♦ how to prepare an injection

♦ how to give an intradermal injection

♦ how to give a subcutaneous injection

♦ how to give an intramuscular injection.

Understanding injection

The ability to inject drugs into a patient's skin, subcutaneous tissue, or muscle is a key nursing skill that you must exercise with great accuracy and care.

Quick and potent

These routes of administration promote a rapid onset of drug action and high drug levels in a patient's blood, in part because they sidestep the breakdown that can take place in the GI tract and liver.

It calls for preparation

To prepare for an injection, you need to know how to correctly choose a needle and withdraw liquid drug from a vial or an ampule. You may need to reconstitute the drug or combine drugs in a single syringe. Then you'll need to administer the injection to the appropriate site using proper techniques.

After administering the injection, don't recap the needle. Dispose of the syringe in the nearest sharps container.

Preparing an injection

Typically, unless you're using one of the special needleless injection systems described later in this chapter, the first step in preparing for an injection is to choose the proper syringe and needle. Consider the route of administration, the size of the patient, and the most likely injection site when you select a syringe and needle. (See *Selecting syringes and needles*.)

Next, you'll need to withdraw the drug from its vial or ampule into a syringe—possibly together with another drug.

Withdrawing a drug from a vial

Withdrawing a drug from a vial may require you to perform two steps: reconstitution and withdrawal.

What you need

Medication vial ✳ vial or ampule of an appropriate diluent ✳ alcohol pads ✳ syringe ✳ two needles of appropriate size ✳ filter needle (if indicated, to screen particles that may be created during reconstitution)

Getting ready

• Verify the order on the patient's chart.
• Wash your hands.

How you do it

• Place the vial on a countertop.
• Wipe the rubber diaphragm on top of the vial with an alcohol pad.
• Avoid rubbing the diaphragm vigorously because doing so can move bacteria from the nonsterile rim of the vial onto the diaphragm.
• Next, wipe the rubber diaphragm on the top of the diluent vial with a fresh alcohol pad.

Give it some space

• Pick up the appropriate syringe, uncap the needle, and pull back on the plunger until the air-filled space inside the syringe equals the amount of diluent desired.

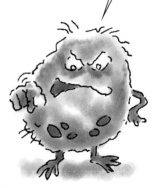

Use care when rubbing the diaphragm—otherwise, you'll move me from the nonsterile rim of the vial onto the diaphragm and then you'll have trouble!

Gear up!

Selecting syringes and needles

Success at giving injections greatly improves with your ability to choose the proper syringe and needle for the task.

Syringes
Illustrated below are four types of commonly used syringes.

Standard syringe
A standard syringe is available in 3-, 5-, 10-, 20-, 25-, 30-, 35-, and 50-ml sizes. It's used to administer numerous drugs in various settings. It consists of a plunger, barrel, hub, and needle. The dead space is the volume of fluid remaining in the syringe and needle when the plunger is depressed completely.

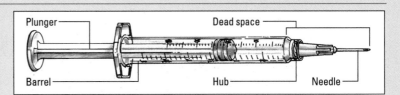

Insulin syringe
An insulin syringe has an attached 25-gauge (25G) needle and no dead space. It's divided into units rather than milliliters and should be used only for insulin administration.

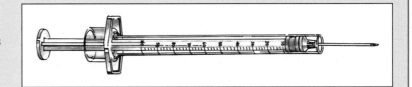

Tuberculin syringe
A tuberculin syringe holds up to 1 ml and typically is used for intradermal (I.D.) injections. It can also be used to give small doses, as might be required in pediatric and intensive care units.

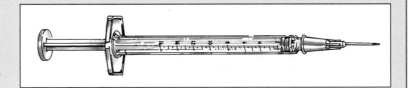

Unit-dose syringe
A unit-dose syringe is prefilled with a measured drug dose in a ready-to-dispense plastic cartridge. You need only to attach a needle.

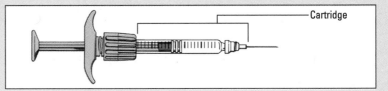

(continued)

Selecting syringes and needles (continued)

Needles

You'll choose different types of needles based on whether you're giving an I.D., subcutaneous (S.C.), or I.M. injection. Needles come in various lengths, diameters (or gauges), and bevel designs.

Intradermal needle

For an I.D. injection, select a needle ⅜" to ⅝" in length and 25G in diameter, with a short bevel.

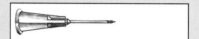

Subcutaneous needle

For an S.C. injection, select a needle ⅝" to ⅞" in length and 23G to 25G in diameter, with a medium bevel.

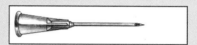

Intramuscular needle

For an I.M. injection, select a needle 1" to 3" in length and 18G to 23G in diameter, with a medium bevel.

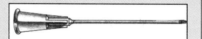

Shielded needle

To reduce the risk of needle-stick injury and the disease transmission that could result, consider choosing a shielded needle when you give injections. A safety device built onto the syringe, shown in the illustrations below, can be used to cover the needle when you're finished giving an injection, thus eliminating the temptation to recap a used needle.

After you've completed an injection, simply grasp the syringe flanges with one hand and push the shield forward with the other hand until it clicks, as shown below. The shield is now locked firmly in place over the needle.

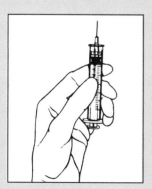
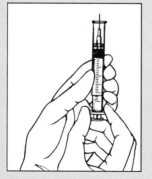
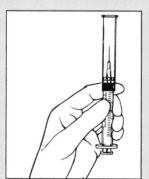

• While holding the base of the vial to keep it steady, puncture the rubber diaphragm of the diluent vial with the needle, as shown below, and inject the air from the syringe into the vial.

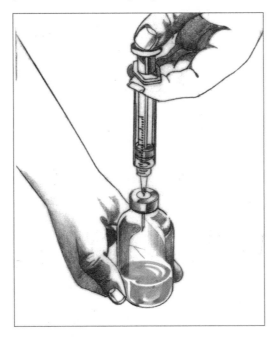

• Draw up the appropriate amount of diluent into the syringe.
• Next, turn to the drug vial. While holding the base to keep the vial steady, inject the diluent into it and withdraw the needle.

Shake and roll

• Shake the vial or roll it between your hands to mix the drug and diluent thoroughly.
• If the drug vial contains its own diluent compartment, remove the protective cap and use your finger to depress the rubber plunger. This forces the lower stopper to fall to the bottom of the vial along with the diluent. Gently roll the vial between your hands to mix the drug and diluent.
• If you need to draw the drug through a filter needle, remove the original needle from the syringe, attach the filter needle, and then uncap it. If you don't need a filter needle, simply leave the original needle on the syringe.

Pump up the volume

• Pull back on the plunger until the volume of air in the syringe equals the volume of drug to be given.
• Puncture the diaphragm of the drug vial, and inject the air.

• Invert the vial, as shown below, and withdraw the amount of drug to be given.

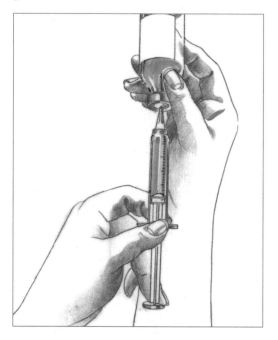

New needle needed

• Remove the needle from the syringe, and replace it with a new sterile needle. You should do so because puncturing a rubber diaphragm can dull a needle and increase the pain of injection, and also because drug stuck to the outside of the used needle could irritate the patient's tissues.
• Label the drug-filled syringe to finish preparing it for administration.

Practice pointers

• When inserting a needle through a rubber diaphragm, hold the needle bevel-up and exert slight lateral pressure as the needle penetrates the diaphragm. By using this technique, you'll avoid cutting a piece of rubber out of the stopper and pushing it into the vial.

Withdrawing a drug from an ampule

You may be required to withdraw a drug from an ampule.

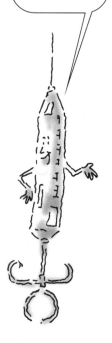

Don't forget to remove the needle from me and replace it with a new sterile needle before injection.

What you need

Medication ampule ✳ dry 2″ × 2″ gauze pad ✳ syringe ✳ filter nee-dle ✳ needle for injecting the drug

Getting ready

- Verify the order on the patient's chart.
- Wash your hands.

How you do it

- Check to make sure all of the fluid is in the bottom of the am-pule. If you see fluid in the stem or the top of the ampule, gently flick the stem to knock the fluid out of the stem and into the bot-tom of the ampule.
- If flicking the stem doesn't force all of the fluid to the bottom of the ampule, try holding the ampule by the stem, raising it to about eye level, and then quickly and carefully swinging it downward at arm's length.

Bottom of the ampule

- Once all of the fluid is in the bottom of the ampule, wrap it in a dry 2″ × 2″ gauze pad so the pad covers the ampule's stem.
- Hold the body of the ampule with one hand and the top portion of the ampule between the thumb and first two fingers of your other hand.

It's a snap!

- While pointing the ampule away from you and others, snap off the top, as shown below.

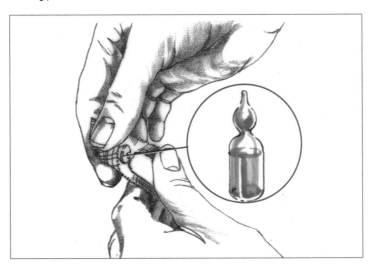

• With a filter needle on the syringe, aspirate the correct amount of drug from the open ampule. The filter needle strains out small pieces of glass that might have fallen into the drug.

New needle needed (again)

• Replace the filter needle with a fresh needle appropriate for injecting the drug. Changing needles prevents a drug on the outside of the filter needle from irritating the patient's tissues.
• Label the drug-filled syringe to finish preparing it for administration.

Practice pointers

• An opened ampule doesn't contain a vacuum, so you don't have to inject air as you do with a vial.

> Remember to use a filter needle to strain out small pieces of glass that aren't visible to the naked eye.

Combining drugs in a syringe

Combining two drugs in one syringe or cartridge avoids the discomfort of two separate injections. Typically, you can combine drugs from:
• two multidose vials (as with regular and long-acting insulin, for example)
• one multidose vial and one ampule
• two ampules
• a multidose vial or an ampule into a partially filled cartridge-injection system.

Bad combinations

Don't combine drugs in a syringe if the drugs are incompatible or if the combined doses exceed the amount of solution that can be absorbed from a single injection site.

What you need

Drug vials or ampules ✳ alcohol pads ✳ syringe ✳ one or more needles of appropriate size

Getting ready

• Verify the order on the patient's chart.
• Wash your hands.

For two multidose vials

• Using an alcohol pad, wipe the rubber stopper on the first vial.

• Pull back the plunger of the syringe until the volume of air in the syringe equals the volume of drug to be withdrawn from the first drug vial.

Don't touch!

• Without inverting the first drug vial, insert the needle into the vial. Make sure the needle tip doesn't touch the liquid in the vial.
• Inject the air into the vial, and then withdraw the needle.

Moving to vial #2...

• Using an alcohol pad, wipe the rubber stopper on the second drug vial.
• Now, pull back the plunger of the syringe until the volume of air in the syringe equals the volume of drug to be withdrawn from the second vial.
• Insert the needle into the second vial, invert the vial, and withdraw the correct amount of the drug.
• Wipe the rubber stopper of the first vial again, insert the needle, invert the vial, and withdraw the correct amount of the drug.

Change needles if possible

• Ideally, to avoid contaminating the second drug drawn into the syringe, you should change the needle on the syringe. In reality, however, this isn't always possible because many disposable syringes don't have removable needles.
• If possible, replace the needle with a fresh needle before you administer the drug.

For a multidose vial and ampule

• Wipe the vial's rubber stopper with an alcohol pad, inject an amount of air equal to the drug dose to be given, invert the vial, and withdraw the correct dose.
• Place the sterile cover back on the needle, and place the syringe on the counter.

Bottoming out

• Make sure all of the drug is in the bottom of the ampule, wrap the ampule with a dry 2″ × 2″ gauze pad, and snap the neck of the ampule away from you.
• Replace the needle on your syringe with a filter needle, insert the needle into the ampule, and withdraw the correct drug dose into the syringe. Be careful not to touch the outside of the ampule with the needle.
• Change back to a regular needle to give the injection.

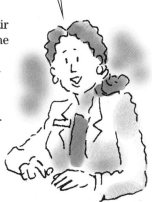

Incompatible drugs or those that combine to form doses exceeding what can be absorbed in a single injection site shouldn't be mixed.

For two ampules

- Make sure all of the fluid is in the bottom of the first ampule, wrap the ampule with a dry $2'' \times 2''$ gauze pad, and snap the neck of the ampule away from you.
- Repeat this process for the second ampule.
- Use a filter needle to draw up the required amount of both drugs, one after the other.
- Change to a regular needle to give the injection.

For a cartridge-injection system

- If the cartridge has a removable needle with a rubber stopper, gently remove the capped needle from the cartridge to expose the rubber stopper.
- Wipe the rubber stopper with an alcohol pad, and insert the needle of an empty syringe into the partly filled cartridge. Don't let the needle touch the drug inside the cartridge.

Equal volume

- Aspirate from the cartridge a volume of air equal to the volume of drug you'll be adding to the cartridge, and then withdraw the needle.
- Draw the correct amount of drug from a vial or an ampule into the syringe.

Rewipe

- Wipe the rubber stopper on the cartridge again, and insert the needle of the syringe into the cartridge.
- Inject the correct amount of compatible drug into the partly filled cartridge.
- Replace the needle on the cartridge using aseptic technique.

In addition...

- If the cartridge doesn't have a rubber stopper, you can add a compatible drug by holding the cartridge needle-up, pulling back the plunger until it reaches a level equal to the combined drug volume, and then inserting the needle into an inverted, single-dose drug vial (after cleaning the diaphragm with an alcohol pad). Advance the needle until the tip is above the liquid in the vial. Inject into the vial an amount of air equal to the volume to be withdrawn from the vial, and then pull the needle into the liquid and withdraw the drug into the cartridge. Remove the needle from the vial, expel excess air, and replace the needle guard.

Irreconcilable differences

- After mixing drugs in a syringe or cartridge, check for signs of incompatibility, such as discoloration and precipitation.

• Label the drug-filled syringe to finish preparing it for administration.

Practice pointers

• Never combine drugs unless you're sure they're compatible, and never combine more than two drugs.
• Although drug incompatibility usually causes a visible reaction — such as clouding, bubbling, or precipitation — it may not. Always check a reputable drug reference or ask a pharmacist if you aren't sure about compatibility.

The clock may be ticking

• Some drugs should be given within 15 minutes after they're mixed; ask a pharmacist if you aren't sure about this timing.
• To reduce the risk of drug contamination, most facilities dispense parenteral drugs in single-dose vials. Insulin is the main exception. Check your facility's policy before you mix insulins.

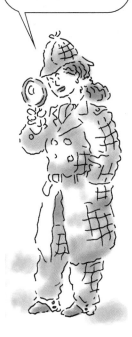

After mixing drugs in a syringe or cartridge, check for discoloration and precipitation.

Administering an intradermal drug

In *intradermal (I.D.) administration*, you inject a small amount of liquid (usually 0.5 ml or less) into the outer layers of a patient's skin. A substance administered in this way undergoes little systemic absorption.

Identifying I.D.

You'll use this route to deliver substances that test for allergies and tuberculosis. You also may use it to deliver a local anesthetic, such as lidocaine, before the patient undergoes a venipuncture procedure. Although the most common site for I.D. injection is the ventral forearm, other sites can be used. (See *Intradermal injection sites*, page 226.)

Giving an I.D. injection

You may be required to give an I.D. injection, such as:
• tuberculosis (TB) testing
• allergy testing
• certain vaccines
• local anesthetics.

Intradermal injection sites

The most common intradermal injection site is the ventral forearm. Other sites (indicated by dotted areas in the illustration below) include the upper chest, upper arm, and shoulder blades. Skin in these areas is usually lightly pigmented, thinly keratinized, and relatively hairless, facilitating detection of adverse reactions.

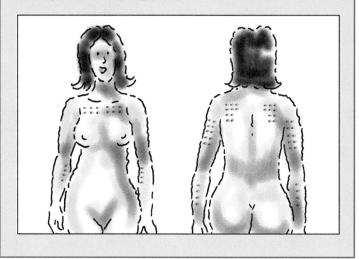

What you need

Tuberculin syringe with a 26G or 27G ½″ or ⅝″ needle ✳ prescribed test antigen (or drug) ✳ gloves ✳ marking pen ✳ alcohol pads

Getting ready

• Verify the order on the patient's chart.
• Check the drug's expiration date.
• Wash your hands.
• Identify the patient by checking his armband.

Stand by please

• Explain the procedure to the patient, and tell him that he'll need to stay nearby for about 30 minutes after the time of injection in case he has a severe allergic reaction to it.

How you do it

• Select an injection site.
• To use the ventral forearm, have the patient sit up and extend one arm. Make sure the arm is supported.

Peak technique

Giving an intradermal injection

To give an intradermal injection, first secure the forearm. Then insert the needle at a 10- to 15-degree angle so that it just punctures the skin's surface, as shown below. The antigen should raise a small wheal as it's injected.

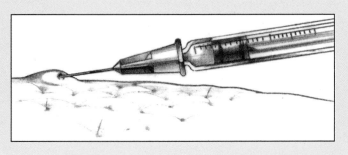

Danger zone

Don't get caught off guard

A patient who is hypersensitive to the test antigen may have an anaphylactic reaction. Be prepared to inject epinephrine immediately and to perform emergency resuscitation procedures.

• Put on gloves. Then use an alcohol pad to clean the ventral forearm two or three fingerwidths distal to the antecubital space. Make sure the site is free from hair and blemishes. Let the skin air-dry.
• While holding the patient's forearm in your nondominant hand, stretch the skin taut. (See *Giving an intradermal injection.*)
• Withdraw the needle at the same angle you inserted it.

Missing wheals

• If no wheal forms, you've probably injected the antigen too deeply. Give another dose at least 2″ (5 cm) from the first site.
• If you're giving more than one I.D. injection, space them about 2″ apart.

Keeping track

• Circle and label each test site with a marking pen so you can track the response to each substance given.
• Dispose of your gloves, needles, and syringes according to standard precautions.

Practice pointers

• Be prepared to deal with a possible anaphylactic reaction. (See *Don't get caught off guard.*)

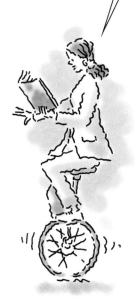

If you don't see a wheal form after injection, you went in too deeply. Try again!

- Notify a doctor immediately if an allergic reaction occurs.
- Don't rub the site after you give an I.D. injection. Doing so could irritate the underlying tissue and alter test results.
- Assess the patient's response to the skin testing in 24 to 48 hours.

Check the response

- When interpreting the patient's response, keep in mind that erythema without induration (a hard, raised area) isn't significant. If the test area is indurated, measure the diameter in millimeters.
- Induration of more than 5 mm after a tuberculin test may indicate a positive test result. After allergy tests, induration and erythema of more than 3 mm may indicate a positive result. The larger the affected area, the stronger the allergic reaction.

What to teach

- Tell the patient not to remove the skin labels until the test period ends and not to cover the sites with bandages.
- Advise him not to scratch the injection sites; if they itch, he should apply cold compresses to dull the itch. Also, warn him not to rub the area while drying it, but rather to pat it dry.

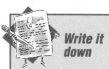

Write it down

Documenting intradermal injections

Be sure to record:
- name of the drug or antigen given
- amount given
- site or sites used
- patient's response
- result at each injection site.

Administering subcutaneous drugs

In *subcutaneous (S.C.) administration*, you inject a small amount of liquid drug (usually 0.5 to 2 ml) into the subcutaneous tissue beneath the patient's skin. From there, the drug is absorbed slowly into nearby capillaries.

Steady and safe

As a result, a dose of concentrated drug can have a longer duration of action than it would by other injection routes. Plus, S.C. injection causes little tissue trauma and offers little risk of striking large blood vessels and nerves.

When S.C. isn't OK

Typically, heparin and insulin are given by S.C. injection. However, an S.C. injection is contraindicated in areas that are inflamed, edematous, scarred, or covered by a mole, birthmark, or other lesion. It may also be contraindicated in patients with impaired coagulation.

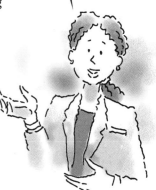

Give a drug S.C. and the patient enjoys the benefit of a longer duration of action.

Giving an S.C. injection

You may be required to give a drug subcutaneously, such as:
- heparin
- insulin
- ovulation stimulating drugs (or fertility drugs).

What you need

Prepared drug (with an appropriate syringe) ✱ needle of appropriate size (usually 25G to 27G and ⅝″ or ½″) ✱ gloves ✱ two alcohol pads

For insulin administration

Insulin infusion pump or S.C. injector optional (see *Understanding insulin administration aids*)

Getting ready

- Verify the order on the patient's chart.

Gear up!

Understanding insulin administration aids

These days, patients have insulin delivery options beyond standard subcutaneous (S.C.) injections, such as S.C. infusion, an implanted catheter, or needle-free insulin delivery.

S.C. infusion

In continuous S.C. insulin infusion, the patient carries a portable infusion pump that holds insulin and is programmed to deliver precise insulin doses—both baseline and bolus—over a 24-hour period. (The device can be used for pain management as well.) Some insulin pumps allow you to track daily bolus doses, to review the last 12 alarms, and to download the device's long-term memory.

To deliver the infusion, the patient will need a 25G to 27G subcutaneous needle inserted at a 30- to 45-degree angle into the abdomen, thigh, or arm. The insertion site should be rotated every 2 to 3 days according to standard precautions. After needle insertion, cover the site with a transparent adhesive dressing. Teach the patient how to recognize and when to report possible problems with the device insertion site.

Implanted catheter

Some patients may prefer an indwelling subcutaneous catheter, such as an Insuflon catheter, rather than a needle. After insertion, the catheter remains in the fatty tissue of the abdomen. A small adhesive foam pad protects the insertion site and catheter and allows the patient to bathe, shower, and engage in sports or other activities. After 3 to 7 days, the catheter should be removed and inserted in the opposite side of the abdomen, 1″ to 2″ (2.5 to 5 cm) away from previously used sites.

Needle-free insulin delivery

Needle-free insulin delivery uses a device that looks something like a syringe without a needle. A spring inside the device triggers a plunger that expels a prescribed dose of insulin through a tiny hole at the tip. When the patient holds the device against the skin surface and discharges it, a thin column of insulin penetrates the skin and disperses within the subcutaneous tissue. This device is popular for home use, especially by patients (including children) who are afraid of needles.

Subcutaneous injection sites

Potential subcutaneous (S.C.) injection sites (as indicated by the dotted areas in the illustration below) include the fat pads on the abdomen, upper hips, upper back, and lateral upper arms and thighs.

Preferred injection sites for insulin are the arms, abdomen, thighs, and buttocks. The preferred injection site for heparin is the lower abdominal fat pad, just below the umbilicus.

When you repeat, rotate

For S.C. injections administered repeatedly, such as insulin, rotate sites. Choose one injection site in one area, move to a corresponding injection site in the next area, and so on. When returning to an area, choose a new site in that area.

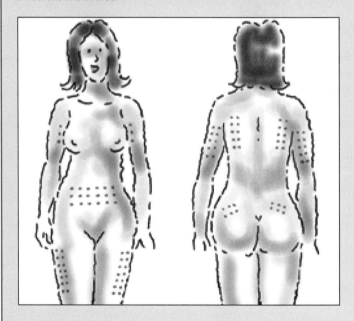

- Check the drug's color, clarity, and expiration date.
- Identify the patient by checking his armband.
- Explain the procedure to the patient.
- Select an appropriate injection site. (See *Subcutaneous injection sites*.)

Give your patient the cold shoulder

- Before giving the injection, you may apply a cold compress to the injection site to minimize pain.
- Wash your hands and put on gloves.

How you do it

• Position and drape the patient, if necessary.

Bubble trouble

• If you're giving insulin, gently invert and roll the vial to mix the drug. Don't shake the vial because air bubbles could get into the syringe and reduce the dose given.
• Clean the injection site with an alcohol pad, starting at the center of the site and moving outward in a circular motion. Let the skin air-dry to avoid stinging.
• If you wish, open a second alcohol pad and place it between the index and middle fingers of your nondominant hand.
• Remove the protective needle sheath.

Hold the fat

• With your nondominant hand, grasp the skin around the injection site and firmly elevate the subcutaneous tissue to form a 1″ (2.5-cm) fat fold (½″ [1.3-cm] for heparin). If the patient is large, you may be able to spread the skin taut rather than forming a fold. (See *Technique for subcutaneous injections.*)
• Position the needle with the bevel up, and tell the patient that he'll feel a prick as you insert it quickly—in one motion—at a 45-degree angle.
• Pull back the plunger slightly to check for blood return; if none returns, inject the drug slowly.

Try not to be irritating

• After injection, remove the needle gently but quickly at the same angle used for injection. However, when injecting heparin, leave the needle in place for 10 seconds; then withdraw it.
• Cover the injection site with an alcohol pad, and massage gently.

Just checking

• Check the injection site for bleeding or bruising. If bleeding continues, apply pressure. If a bruise develops, apply ice. Watch for adverse reactions at the injection site for 30 minutes.
• Dispose of the equipment according to standard precautions. To avoid needle-stick injuries, don't recap the needle.

Practice pointers

• If your patient is of average weight, you can reach subcutaneous tissue by using a ½″ needle and inserting it at a 90-degree angle; if your patient is thin, use a ⅝″ needle and insert it at a 45-degree an-

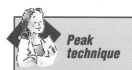

Peak technique

Technique for subcutaneous injections

Before giving the injection, elevate the subcutaneous tissue at the site by grasping it firmly, as shown below. Insert the needle at a 45- or 90-degree angle to the skin surface, depending on needle length and the amount of subcutaneous tissue at the site. Some medications, such as heparin, should always be injected at a 90-degree angle.

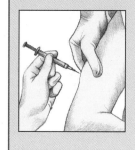

Ages and stages

Giving a child an S.C. or I.D. injection

You may give certain drugs to children by the subcutaneous (S.C.) or intradermal (I.D.) route. For example, insulin, hormone replacement, allergy desensitization, and some vaccines are given by S.C. injection. Tuberculin testing, local anesthesia, and allergy testing are given by I.D. injection. The procedure for S.C. or I.D. injection differs little from that used for an adult patient.

In a child, you can reach subcutaneous tissue by using a ⅝" needle and inserting it at a 45-degree angle.

gle. If your patient is a child, you may also give certain drugs by the S.C. route. (See *Giving a child an S.C. or I.D. injection.*)

Do a double take

• If you're giving insulin, double-check that you have the correct type, unit dose, and syringe. Before mixing insulins in a syringe, make sure they're compatible and that you have a doctor's order to do so. Follow your facility's policy about which insulin to draw up first. Don't mix insulins of different purities or origins.

Remember to rotate

• If you'll be giving repeated S.C. injections, as with insulin, rotate the injection sites.
• Don't administer heparin injections within 2" (5.1 cm) of a scar, a bruise, or the umbilicus.
• Don't aspirate for blood when giving insulin or heparin. This is unnecessary with insulin and may cause a hematoma with heparin.
• Don't massage the site if you've given insulin or heparin. With other drugs, however, gentle massage may help to distribute the drug and enhance absorption.

What to teach

• If the patient will be giving himself S.C. injections at home, teach him the correct way to perform the procedure. Send him home with written instructions to support your teaching.
• Teach your patients, especially the older adults, how to use compliance aids. (See *Using compliance aids.*)

No place like home

Using compliance aids

To help your patient safely comply with injectable drug therapy, you or a family member or other caregiver can premeasure doses for him using compliance aids such as the ones shown below. Most pharmacies or community service agencies can supply similar aids.

Syringe-filling device

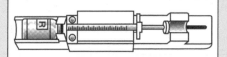

A syringe-filling device precisely measures insulin doses for a visually impaired person with diabetes. Designed for use with a disposable U-100 syringe and an insulin bottle, the device is set by the caregiver to accommodate the syringe's width. The patient then positions the plunger at the point determined by the dose and tightens the stop. When the device is set, he can draw up the precise dose ordered for each injection.

Drawbacks

The device has several drawbacks: It can't be used if insulin must be mixed or if doses vary;

the settings must be checked and adjusted whenever the syringe size or type is changed; and the screws must be checked regularly because they loosen with repeated use.

Syringe scale magnifier

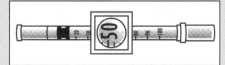

A syringe scale magnifier helps a visually impaired patient with diabetes read syringe markings, thereby enabling him to fill his own syringe. The plastic magnifier snaps onto the syringe barrel. This device may be impractical for a patient with arthritis who can't easily attach the magnifier to the syringe.

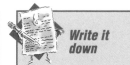

Write it down

Documenting subcutaneous injections

Be sure to record:
• date and time of the injection
• drug and dose given
• injection site used
• patient's reaction to the drug.
• teaching and written materials provided, the patient's response to your teaching, return demonstrations given, questions answered, and follow-up plans made for the patient, when necessary.

• Inform the patient that different brands of syringes have differing amounts of space between the bottom line and the needle. Suggest that he tell his doctor or pharmacist if he changes the brand of syringe he uses.

Administering intramuscular drugs

An *intramuscular (I.M.) injection* deposits drug deep into muscle tissue that's richly supplied with blood. As a result, the injected drug moves rapidly into the systemic circulation. Other advantages include:
• bypassing damaging digestive enzymes
• relatively little pain (because muscle tissue contains few sensory nerves)

- delivery of a relatively large volume of drug (the usual dose is 3 ml or less, but you may give up to 5 ml into a large muscle).

Be able to I.D. the candidate for I.M.

Children, elderly patients, or thin people may tolerate less than 2 ml. For some drugs, you may give I.M. injections using a Z-track technique or a needle-free injection system.

Giving an I.M. injection

Getting ready

You may be required to inject drugs intramuscularly, such as pain medications (narcotics) or gold injections for arthritis.

What you need

Prescribed drug ✳ 3- to 5-ml syringe ✳ 20G to 25G needle (smaller gauge for a thicker drug) about 1″ to 3″ (depending on the site used and the amount of fat present) ✳ gloves ✳ alcohol pads ✳ small bandage

The needle may be packaged separately, or it may come attached to the syringe. Most often, you'll use a 1½″ to 2″ needle. Your technique and all equipment must be sterile.

Reflection before injection

Some situations will prevent I.M. administration of drugs. (See *Precautions for I.M. injections*.)

Danger zone

Precautions for I.M. injections

Before you give your patient an I.M. injection, remember these precautions:
- Don't give I.M. injections into inflamed, edematous, or irritated sites or sites with moles, birthmarks, scar tissue, or other lesions.
- I.M. injections may be contraindicated in patients who have impaired coagulation or conditions that hinder peripheral absorption, such as peripheral vascular disease, edema, or hypoperfusion; and during an acute myocardial infarction.
- Never give an I.M. injection into an immobile limb because the drug will absorb poorly and a sterile abscess could develop.

Getting ready

- Verify the order on the patient's chart.
- Reconstitute the drug, if necessary; then check the drug's color, clarity, and expiration date.
- Draw the correct amount into the syringe.
- Identify the patient by checking his armband.
- Explain the procedure to the patient.
- Wash your hands.

Muscling up

- If your patient is elderly, additional points need to be considered. (See *I.M. injections in elderly patients.*)
- If your patient is an adult, consider using the dorsogluteal, ventrogluteal, vastus lateralis, or deltoid muscle. (See *Locating I.M. injection sites*, page 236.)
- If your patient is an infant or a child, consider using the vastus lateralis muscle. (See *I.M. injection sites in infants and children*, page 237).

How you do it

- Position and drape the patient so you have easy access to the chosen site. Locate the specific insertion site, and choose the proper needle angle.
- Check the injection site to make sure it has no lumps, depressions, redness, warmth, or bruising.
- Put on gloves.
- Clean the site with an alcohol pad, starting at the center of the site and spiraling outward about 2″ (5 cm). Let the skin air-dry.
- Remove the needle cover, and expel all air bubbles from the syringe.
- Urge the patient to relax the muscle that will receive the injection. A tense muscle increases pain and bleeding.
- With the thumb and index finger of your nondominant hand, gently stretch the skin taut at the injection site.
- Position the syringe at a 90-degree angle to the skin surface, with the needle a few inches away from the skin.
- Tell the patient that he'll feel a prick, and then quickly thrust the needle into the muscle.

Seeing red? Stop!

- While supporting the syringe with your nondominant hand, use your dominant hand to aspirate for blood. If blood appears in the syringe, the needle is in a blood vessel. Withdraw it, discard it, and prepare another injection with a new syringe and fresh medication. *(Text continues on page 238.)*

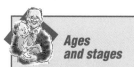

Ages and stages

I.M. injections in elderly patients

If your patient is elderly, consider using a shorter needle for I.M. injections. Also, because elderly people have less subcutaneous tissue and more fat around the hips, abdomen, and thighs, consider using the vastus lateralis or ventrogluteal area (gluteus medius and minimus, but not gluteus maximus).

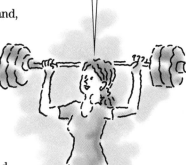

A tense muscle increases pain and bleeding. Tell your patient to relax!

Locating I.M. injection sites

The most common I.M. injection sites used in adults are discussed below.

Deltoid

Find the lower edge of the acromial process and the point on the lateral arm in line with the axilla. Insert the needle 1″ to 2″ (2.5 to 5 cm) below the acromial process, usually two or three fingerwidths, at a 90-degree angle or angled slightly toward the process. Typical injection: 0.5 ml (range: 0.5 to 2 ml).

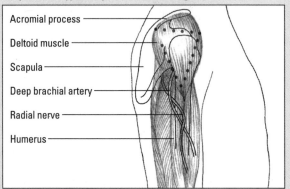

Acromial process
Deltoid muscle
Scapula
Deep brachial artery
Radial nerve
Humerus

Dorsogluteal

Inject above and outside a line drawn from the posterior superior iliac spine to the greater trochanter of the femur. Or divide the buttock into quadrants, and inject in the upper outer quadrant, about 2″ to 3″ (5 to 7.5 cm) below the iliac crest. Insert the needle at a 90-degree angle. Typical injection: 1 to 4 ml (range: 1 to 5 ml).

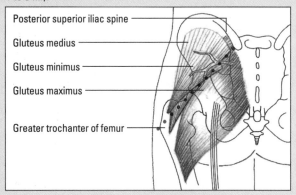

Posterior superior iliac spine
Gluteus medius
Gluteus minimus
Gluteus maximus
Greater trochanter of femur

Ventrogluteal

Locate the greater trochanter of the femur with the heel of your hand. Then spread your index and middle fingers from the anterior superior iliac spine to as far along the iliac crest as you can reach. Insert the needle between the two fingers at a 90-degree angle to the muscle. (Remove your fingers before inserting the needle.) Typical injection: 1 to 4 ml (range: 1 to 5 ml).

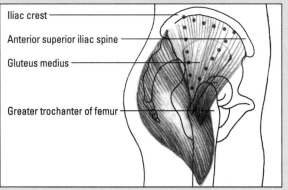

Iliac crest
Anterior superior iliac spine
Gluteus medius
Greater trochanter of femur

Vastus lateralis

Use the lateral muscle of the quadriceps group, from a handbreadth below the greater trochanter to a handbreadth above the knee. Insert the needle into the middle third of the muscle parallel to the surface on which the patient is lying. You may have to bunch the muscle before insertion. Typical injection: 1 to 4 ml (range: 1 to 5 ml; 1 to 3 ml for infants).

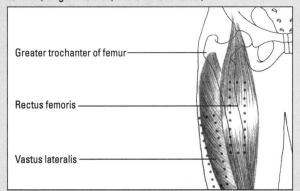

Greater trochanter of femur
Rectus femoris
Vastus lateralis

Ages and stages

I.M. injection sites in infants and children

When selecting the best site for a child's I.M. injection, consider the child's age, weight, and muscular development; the amount of subcutaneous fat over the injection site; the type of drug you're administering; and the drug's absorption rate.

Vastus lateralis and rectus femoris injections

For a child under age 3, you'll typically use the vastus lateralis or rectus femoris muscle for an I.M. injection. Constituting the largest muscle mass in this age-group, the vastus lateralis and rectus femoris have few major blood vessels and nerves.

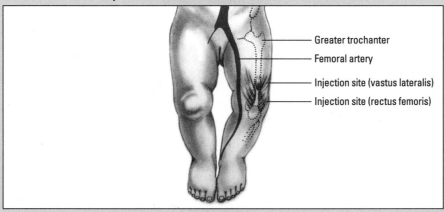

Greater trochanter

Femoral artery

Injection site (vastus lateralis)

Injection site (rectus femoris)

Ventrogluteal and dorsogluteal injections

For a child over age 3 who has been walking for at least 1 year, you'll probably use the ventrogluteal or dorsogluteal muscle. These muscles are relatively free from major blood vessels and nerves.

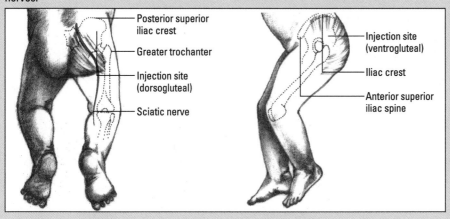

Posterior superior iliac crest

Greater trochanter

Injection site (dorsogluteal)

Sciatic nerve

Injection site (ventrogluteal)

Iliac crest

Anterior superior iliac spine

• If you aspirate no blood, then inject the drug slowly and steadily into the muscle, allowing it to distend and accept the drug gradually. You should feel little or no resistance.

Quickly yet gently

• After you have injected the drug, remove the needle quickly but gently, at a 90-degree angle.
• Using a gloved hand, immediately cover the injection site with an alcohol pad. Apply gentle pressure and, unless contraindicated, massage the relaxed muscle to help distribute the drug and promote absorption.

Inspection of injection

• Remove the alcohol pad, and inspect the site for bleeding or bruising. If bleeding continues, apply pressure. If a bruise develops, apply ice. Watch for adverse reactions at the site for 30 minutes after the time of injection.
• Discard all equipment according to standard precautions.

Practice pointers

• If your patient complains of pain and anxiety from repeated I.M. injections, numb the site with ice for several seconds before you give the injection.
• If you need to inject more than 5 ml of drug, split it between two different sites.

A pinch of gentleness

• If the patient is extremely thin, pinch the muscle gently to elevate it, so you won't push the needle completely through the muscle.
• For an infant or toddler, use a 25G to 27G ½″ to 1″ needle. Also, don't exceed recommended volumes when giving the injection. (See *Adapting injections for children.*)
• If necessary, when giving an I.M. injection to a child under age 5, stand on the side opposite his vastus lateralis muscle and bend over him so your torso acts as a restraint.
• Elderly patients have a higher risk of hematoma and may need direct pressure over the puncture site for a longer time than usual.

Rubbing it in

• Unless contraindicated, gently massage the injection site to aid drug absorption and distribution.
• Rotate sites if your patient needs repeated injections.

Danger zone

I.M. injection complications

Accidentally injecting concentrated or irritating medications into subcutaneous tissue or other areas where they can't be fully absorbed can cause sterile abscesses to develop.

In addition, failing to rotate sites in patients who require repeated injections can lead to deposits of unabsorbed medications. Such deposits can reduce the desired pharmacologic effect and may lead to abscess formation or tissue fibrosis.

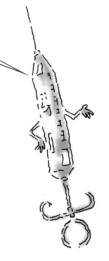

When injecting more than 5 ml of drug, split it between two different sites.

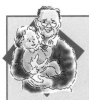

Ages and stages

Adapting injections for children

When giving an intramuscular (I.M.) injection to a child, you'll need to adapt your approach to accommodate the child's age, the injection site, and the volume of drug you need to give. Use the table below as a guide.

Deltoid	• Not recommended for children under age 3. • Can be used to give 0.5 ml or less in children ages 18 months to 3 years if no other site is available. • Give 0.5 ml or less in patients ages 3 to 15. • Give 1.0 ml or less in patients ages 15 to adulthood.
Gluteus maximus or ventrogluteal site	• Not recommended for children under age 3. • Can be used to give 1.0 ml or less in children ages 18 months to 3 years if no other site is available. • Give 1.5 ml or less in patients ages 3 to 6. • Give 2.0 ml or less in patients ages 6 to 15. • Give 2.5 ml or less in patients ages 15 to adulthood.
Vastus lateralis or rectus femoris	• Give 1.0 ml or less in children under age 3. • Give 1.5 ml or less in patients ages 3 to 6. • Give 2.0 ml or less in patients ages 6 to 15. • Give 2.5 ml or less in patients ages 15 to adulthood.

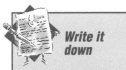

Write it down

Documenting I.M. injections

Be sure to record:
• name of the drug given
• dose given
• date and time of the injection
• site used
• patient's response
• condition of the site after the injection
• patient teaching and any written instructions provided, the patient's and caregiver's responses to your teaching, their ability to perform the procedure, and any follow-up plans that have been made, when necessary.

• Prevent complications associated with I.M. injections. (See *I.M. injection complications.*)

What to teach

• Explain the procedure and its purpose to the patient.
• Tell the patient to report any reactions that develop at the site, such as swollen areas or local irritation.
• If the patient will be receiving I.M. injections at home, make sure that he or a caregiver can administer them correctly.

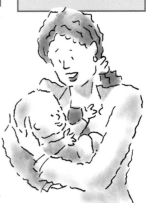

Giving a Z-track injection

If you need to give an irritating drug (such as iron dextran) or if you need to give an injection to an elderly patient with decreased muscle mass, use the Z-track method of I.M. administration. A *Z-track injection* is a method of displacing the tissues before you insert the needle for an I.M. injection. Afterward, restoring the tissues to their normal positions traps the drug inside the muscle.

What you need

Ordered drug ✳ syringe of appropriate size ✳ two needles (one of which should be 3″) ✳ alcohol pads ✳ gloves

Getting ready

- Verify the order on the patient's chart.
- Reconstitute the drug as needed. Check the drug's color, clarity, and expiration date.
- Draw the correct amount into the syringe.
- After drawing up the ordered dose, add 0.3 to 0.5 ml of air into the syringe. Then replace the original needle with a sterile one that's 3″.
- Identify the patient by checking his armband.
- Explain the procedure to the patient.
- Wash your hands and put on gloves.

How you do it

- Select an injection site, usually the buttock.
- Use an alcohol pad to clean the site, starting at the center and spiraling outward about 2″ (5 cm). Let the skin air-dry.

Here's the skinny

- Place the index finger of your nondominant hand on the injection site, and drag the skin about ½″ (1.5 cm) to one side.
- Insert the needle at a 90-degree angle into the site on which you originally placed your finger.
- Inject the drug, and withdraw the needle.
- Then release the skin, allowing the displaced layers to return to their original positions. (See *Displacing the skin for Z-track injection.*)

Practice pointers

- Never inject more than 5 ml into a single site using the Z-track method.

Here's a new message: Don't massage!

- Never massage a Z-track injection site because you could cause irritation or force the drug into subcutaneous tissue.
- To increase the rate of absorption, encourage such physical activity as walking.
- For subsequent injections, alternate buttocks.

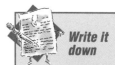
Write it down

Documenting Z-track injections

Be sure to record:
- name of the drug and dose given
- date and time of the injection
- site and method (Z-track) used
- patient's response
- site condition after the injection
- patient teaching and written instructions provided, the patient's and caregiver's responses to your teaching, their ability to perform the procedure, and follow-up plans that have been made, when necessary.

Peak technique

Displacing the skin for Z-track injection

Discomfort and tissue irritation may result from drug leakage into subcutaneous tissue. Displacing the skin helps prevent these problems.

By blocking the needle pathway after an injection, the Z-track technique allows I.M. injection while minimizing the risk of subcutaneous irritation and staining from such drugs as iron dextran.

How to do it

To begin, place your finger on the skin surface, and pull the skin and subcutaneous layers out of alignment with the underlying muscle, as shown below. You should move the skin about ½″ (1.5 cm).

Insert the needle at a 90-degree angle at the site where you initially placed your finger, as shown below. Inject the drug, and withdraw the needle.

Finally, remove your finger from the skin surface, allowing the layers to return to their normal positions. The needle track (shown by the dotted line below) is now broken at the junction of each tissue layer, trapping the drug in the muscle.

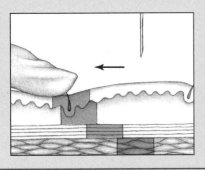

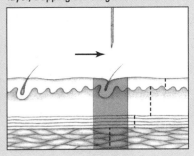

What to teach

- Tell the patient not to wear tight-fitting clothes over the site; doing so could cause irritation or could force the drug into subcutaneous tissue.
- Advise him to report swelling, irritation, or other problems at the injection site.
- If the patient will continue to receive Z-track injections at home, make sure that he or a caregiver can administer them correctly.

Giving a needle-free I.M. injection

A *needle-free injection system* eliminates the risk of needle-stick injuries and possible transmission of hepatitis B, human immunodeficiency virus, and other bloodborne pathogens.

To deliver needle-free injections, you may use a device such as the Biojector 2000. This injector uses carbon dioxide (CO_2) to drive a plunger that propels the drug through micro-orifices and into the muscle. The CO_2 never comes in contact with the drug. Each drug dose is given with a separate sterile syringe, thereby eliminating the risk of cross-contamination among patients.

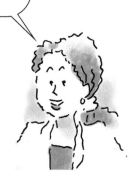

> No more tears! Needle-free injection technology allows for vaccines and other drugs to be administered through the skin without the use of conventional needles.

A unique system for common drugs

Most commonly injected drugs can be administered with the needle-free injector. Just make sure you select the proper syringe that has been designed for the drug you'll be giving and the site you'll be using.

What you need

Biojector 2000 ✳ appropriate syringe device (which contains a disposable syringe and a fill tube with needle) ✳ special syringe cap ✳ CO_2 cartridge ✳ vial of the prescribed drug ✳ gloves ✳ alcohol pads ✳ several 3″ × 3″ gauze pads ✳ bandage

Getting ready

• Verify the order on the patient's chart.
• Wash your hands.
• Identify the patient by checking his armband.
• Explain the procedure to the patient.

How you do it

• Check the indicator needle on the pressure gauge at the rear of the injector. The needle should rest in the positive (green) section of the pressure gauge. If not, you'll need to replace the CO_2 cartridge.
• Check the drug's expiration date.
• Next, carefully open the syringe package, and remove the syringe assembly and the safety cap.
• Remove the protective cover from the fill tube needle.

Stop at the 1-ml line

• Draw the prescribed drug from the vial into the syringe, just as you would with a standard syringe. Don't fill the syringe beyond the 1-ml line.
• Replace the needle cover using a one-handed technique, and then remove the needle from the syringe and discard the needle into a sharps container.

Protecting tip

- To avoid touching and contaminating the syringe while inserting it into the injector, put the protective cap over the tip of the syringe.
- Next, place the cap on a firm, level surface, and lower the syringe barrel into the cap. Insert the filled syringe into the injector, aligning the notches in the top of the syringe barrel with the matching grooves in the collar of the device.

Green means go

- Turn the syringe about one-quarter turn clockwise to lock it in place. Then check the syringe lock indicator to make sure that green appears in the window.
- Put on gloves.
- Use an alcohol pad to clean the injection site, starting in the center and spiraling outward about 2″ (5 cm). Let the skin air-dry to avoid stinging and possible slipping of the injector.
- To inject the drug, hold the patient's skin firmly enough to keep it from moving during the injection.
- Press the device firmly against the patient's skin at a 90-degree angle to the skin surface. Remind the patient to relax his muscle and to hold still.

Hear a hiss? There's nothing amiss.

- Using one slow, smooth motion, press and release the actuator lever on the underside of the injector device. You may hear a hissing sound. This is the normal sound of CO_2 escaping from the device.
- Hold the injector in place for 1 or 2 seconds after the drug is delivered; then remove the device.
- Use a 2″ × 2″ gauze pad to immediately apply pressure to the site for about 1 minute to minimize bleeding and bruising.
- Apply a bandage to the site.
- Remove the syringe from the injector, and discard it.

Practice pointers

- When the filled syringe has been locked in place, you can press the actuator to expel the drug. Be careful not to press it until the injector is in position because the stream of medication can penetrate soft tissue even a few centimeters away.

So there was no needle, but the care's the same...

- Although you have used no needle to deliver the drug, the site must be managed as if you had.
- Don't rub or massage the site after the injection.

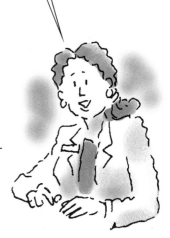

Don't press the actuator too soon. A stream of medication can penetrate soft tissue even a few centimeters away.

• Watch for any reactions, such as tenderness, redness, wheals, or lumps, which may follow the injection. They should resolve within 1 hour.

What to teach

• Tell the patient that local reactions, such as burning, stinging, skin irritation, induration, bleeding, and ecchymosis, may occur at the injection site, just as they can with an injection given by syringe and needle.
• Warn him that the Biojector 2000 makes a hissing sound as it delivers the drug.

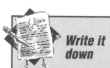

Write it down

Documenting needle-free I.M. injections

Be sure to record:
• name of the drug given
• dose given
• date and time it was given
• method used to inject it
• site into which you injected it
• patient's response to the procedure.

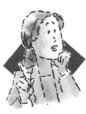

Quick quiz

1.   Which of the following routes of administration would you use if you wanted to inject a small amount of liquid drug (usually 0.5 ml or less) into the outer layers of a patient's skin?
  A.   Intradermal (I.D.)
  B.   Subcutaneous
  C.   Intramuscular
  D.   Intravenous

Answer: A. An I.D. injection allows injection of a small amount of liquid drug (usually 0.5 ml or less) into the outer layers of a patient's skin.

2.   Which of the following statements best describes a Z-track injection?
  A.   It's a method of depositing a drug deep into muscle tissue that's richly supplied with blood.
  B.   It's a method of injecting a small amount of liquid drug (usually 0.5 to 2 ml) into the subcutaneous tissue beneath the patient's skin.
  C.   It's a method of displacing the tissues before you insert the needle for an I.M. injection.
  D.   It's a method of aligning the tissues before you insert the needle for a subcutaneous injection.

Answer: C. A Z-track injection is a method of displacing the tissues before you insert the needle for an I.M. injection. Afterward, restoring the tissues to their normal positions traps the drug inside the muscle.

3. To give an I.D. injection, you should insert the needle at a:
   A.   10- to 15-degree angle.
   B.   45-degree angle.
   C.   90-degree angle.
   D.   20- to 30-degree angle.

Answer: A. To give an I.D. injection, after securing the forearm you insert the needle at a 10- to 15-degree angle so that it just punctures the skin's surface. The antigen should raise a small wheal as it's injected.

4. Which of the following I.M. injection sites would you typically select for a child under age 3?
   A.   Ventrogluteal muscle
   B.   Deltoid muscle
   C.   Dorsogluteal muscle
   D.   Vastus lateralis muscle

Answer: D. For a child under age 3, you'll typically use the vastus lateralis or rectus femoris muscle for an I.M. injection. Constituting the largest muscle mass in this age-group, the vastus lateralis and rectus femoris have few major blood vessels and nerves.

5. When giving an S.C. injection to a patient of average weight, you can reach subcutaneous tissue by using:
   A.   A ⅝″ needle inserted at a 45-degree angle.
   B.   A ½″ needle inserted at a 90-degree angle.
   C.   A 1″ needle inserted at a 45-degree angle.
   D.   A 1″ needle inserted at a 90-degree angle.

Answer: B. If your patient is of average weight, you can reach subcutaneous tissue by using a ½″ needle and inserting it at a 90-degree angle.

Scoring

☆☆☆   If you answered all five questions correctly, sensational! Needle-less to say, you're in the top of your class!

☆☆   If you answered two or three correctly, great! It's a reflection on your injection know-how!

☆   If you answered fewer than two correctly, it looks like you might need a shot in the arm. Review the chapter, and you'll soon feel sharp!

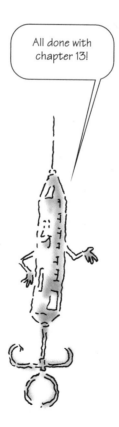

Intravenous administration

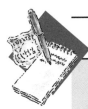

Just the facts

In this chapter, you'll learn:

♦ the principles of I.V. administration

♦ how to give a bolus I.V. injection

♦ how to give an intermittent I.V. infusion

♦ how to administer a continuous I.V. infusion

♦ how to use special I.V. catheters

♦ how to give medications using a vascular access port.

Understanding I.V. administration

The I.V. route of drug administration offers an almost immediate onset of drug action, complete drug availability, and close control over the amount of drug given and the level maintained in the patient's blood.

For starters

Before administering a drug by the I.V. route, make sure it has been approved by your facility for I.V. use. Prepare the drug correctly before use as recommended by the manufacturer. Don't give a cloudy or discolored drug or any fluid that has particles floating in it. When you give more than one drug, flush the line with one and one-half times the volume capacity between drugs unless you know that the drugs are compatible.

In the I.V. league

You may give an I.V. drug by bolus injection, intermittent infusion, or continuous infusion into a peripheral I.V. line, a central I.V. line, or an implanted vascular access port. In all cases, you need considerable clinical expertise, sound preparation, and meticulous technique to excel at this advanced form of drug administration.

Giving a bolus injection

An I.V. bolus injection, commonly known as I.V. push, produces a peak drug level almost immediately in the patient's blood. Usually, you'll administer a bolus injection into an existing peripheral primary I.V. line, into an intermittent infusion device, or directly into a vein.

> Administering some drugs, such as potassium chloride, by I.V. bolus can be dangerous.

> Know which drugs can and can't be given rapidly.

Don't get too pushy

Don't give an I.V. bolus if rapid administration of the drug could be life-threatening, as with potassium chloride. Also, don't give a drug by I.V. bolus if you need to dilute it first in a large amount of fluid. Finally, keep in mind that drug tolerance declines in patients who have decreased cardiac output, diminished urine output, pulmonary congestion, or systemic edema. To compensate, you may need to dilute the drug more than usual for these patients and give it at a slower rate.

Lining up your patients

If you need to insert an I.V. line in your patient, the process will differ if your patient is elderly (see *Inserting an older adult's I.V. line*) or if your patient is a child (see *Inserting a neonate's or a child's I.V. line*, page 250).

Giving a bolus through a peripheral line

You may need to give a drug by I.V. bolus, such as atropine, especially in emergency situations.

What you need

Prescribed drug ✳ syringe of appropriate size (either a needle–less system or one with a 20G or 22G 1″ needle) ✳ alcohol or povidone-iodine pads ✳ gloves

Getting ready

• If the drug isn't compatible with the patient's I.V. solution, also get two 3-ml syringes with 20G or 22G 1″ needles and fill them with normal saline solution.
• Check your facility's policy to see if you need another 3-ml syringe with heparin flush solution.
• Verify the order on the patient's chart.
• Make sure the drug is compatible with the I.V. solution.

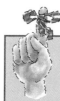

Memory jogger

In selecting the best site for a venipuncture, think like a **VIP**:

For the **V**ein, consider its location, condition, and physical path along the extremity.

For the **I**nfusion, consider its purpose and duration.

For the **P**atient, consider his degree of cooperation and compliance, along with his preference.

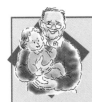

Ages and stages

Inserting an older adult's I.V. line

When inserting an older adult's I.V. line, remember these tips:

• Use warm compresses to dilate the patient's veins, especially if he's cold or peripherally constricted.

• Use a 24G or 22G catheter to avoid trauma.

• When inserting the catheter, use the patient's nondominant arm, if possible.

• Use little tourniquet pressure to avoid tissue trauma, especially if the patient takes a corticosteroid or an anticoagulant.

• Avoid inserting the line in areas where valves are located.

• Maintain tension on the skin during the venipuncture. Consider using a one-handed technique.

• Release the tourniquet as soon as you get a blood return.

• Use as little tape as possible, preferably silk or paper tape. Removing the tape can easily tear the patient's skin, so moisten it thoroughly before removing it.

• Consider using a protective polymer solution under the tape around the site.

• Use a padded arm board, stretch netting, or stockinette dressing to protect the site.

• Check the expiration date, and reconstitute or dilute the drug as needed.

• Identify the patient by checking his armband.

• Wash your hands and put on gloves.

How you do it

• Close the flow-control clamp on the existing I.V. line.

• Clean the Y-port closest to the venipuncture site with an alcohol pad or a povidone-iodine pad.

• Insert the needle of the syringe or the needleless system into the Y-port, and inject the drug, as shown below, at the prescribed rate.

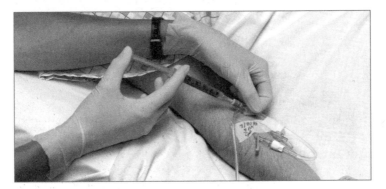

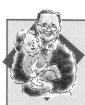

Ages and stages

Inserting a neonate's or a child's I.V. line

This table summarizes key points to remember when inserting an I.V. line in a neonate or a child.

Patient	Finding a vein	Type of catheter	Inserting the catheter	Essential tips
Neonate	• Use a heel warmer to dilate the neonate's veins. • Check these major veins in the neonate: dorsal metacarpals in the hand, saphenous vein in the foot, and temporal, frontal, and posterior auricular veins in the scalp. • Transillumination can help in identifying veins in neonates.	• Use a 24G over-the-needle catheter. • The most common length is ½" to ⅝".	• Get help to hold the neonate; use a papoose board, if needed. • Take steps to maintain the neonate's temperature. • Use no tourniquet or minimum pressure for fragile veins. A rubber band may work well. • Clean the site with alcohol. Iodine tincture, which may affect thyroid function if absorbed through the neonate's thin skin, isn't recommended. • Insert the catheter gently and slowly. • Expect scant blood return in the flashback chamber.	• Using a gauze pad, pad the area under the catheter hub, where a pressure sore might occur. • Use a minimum amount of tape on fragile skin. • Cover the skin over the cannula tip with a transparent dressing so you can check the site. • Use a padded tongue blade or rolled gauze as an arm board.
Child	• Veins in the hands, forearms, or antecubital fossa are preferred. • Avoid the saphenous vein if the child is ambulating. • Use the nondominant arm so a young child can suck his thumb and an older child can do crafts or schoolwork.	• Use the smallest possible catheter for the vein and the viscosity of the solution: 24G, 22G, or 20G. • Thin-walled I.V. catheters provide excellent flow rates, even at smaller gauges.	• Use toys or bubbles to distract the child during insertion. • Get help to hold the child; use a papoose board, if needed. • Use local anesthesia (lidocaine injection or EMLA cream [lidocaine 2.5% and prilocaine 2.5%]) if your facility's policy allows it. • Use positioning for comfort techniques whenever possible.	• Pin the arm board to the bed or use Velcro restraints to limit the mobility of the limb with the I.V. line. • Use a padded board if the I.V. site is over an area of flexion. • Use a sterile, transparent, semipermeable membrane dressing and, if needed, a clear plastic cup so you can see the site. Consider using stockinette or elastic gauze to wrap and cover the I.V. site and board, if it's on an active limb. Be sure to leave the skin over the cannula tip visible so you can check the site. • Secure the tubing to the site. • Allow toddlers, older children, and adolescents to participate. For example, allow them to handle the equipment, clean the site, or place a make-believe I.V. line in a doll (with supervision) to help them cope.

• Remove the syringe from the Y-port, open the flow-control clamp, and set the primary flow rate as prescribed.

Don't push your luck

• If the bolus drug isn't compatible with the primary I.V. solution, ask a pharmacist what you should do. You may need to flush the line with 2 to 3 ml of normal saline solution before and after giving the bolus dose. Or, you may need to use a T-connector to give the drug.
• Discard used items according to standard precautions.

Practice pointers

• Because a bolus drug takes effect rapidly, you'll need to monitor the patient carefully for adverse reactions, such as hypersensitivity, hypotension, or cardiac arrhythmias.
• Make sure the I.V. line is still patent after you've given a bolus dose.

What to teach

• Tell the patient the name of the bolus drug, why you're giving it, and any adverse effects he may experience or should report.
• Advise him to report pain, redness, swelling, or other problems with the insertion site.

> Carefully monitor your patient for adverse reactions when giving a drug bolus. They can be fast-acting.

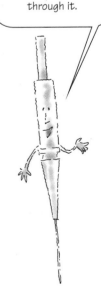

> To check if a saline lock is patent, try to aspirate blood through it.

Giving a bolus through a saline lock

A *saline lock* converts an I.V. line into an intermittent infusion device. It connects to the venous access device by luer-lock, and it has a latex cap through which you can give repeated bolus doses using either a needle or a needleless system. (If the patient has a latex allergy, use a latex-free device.)

A leaky lock

A needleless saline lock may leak if you puncture it with a needle. If you must use a needle, choose the smallest one possible (1″ or less, but no smaller than 25G). If the device leaks after the injection, you'll need to replace it.

What you need

Prescribed drug ✳ syringe of appropriate size (either a needleless system or one with a 20G or 22G 1″ needle) ✳ alcohol or povidone-iodine pads ✳ gloves ✳ two 3-ml syringes with 20G or 22G 1″ needles (fill them with normal saline solution)

Getting ready

• Check your facility's policy to see if you need another 3-ml syringe with heparin flush solution.
• Verify the order on the patient's chart.
• Check the drug's expiration date, and reconstitute the drug, if necessary.
• Identify the patient by checking his armband.
• Wash your hands and put on gloves.

How you do it

• Clean the infusion port of the saline lock with an alcohol pad or a povidone-iodine pad.

Proving patency

• If the saline lock is patent, you should be able to aspirate blood through it. To do so, insert the needle of a saline-filled syringe and aspirate.
• If no blood appears, apply a tourniquet above the site for about 1 minute. Aspirate again.
• If blood still doesn't appear, remove the tourniquet and slowly inject the normal saline solution. If you feel resistance, stop. The device is probably occluded and will need to be replaced.
• Once you can aspirate blood, slowly inject normal saline solution and watch for signs of infiltration, such as puffiness or pain at the site.

If you see swelling — stop!

• If infiltration occurs, remove the saline lock and insert a new one.
• After you've flushed the saline lock, maintain positive pressure and withdraw the syringe and the needle.
• Insert the drug-filled syringe into the infusion port, and inject the drug at the prescribed rate and volume.

Finish with a flush

• Flush the lock with the second saline syringe and then heparin, if needed.
• Discard used items according to standard precautions.

Practice pointers

• Because a bolus drug takes effect rapidly, you'll need to monitor the patient carefully for adverse reactions, such as hypersensitivity, hypotension, or cardiac arrhythmia.

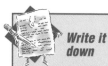

Write it down

Documenting bolus injection administration

Be sure to record:
• type and amount of drug given
• date and time you gave it
• confirmation that the I.V. line was patent
• all solutions used to dilute the drug and flush the I.V. line on the patient's intake and output record
• patient's response to the drug
• condition of the insertion site
• ongoing monitoring that you provided.

Twice is nice

- To keep the device patent, flush it twice—according to your facility's policy—with enough solution to fill the saline lock and to clear residual blood.
- A saline lock can be used for up to 72 hours if it functions properly and if your facility's policy allows.

What to teach

- Tell the patient the name of the bolus drug, why you're giving it, and any adverse effects he may experience or should report.
- Advise him to report pain, redness, swelling, or other problems with the insertion site.

Giving a bolus directly into a vein

If your patient needs rapid drug action—for example, in emergencies—you may need to inject the drug directly into a vein.

What you need

Winged venipuncture device ✳ tourniquet ✳ alcohol pads ✳ povidone-iodine pads ✳ two syringes filled with normal saline solution ✳ one syringe filled with the prescribed drug ✳ appropriate bandage ✳ sterile 2″ × 2″ gauze pads ✳ gloves (see *Winging it with a winged device*, page 254)

Getting ready

- Verify the order on the patient's chart.
- Identify the patient by checking his armband.
- Explain the procedure to the patient.
- Wash your hands and put on gloves.

How you do it

- Select the largest suitable vein, keeping in mind the number of injections the patient may be receiving and the need to preserve proximal veins for future use. The smaller the vein you use for an injection, the more the drug must be diluted to minimize irritation.
- Apply a tourniquet above the injection site to distend it.
- Clean the injection site according to your facility's policy. If you use both alcohol and povidone-iodine, apply the alcohol first. Start at the site, and spiral outward about 2″ (5 cm).

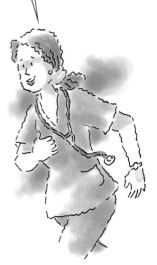

In an emergency, you may need to inject the drug directly into a patient's vein.

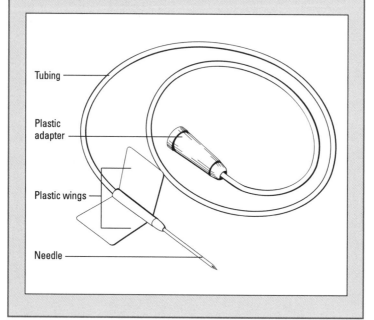

Winging it with a winged device

You may be called upon to administer a drug directly into a patient's vein. To accomplish this, you'll need to insert a winged venipuncture device (as shown below).

Tubing

Plastic adapter

Plastic wings

Needle

Oh, wow! Flashback!

- Insert the venipuncture needle, bevel up, into the vein. You should see blood flashback.
- Tape the wings of the device to the patient's skin.
- Insert a syringe of normal saline solution into the device.
- Withdraw the plunger to check again for blood flashback.
- After you see blood backflow, remove the tourniquet and slowly inject normal saline solution into the vein. Watch for signs of infiltration, such as puffiness or pain.
- Remove the saline-filled syringe, and insert the drug-filled syringe into the venipuncture device.
- Inject the drug as prescribed.

Be very vigilant with vesicants

- If the drug is a vesicant, double-check the patency of the device after injecting every 2 to 3 ml of the drug.

• Withdraw the empty syringe, and insert the second syringe filled with normal saline solution. Flush the venipuncture device to ensure delivery of the full drug dose.
• Another method is to attach a 3-ml syringe filled with normal saline solution to one side of a three-way stopcock and the drug-filled syringe to the other side. Then attach the stopcock to the venipuncture device. You can check for blood backflow, inject the drug, and flush the device by turning the stopcock to the appropriate positions.
• Remove the venipuncture device from the vein, and cover the site with a sterile 2″ × 2″ gauze pad.

3-minute drill

• Apply pressure to the site for at least 3 minutes to prevent formation of a hematoma.
• After the bleeding stops, apply a dressing.
• Discard used items according to standard precautions.

Practice pointers

• Certain drugs are packaged by the manufacturer with specific administration guidelines, such as the appropriate injection rate. Make sure you follow these directions.
• Because a bolus drug takes effect rapidly, you'll need to monitor the patient carefully for adverse reactions, such as hypersensitivity, hypotension, or cardiac arrhythmia.
• Make sure your facility has a written policy concerning direct I.V. bolus injection, and follow it carefully.

What to teach

• Tell the patient the name of the bolus drug, why you're giving it, and any adverse effects he may experience or should report.
• Advise him to report pain, redness, swelling, or other problems with the insertion site.

Giving intermittent infusion

Usually, intermittent drug infusion is given through a secondary administration set or a volume-control set.

Giving intermittent infusion through a secondary line

Most primary administration sets have one or two Y-sites that allow secondary administration—commonly known as a piggyback infusion.

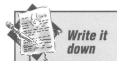

Write it down

Documenting I.V. bolus administration directly into a vein

Be sure to record:
• type and amount of drug given
• date and time you gave it
• patient's response to the drug
• condition of the insertion site
• any ongoing monitoring you provided.

Always follow the specific administration guidelines from the manufacturer when administering a drug.

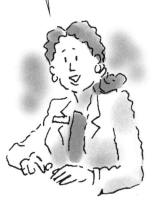

Jump on for a piggyback ride

When a piggyback infusion runs for several hours, it's known as a continuous secondary infusion. When it runs for less time, it's known as an intermittent secondary infusion.

What you need

Prescribed drug (usually premixed in a minibag) ✳ continuous secondary tubing or piggyback extension tubing ✳ extension hook ✳ 20G or smaller 1″ needle or needleless system ✳ medication label (if you aren't using a premixed solution) ✳ alcohol pads ✳ 1″ adhesive tape ✳ gloves

Getting ready

• If the drug is incompatible with the primary I.V. solution, also get two 3-ml syringes with 22G 1″ needles; fill them with normal saline solution.
• Check your facility's policy to see if you need another 3-ml syringe with heparin flush solution.
• You may also need an infusion pump or a time tape.
• Verify the order on the patient's chart.
• Identify the patient by checking his armband.
• Wash your hands.

How you do it

• If you need to add a drug to a secondary I.V. solution, remove any seals from the secondary container. Most solution bags have a sealed outlet and unsealed injection ports, whereas most bottled solutions have a seal covering their dual-outlet port.
• Clean the injection port with an alcohol pad.
• Inject the prescribed drug into the solution, and gently agitate the container to thoroughly mix the solution.

Always be able to label

• Label the container with the patient's name, the date and time, the drug and amount mixed, and your initials.
• Remove the secondary administration set from its packaging.
• Straighten the tubing, and close the roller clamp.
• Remove the protective cap from the distal end of the tubing, and attach the 20G (or smaller) needle or needleless adapter.
• Remove the protective cap from the infusion (outlet) port of the drug container; then remove the cap from the I.V. piercing spike.

Spike it

• Insert the spike into the port of the drug container.

• If the drip chamber has a vent on the side, close it if you're using a bag and open it if you're using a bottle.
• If you haven't already done so, take the equipment and the prepared I.V. solution to the bedside.
• Examine the primary I.V. container for cracks or leaks.
• Locate the Y-port on the primary line.

Piggyback vs. continuous

• For an intermittent piggyback infusion, the port should be positioned above the roller clamp. For a continuous secondary infusion, it should be near the lower end of the primary line.
• Hang the secondary setup on the I.V. pole.
• Using an alcohol pad, clean the selected Y-port on the primary I.V. tubing.
• Insert the needle or needleless adapter from the secondary line into the Y-port of the primary line. (See *Setting up a piggyback set*, page 258.)
• Securely tape the connection, unless you're using a click-lock device with a recessed needle. This device doesn't require taping because a plastic covering locks the needle in place.

Giving a piggyback infusion

• To infuse a piggyback drug without also infusing the primary solution, hang the piggyback container above the level of the primary I.V. solution, using the extension hook that's supplied with the piggyback infusion set.
• Open the roller clamp on the piggyback tubing; then adjust the roller clamp of the primary set to regulate the infusion rate of the piggyback infusion. The primary I.V. solution won't run while the piggyback drug infuses. (To infuse primary and secondary solutions simultaneously, hang them at the same height.)
• If the secondary solution isn't compatible with the primary solution, flush the primary line before and after the piggyback solution is infused.

Giving a continuous secondary infusion

• For a continuous secondary infusion, adjust the roller clamp on the secondary line to the desired drip rate. Then adjust the roller clamp on the primary line to achieve the desired total infusion rate.

Pump it up

• If your facility policy allows, use a pump on the secondary line to maintain a steady flow rate (or a time tape to verify a steady rate).
• If you're using a continuous secondary setup and the primary and secondary solutions are incompatible, stop the primary infu-

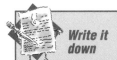
Write it down

Documenting I.V. infusion through a secondary line

Be sure to record:
• type and amount of drug given
• rate and duration of infusion
• date and time you administered the infusion
• amounts and types of solution given on the patient's intake and output record
• patient's response to the infusion
• condition of the insertion site
• any ongoing monitoring you provided.

Peak technique

Setting up a piggyback set

A piggyback set includes a secondary container (a small I.V. bag or bottle) and short tubing with a drip chamber. To use it, connect the piggyback set to a primary line with a Y-port (or piggyback port), as shown below. You must use an extension hook to position the primary I.V. container below the secondary container.

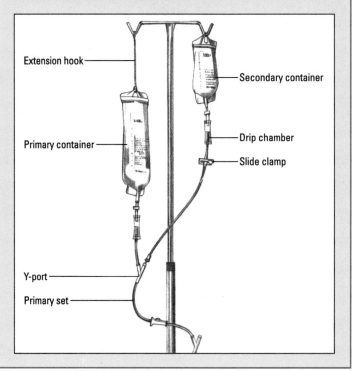

sion. Flush the line with 2 or 3 ml of normal saline solution. Then start the secondary infusion. At the end of the secondary infusion, flush the line again before restarting the primary infusion.

A second-line approach

• If you can't interrupt the primary infusion to run an incompatible secondary infusion, consider a double-lumen catheter or starting another I.V. line.

Finishing the infusion
- If you won't be reusing the tubing from the secondary line, discard it with the empty solution container.

Recycling

- If you'll be reusing the tubing from the secondary infusion set on the same patient, close the clamp on the tubing. Then either replace the used needle or needleless device with a new one, or leave it securely taped or locked in the injection port as a closed system.
- According to policy, label the tubing with the time it was first used. Leave the empty secondary solution container in place until you replace it with a new one.
- Discard used items according to standard precautions.

Practice pointers
- During the infusion, frequently check that the drug in the secondary line is infusing at the desired rate.
- When a continuous secondary infusion ends, the primary infusion will continue. Likewise, when a piggyback infusion ends, the primary infusion will resume. In either case, adjust the drip rate of the primary solution, as needed, when the secondary infusion finishes.

Check for a backcheck

- If you give a piggyback infusion, make sure the primary line has a backcheck valve either in the Y-port or above it. If the tubing doesn't have such a valve and you'll be infusing drugs regularly, replace the tubing with a set that has a backcheck valve.
- Change primary and secondary administration sets every 72 hours (right away if you suspect a problem) or as directed by your facility's policy. Intermittent administration sets should be changed every 24 hours.
- Primary and secondary administration sets commonly include in-line filters to remove particles and pathogens and to keep air out of the line. Change filters when you change the administration set, as directed.

What to teach
- Tell the patient the name of the drug, why you're giving it, and any adverse effects he may experience or should report.
- Tell him to report pain, redness, swelling, or other problems with the insertion site.

If the secondary solution isn't compatible with the primary solution...

...flush the primary line before and after the piggyback solution is infused.

Using a volume-control set for intermittent infusion

A *volume-control set* allows you to give a relatively small volume of fluid in precise amounts—a necessity when treating a child. (See *Volume-control set.*)

The device uses an in-line chamber graduated in milliliters and a rubber float or microporous filter that keeps air from entering the tubing after the chamber is empty.

What you need

Volume-control set ✻ prescribed fluid ✻ syringe (needleless or with an appropriate needle) filled with the prescribed drug ✻ alcohol pad or antiseptic specified by your facility ✻ gloves

Getting ready

• Verify the order on the patient's chart.
• Identify the patient by checking his armband.
• Wash your hands and put on gloves.
• Remove the volume-control set from its packaging.

Prime time

• Prime the set with I.V. fluid.
• Clean the injection port on top of the chamber, and inject the drug into the chamber.
• Gently rotate the chamber to mix the drug.
• Place a label on the chamber that identifies the drug, dose, time, and date.
• Fasten the tubing to the injection port of the primary line.

Stop or go slow

• Either stop the primary infusion or set a low drip rate so the line will be open when the secondary infusion stops.
• Open the lower clamp of the volume-control set, and start the infusion at the desired rate.
• When the chamber is empty, allow about 10 ml of I.V. solution to flow into it and through the tubing to flush the system, unless contraindicated.
• Discard used items according to standard precautions.

Practice pointers

• Make sure you know how to calculate and control the rate of the prescribed therapy.
• Refill the chamber for the next infusion.
• A volume-control set can be used for continual flow by clamping the air vent tube.

Ages and stages

Volume-control set

Infants, small children, and children with cardiopulmonary problems are particularly vulnerable to fluid overload and drug toxicity with I.V. administration. To prevent fluid overload and to make sure the child receives a precise volume of fluid, use a volume-control set on the infusion pump, as shown below.

A calibrated chamber

A volume-control set has a calibrated fluid chamber positioned between the I.V. bag and the drip chamber in the I.V. tubing, as shown below. It can help prevent fluid overload in your pediatric patients, but remember not to place more than 2 hours' worth of I.V. fluid in it at one time.

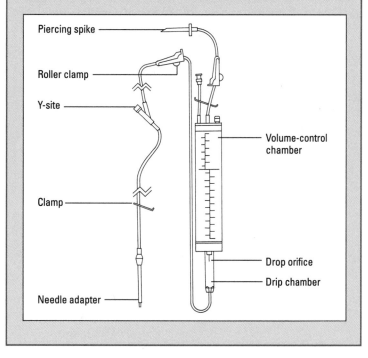

Memory jogger

To remember how to prime the volume-control set, fill the chamber with at least 20 ml of fluid; then use the mnemonic **OSCAR** (after all, you deserve an award):

Open the flow-regulating clamp,

Squeeze and hold the drip chamber,

Close the regulating clamp directly below the drip chamber,

And...

Release the drip chamber.

Child watch

• Because children are prone to fluid overload and their immature body systems may have difficulty metabolizing drugs, they need more frequent monitoring than adults do, to prevent potential complications of medications administered I.V.

What to teach

- Tell the patient the name of the drug, why you're giving it, and any adverse effects he may experience or should report.
- Tell him to report pain, redness, swelling, or other problems with the insertion site.

Administering a continuous infusion

The continuous infusion method allows a drug to be administered over an extended period. You may give a bolus dose first, then switch to a continuous infusion to maintain drug levels in the patient's blood.

Tool time

This precise therapy may require you to use special connectors, anchoring devices, filters, and one of a wide selection of pumps to manage the rate of infusion and reduce the risk of complications. (See *Understanding I.V. pumps*.)

Using an infusion pump

You may need to give your patient a continuous infusion of a drug after a bolus dose such as heparin.

What you need

Pump ✳ drug administration set compatible with the device ✳ 3-ml syringe with a needleless system or a 25G ⅝″ needle ✳ flushing solution ✳ alcohol pads ✳ patency solution (if indicated) ✳ gloves

Getting ready

- Verify the order on the patient's chart.
- Identify the patient by checking his armband.

A programming note

- Set up the pump according to the manufacturer's instructions and your facility's policy. Program the infusion as prescribed.
- Wash your hands and put on gloves.

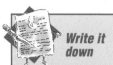

Write it down

Documenting volume-control set administration

Be sure to record:
- types and amounts of drugs and solutions given
- rate and duration of infusion
- date and time you administered the infusion
- amounts and types of solution given on the patient's intake and output record
- patient's response to the infusion
- condition of the insertion site
- ongoing monitoring you provided.

Gear up!

Understanding I.V. pumps

When administering I.V. drugs, you'll need to be familiar with a wide range of pumps, all of which are designed to infuse I.V. fluids and drugs at precise rates.

Infusion pumps use positive pressure, measured in pounds per square inch, to propel solution through I.V. tubing. They're more precise than controllers, and they can overcome resistance—which reduces occlusion and allows arterial infusion.

• An *elastomeric pump* has a bladder reservoir filled with infusate. As the bladder collapses, pressure increases and propels remaining fluid from the reservoir. This single-use, disposable pump simplifies delivery of single-dose infusions of drug solutions.

• A *pressure-controlled pump* contains a mechanical arm or spring that presses on a reservoir. The pressure forces solution from the reservoir into the attached tubing. A restriction component controls the flow rate.

• A *volumetric infusion pump* uses pressure to move solution through tubing at a preselected, completely controlled flow rate. It can overcome resistance caused by filters, viscous fluids, a narrow-lumen I.V. catheter, and patient movement.

• A *syringe pump* typically is used for slow but precise infusion of a small volume of solution over a long period. You fill a 5- to 60-ml syringe with solution and place it into the pump.

• A *peristaltic pump* is so named because it applies intermittent pressure to the tubing. It's usually used for enteral feedings.

• A *membrane infusion pump,* a combination controller and infusion pump, uses gravity to propel solution and a membrane to filter particulates, bacteria, and endotoxins.

• A *patient-controlled analgesia pump* lets the patient control the delivery of pain medication, usually morphine. It prevents accidental overdose with a lockout mechanism during which the pump won't dispense the drug.

• An *ambulatory infusion pump,* a small, battery-powered device, has internal storage for small volumes of solution. For larger volumes, the pump connects to a reservoir with short tubing. Either way, the patient can go out in public with little disruption or restriction of movement.

• A *special program pump* can be programmed to deliver solutions in selected patterns. For example, a pump can gradually start and stop total parenteral nutrition. Or, it can deliver chemotherapy by circadian rhythm.

• A *multichannel pump* can deliver two to four infusions at the same time using varying rates, volumes, and times.

How you do it

• Make sure the clamp on the administration set is closed and the line has no air bubbles in it.

Always check for patency

• Inject normal saline solution into the patient's vascular access device to make sure it's patent.
• Wipe the port again with a clean alcohol pad.
• Connect the tubing of the administration set to the device.

No place like home

Using an I.V. pump in the home

Make sure the patient and his family understand the purpose of using the pump. Demonstrate how the device works and how to maintain the system (tubing, solution, and site assessment and care) until you're confident that the patient and family can proceed safely. As time permits, have the patient repeat the demonstration.

Get complicated

Discuss which complications to watch for, such as infiltration, and review measures to take if complications occur. Schedule a teaching session with the patient and his family so you can answer questions they may have about the procedure before the patient's discharge.

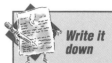

Write it down

Documenting I.V. infusion using a pump

Be sure to record:
• types and amounts of drugs and solutions given
• rate and duration of infusion
• equipment used
• date and time you administered the infusion
• amounts and types of solution given on the patient's intake and output record
• patient's response to the infusion
• condition of the insertion site
• ongoing monitoring that you provided.

• Open the clamp and begin the infusion.
• Discard used items according to standard precautions.

Practice pointers

• Make sure you know how to troubleshoot the device you're using and that you know your facility's policy about it.
• The amount or type of infusion to be administered, the patient's age and condition, and the care setting may influence the infusion device you use. If the patient needs to receive infusions at home, consider his lifestyle, his use of ambulatory devices, and the level of family support available to him. (See *Using an I.V. pump in the home.*)

What to teach

• Tell the patient the name of the drug, why you're giving it, and about adverse effects he may experience or should report.
• Advise him to report pain, redness, swelling, or other problems with the insertion site.
• If the patient will receive infusions at home, make sure he or a caregiver can administer them safely and correctly. Also make sure you teach how to care for the I.V. site and identify certain complications. (See *I.V. therapy in the home.*)

No place like home

I.V. therapy in the home

Most patients who receive I.V. therapy at home have a central venous line. But if you're caring for a patient going home with a peripheral line, you should teach him how to care for the I.V. site and identify and report such problems as redness, swelling, or discomfort; if the dressing becomes moist; or if blood appears in the tubing. Also, tell the patient to report any problems with the I.V. line—for instance, if the solution stops infusing or if an alarm goes off on an infusion pump. Explain that the I.V. site will be changed at established intervals by a home care nurse. If the patient must observe movement restrictions, make sure he understands them.

Intermittent instruction

If the patient is using an intermittent infusion device, teach him how and when to flush it. Finally, teach the patient to document daily whether the I.V. site is free from pain, swelling, and redness.

Understanding special I.V. catheters

One way to avoid the trauma of repeated venipuncture is by using an I.V. catheter, such as a midline catheter, a peripherally inserted central catheter, or a traditional central venous catheter.

Using a midline catheter

A *midline catheter* is a special I.V. catheter inserted peripherally into a vein in the antecubital space; its tip lies 1″ (2.5 cm) or more below the axillary vein, as shown at top of page 266.

Middle management

Made of Silastic or polyurethane, a midline catheter may have one or two lumens that range in size from 2F to 6F (about 14G to 22G). Some catheters have a built-in extension set to reduce jostling and site irritation. Most midline catheters are open at the tip and require instillation of heparin or saline to remain patent.

Decreased extravasation is an extra bonus

Unlike a typical I.V. line, a midline catheter can be left in place for up to 4 weeks. It's much less likely to dislodge than a typical I.V. line, thus reducing the risk of extravasation.

However, you can't use a midline catheter for continuous vesicant chemotherapy, central total parenteral nutrition, solutions or drugs with a pH below 5 or above 9, or solutions or drugs with a

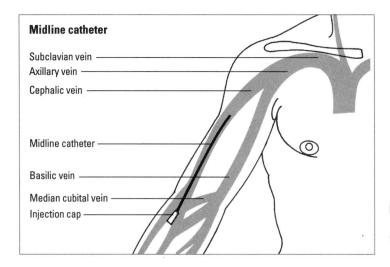

Midline catheter

Subclavian vein

Axillary vein

Cephalic vein

Midline catheter

Basilic vein

Median cubital vein

Injection cap

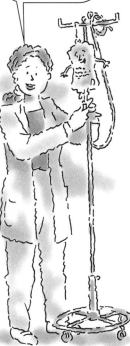

Unlike a typical I.V. line, a midline catheter can be left in place for up to 4 weeks.

serum osmolality above 500 mOsm/L. Doing so could raise the risk of phlebitis, thrombosis, or sclerosis.

What you need

Sterile gloves (preferably powder-free) ✳ mask ✳ drug or solution to be infused ✳ alcohol pads or another cleaner specified by your facility ✳ 5-ml syringe and a 10-ml syringe filled with normal saline solution ✳ two 25G 1″ needles ✳ sterile drape ✳ adhesive dressing

Getting ready

- Verify the order on the patient's chart.
- Identify the patient by checking his armband.
- Explain the procedure to the patient.
- Help the patient into a comfortable reclining position with his arm extended at a 45- to 90-degree angle.
- Wash your hands and put on gloves.
- Set up a sterile field.

For good measure

- Measure the length of catheter extending from the patient's arm to confirm that it hasn't migrated since being inserted.
- Locate the injection cap on the catheter hub. Clean it with three alcohol pads (or other cleaner). Let the cap air-dry between each wipe.
- Attach the 5-ml syringe, and aspirate for patency.
- If you're starting an infusion, connect the I.V. tubing.

- Secure the hub with sterile stabilizing strips or a commercial securing device (StatLock or K-LoK, for example) so it won't be pulled during the infusion.

Be extra careful of extravasation

- Watch the patient's upper arm to detect swelling as the fluid starts infusing; swelling suggests extravasation.
- After you give a drug or solution through a midline catheter, flush the catheter with 5 to 10 ml of normal saline solution.
- Discard used items according to standard precautions.

Practice pointers

- Check your facility's policy when determining which flush solution to use to keep the line patent. You may use a heparin flush (usually 2 to 3 ml of a 1:100 U/ml solution) during intermittent therapy.
- If the patient is allergic to heparin or has a condition that contraindicates its use, consider using a valved catheter, for which you can use a saline flush.

Clot buster

- Pediatric midline catheters are small and clot easily. Use a continuous low-volume flush system as specified by your facility's pediatric protocols.
- Change the dressing at established intervals—48 hours to 7 days, depending on the dressing being used. Assess the site for bleeding, signs of phlebitis, or other complications.
- When changing tubing or the injection cap, keep the hub at or below the patient's heart level to reduce the risk of air embolism.
- Regularly assess the site for complications, especially mechanical or chemical phlebitis.
- Don't take blood pressure measurements in an arm that has a midline catheter in it.
- Don't use hemostats or clamps on the catheter if they have teeth and sharp edges.
- Don't use a needle longer than 1″ to flush the catheter because it could puncture the lumen. Use a needleless system, if possible.

> Keep the hub level with the patient's heart or lower to prevent air embolism when changing tubing.

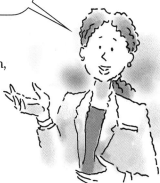

What to teach

- Teach the patient about the catheter, why he has one, and how to assess the insertion site.

• Tell him not to apply pressure to the axilla or inner surface of the upper arm (as from a crutch) because this could dislodge the catheter or irritate the vein.

Using a peripherally inserted central catheter

A *peripherally inserted central catheter* (commonly called a PICC) is a special I.V. catheter inserted into a peripheral vein and advanced until the tip of the catheter lies in the superior vena cava, as shown below.

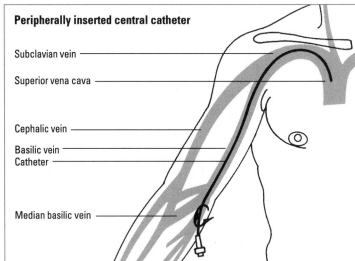

Peripherally inserted central catheter

Subclavian vein

Superior vena cava

Cephalic vein

Basilic vein

Catheter

Median basilic vein

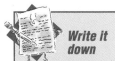

Write it down

Documenting midline catheter medication administration

Be sure to record:
• drug or solution administered
• date and time you administered it
• that the line was patent
• flush procedures administered
• patient's tolerance of the catheter and infusions through it
• condition of the insertion site and dressing
• dressing changes you performed
• patient teaching provided.

Quick PICC info

Typically, a PICC is used for long-term infusion therapy in patients who lack adequate peripheral venous access, are homebound, or require frequent venipunctures to obtain blood for testing. A PICC also may be used for patients receiving chemotherapy, total parenteral nutrition, analgesics, frequent blood transfusions, dobutamine, antibiotics, or other infusions that irritate peripheral vessels. You can use a PICC to infuse solutions with an osmolality of 600 mOsm/L or more and a pH below 6 or above 8.

PICC and choose

Several different PICCs are available. They're made of silicone or polyurethane, and they have one or two lumens. Single-lumen catheters range from 16G to 28G; double-lumen models range from 2F to 5F. They're all about 20″ to 24″ (50 to 61 cm) long; single-lumen catheters can be trimmed to a specified length.

What you need

Three 10-ml syringes—two filled with 3 ml of normal saline solution and one with heparin flush solution (according to facility policy) ✳ gloves ✳ alcohol pads ✳ prescribed drug in a 10-ml syringe

Getting ready

- Verify the order on the patient's chart.
- Identify the patient by checking his armband.

First PICC

- If you're giving the first drug dose through a newly inserted PICC, make sure the patient has had a chest X-ray to confirm correct placement of the catheter.
- Wash your hands and put on gloves.

How you do it

- Measure the length of catheter extending from the patient's arm to confirm that it hasn't migrated since being inserted.
- Clean the injection port with an alcohol wipe.

Blocked!

- Using aseptic technique, flush the tubing with normal saline solution. If you feel resistance, stop. The catheter may be blocked. A doctor may order an X-ray to look for a kink in the catheter, thrombolytic therapy to dissolve a clot, or administration of a drug to alter the pH of a precipitate and bring it back into solution.
- If the port flushes easily, finish the flushing procedure.
- Clean the injection port again with an alcohol wipe.
- Inject the drug as ordered.

Don't forget to flush

- Afterward, flush the catheter with the second saline-filled syringe.
- Repeat the entire procedure for each drug given. Follow the final saline flush with a heparin flush according to facility policy.
- Discard used items according to standard precautions.

Practice pointers

- At 24 hours after insertion, remove the original dressing and replace it with a transparent semipermeable membrane or other dressing specified by facility policy. Change it every 7 days, or right away if it becomes loose, soiled, or wet.

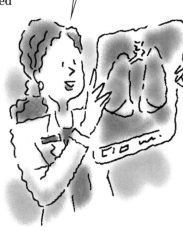

Correct placement of a PICC is confirmed with a chest X-ray.

• Always use aseptic technique when you work with a PICC.
• Carefully secure all junctions between I.V. tubing and devices added for drug administration to reduce the risk of complications.

Stick with PICC

• A PICC can remain in place for months—possibly 1 year or longer if no complications arise.
• Watch for such complications as mechanical phlebitis, bleeding, infection, thrombosis, catheter migration or dislodgment, air embolism, pain, and catheter fracture.

What to teach

• Explain to the patient what a PICC is and why he needs one.
• Instruct him or a caregiver to report changes in the arm (such as numbness, tingling, coolness, or decreased sensation) or the insertion site (such as swelling, warmth, redness, or tenderness).

Using a traditional central venous catheter

A *central venous catheter* is a specialized I.V. catheter with its tip in the superior vena cava, inferior vena cava, or right atrium of the heart. It can be used to deliver fluids and drugs to the superior vena cava (occasionally to the inferior vena cava), monitor central venous pressure and cardiac efficiency, and obtain blood samples.

The solution for pollution is dilution

Fluids and drugs are rapidly diluted in the large vena cava, thereby reducing the risk of chemical phlebitis. Thus, a central line can be used to administer highly osmolar or caustic fluids.

Tunnel vision

A central venous catheter may be nontunneled or tunneled, the former for short-term therapy and the latter for long-term therapy. (See *Comparing central venous catheters*.)

What you need

Prescribed drug ✳ delivery system for the drug ✳ clean gloves ✳ sterile gloves ✳ 10-ml luer-lock syringe of normal saline solution (preservative-free for infants) ✳ 10-ml luer-lock syringe of heparin flush solution ✳ alcohol or povidone-iodine pads ✳ 4″ × 4″ gauze pads ✳ securing device, if needed

Getting ready

• Verify the order on the patient's chart.

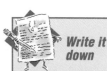

Write it down

Documenting drug administration through a peripherally inserted central catheter

Be sure to record:
• drug or solution administered
• date and time you administered it
• that the line was patent
• flush procedures administered
• patient's tolerance of the catheter and infusions through it
• condition of the insertion site and dressing
• dressing changes you performed
• patient teaching you provided.

Gear up!

Comparing central venous catheters

Each type of central venous catheter offers advantages and disadvantages. This table reviews nontunneled catheters along with Groshong, Hickman, and Broviac tunneled catheters.

Catheter	Advantages	Disadvantages
Nontunneled	• Easily inserted at bedside • Cost effective • Easily removed • Easily changed over guide wire • Stiffness aids central venous catheter monitoring • Allows administration of several solutions at once	• Easily dislodged by patient movement • Limited functions • More thrombogenic because of catheter material • Requires sterile dressing changes • Not flexible; may break • Requires heparin flushes when not in use
Groshong Closed-end tip Dacron cuff	• Valve eliminates need for Valsalva's maneuver and frequent flushing • Doesn't require heparin • Less thrombogenic • Easily repaired • Anchored to chest wall so movement isn't restricted • Cuff decreases chance of infection • Doesn't require clamping • Reduced time and cost for maintenance	• Requires surgical insertion • Fragile; can tear or kink easily • Blunt end makes it difficult to clear substances from tip • Requires doctor for removal • Susceptible to infection • May affect body image
Hickman Large lumen Small lumen Dacron cuff Clamps	• Less thrombogenic • Anchored to chest wall so movement isn't restricted • Cuff decreases chance of infection • Clamp eliminates need for Valsalva's maneuver	• Requires surgical insertion • Difficult to repair • Open end • Requires doctor for removal • Tears and kinks easily • Susceptible to infection • May affect body image
Broviac Lumen Clamp Catheter Dacron cuff	• Small lumen • Less thrombogenic • Anchored to chest wall so movement isn't restricted • Cuff decreases chance of infection • Clamp eliminates need for Valsalva's maneuver	• Requires surgical insertion • Open end • Requires doctor for removal • Tears and kinks easily • Small lumen may limit use • Single lumen limits function • May affect body image • Susceptible to infection • Difficult to repair

• Prepare the prescribed drug as ordered, and check the expiration date.
• Identify the patient by checking his armband.
• Tell the patient what you'll be giving him and why.
• Wash your hands and put on gloves.

How you do it

• Clean the port of the injection cap with an alcohol pad or a povidone-iodine pad. Keep the cap in your hand.

Push, don't pull

• While holding the saline-filled syringe and the cap in the same hand, remove the needle cover with your other hand. Don't pull on the catheter as you do so.
• Push the needle into the port of the injection cap. Stop when you feel resistance. The needle may go all the way into the cap, or some may show.
• Unclamp the catheter.
• Aspirate for blood to ensure patency, and then push the 10-ml saline flush into the catheter using steady pressure. It should flush easily. If it doesn't, make sure the clamp is open and the catheter has no kinks. If you still can't flush it, alert the doctor.

Stay positive

• As you near the end of the flush solution, while you're still pushing it, reclamp the catheter to maintain positive pressure in the catheter. Remove the flush syringe.
• Again, clean the port of the injection cap with an alcohol pad or a povidone-iodine pad.
• Next, insert the needle of the prescribed drug dose.
• Open the clamp, and infuse the ordered drug.
• Appropriately discard the used needle and syringe.
• Clean and flush the port again to remove residual drug. Remember to reclamp the catheter while pushing the flush solution, to keep positive pressure in the catheter.

Finalizing the deal

• Finally, clean the injection port, insert the needle of the syringe filled with heparin flush solution, and flush the catheter using the same steady pressure. As you push the final milliliter of solution, reclamp the catheter.
• Redress the site according to facility policy.
• Discard used items according to standard precautions.
• If you give a fluid or drug that's incompatible with heparin, make sure you flush the line with normal saline solution before flushing it with heparin.

Danger zone

Risks of CV therapy

As with any invasive procedure, central venous (CV) therapy poses risks, including pneumothorax, air embolism, thrombosis, and infection. The chart below highlights the complications.

Pneumothorax, hemothorax, chylothorax, or hydrothorax	Air embolism	Thrombosis	Local infection	Systemic infection
• Chest pain • Dyspnea • Cyanosis • Decreased breath sounds on the affected side • With hemothorax, decreased hemoglobin because of blood pooling • Abnormal chest X-ray	• Respiratory distress • Unequal breath sounds • Weak pulse • Increased central venous pressure • Decreased blood pressure • Churning murmur over the precordium • Change in or loss of consciousness	• Edema at the puncture site • Erythema • Ipsilateral swelling of the arm, neck, and face • Pain along the vein • Fever, malaise • Tachycardia	• Redness, warmth, tenderness, and swelling at the insertion or exit site • Possible exudate of purulent material • Local rash or pustules • Fever, chills, malaise	• Fever, chills without other apparent reason • Leukocytosis • Nausea, vomiting • Malaise • Elevated urine glucose level

Practice pointers

• For the first 24 hours, you may see serosanguineous drainage at a new site.
• Change the dressing at the insertion site according to your facility's policy.
• To prevent I.V.-related infection, maintain strict aseptic technique when giving solutions, changing tubing, and dressing the insertion site.

The center of attention

• Regularly flush a central line—especially before and after giving a drug—to keep it patent. Also, flush the line when you stop an I.V. infusion, whenever the catheter isn't being used, and after you've drawn blood through it. When flushing the catheter with heparin, use the lowest possible concentration (from 1 to 10 U/ml in infants and from 10 to 100 U/ml in children and adults).
• Typically, the appropriate flush volume equals twice the capacity of the cannula and add-on device; thus, the flush amount varies with the catheter being used. As always, follow your facility's policy about flush volumes.

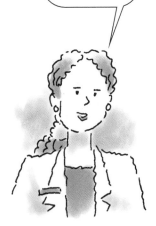

How low can you go? When flushing with heparin, use the lowest possible concentration!

No place like home

CV therapy in the home

Long-term use of a central venous (CV) catheter allows patients to receive caustic fluids and blood infusions at home. These catheters have a much longer life because they are less thrombogenic and less prone to infection than short-term devices.

Buddy system
A candidate for home therapy must have a family member or friend who can safely and competently administer the I.V. fluids, a backup helper, a suitable home environment, a telephone, transportation, adequate reading skills, and the ability to prepare, handle, store, and dispose of the equipment. The care procedures used in the home are the same as those used in the facility.

Learning curve
The overall goal of home therapy is patient safety, so your patient teaching must begin well before discharge. After discharge, a home therapy coordinator will provide follow-up care until the patient or someone close to him can provide catheter care and infusion therapy independently. Many home therapy patients learn to care for the catheter themselves and infuse their own medications and solution.

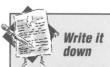

Write it down

Documenting central venous catheter drug administration

Be sure to record:
• date and time
• site used (if the catheter is multilumen)
• medication name and dose
• presence of blood return
• patency of the line
• patient's tolerance of the procedure
• complications noted
• steps taken to resolve complications
• appearance of the insertion site
• patient teaching provided
• patient's or family's response to your teaching.

Clearing up complications

• Complications can occur at any time with a central venous catheter. (See *Risks of CV therapy,* page 273.)
• Besides being susceptible to complications, a central venous catheter can be damaged by frequent manipulation, high flush pressures, and the use of scissors or serrated clamps. A specially trained person can temporarily repair a damaged catheter by using a blunt-tipped needle. Permanent repair kits are available as well.

What to teach

• Explain to the patient the purpose of a central venous catheter.
• If the patient will have central venous therapy at home, make sure he or a caregiver knows how to care for the site, how to flush the line, how to administer drugs or solutions, and how to recognize and respond to complications. If the patient needs them, arrange for him to have follow-up home visits. (See *CV therapy in the home.*)

Understanding vascular access ports

A *vascular access port* (VAP) offers reliable venous access and typically is used for intermittent rather than continuous drug administration. After it's surgically implanted, typically in the chest wall but sometimes in the antecubital space, a VAP can remain in place for years. The tip of an attached catheter empties drug from the VAP into a central vein, usually the superior vena cava near where it enters the right atrium, as shown in the two illustrations below.

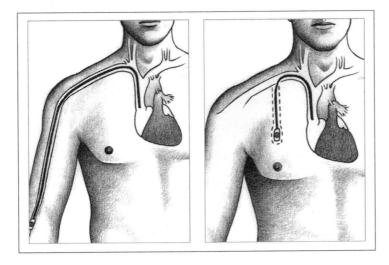

Another implanted device, the implanted infusion pump, offers an avenue for long-term continuous therapy. (See *Using an implanted infusion pump*, page 276.)

A VAP map

A typical VAP has a rigid reservoir with a self-sealing rubber septum on the top or side. (See *Comparing top-entry and side-entry VAPs*, page 277.)

The catheters used with VAPs range from 6F to 10F for one lumen and 10F to 13F for two lumens. The catheter comes either attached to the reservoir or as a two-part system that's connected after insertion. The original catheter ranges in length from about 20″ to 30″ (50 to 76 cm) and is trimmed to fit.

Core concerns

Usually, you'll use a special noncoring needle to inject a drug into a VAP, administer an infusion, or draw blood from a VAP. A noncoring needle has a deflected or angled point, which slices the

Gear up!

Using an implanted infusion pump

If your ambulatory patient needs a low-volume, long-term infusion, he may receive it through a small infusion pump implanted in the subcutaneous tissue of his abdomen or subclavian fossa. A catheter leads from the pump to an artery, vein, or organ into which the drug empties.

Two chambers
As shown in the illustration below, the pump has two chambers separated by a flexible membrane, also called a bellows. One chamber holds the drug solution; the other holds a charging fluid. The charging fluid presses against the flexible membrane, forcing drug out of the pump and into the catheter.

Pressure changes
As the drug infuses, pressure inside the drug chamber drops. The charging fluid expands into vapor, which continues to press against the membrane and force drug out of its chamber and into the catheter. When the drug chamber is refilled, renewed pressure makes the vapor condense back into a liquid, which stores energy for the next cycle.

Special assignment
After receiving special training, you may refill the drug chamber of an implanted infusion pump every 1 to 3 months. Between refills, warn the patient that changes in pressure inside and outside his body can affect the rate of his infusion. For instance, moving from one altitude to another can increase the infusion rate by more than one-third. A fever, a sauna, or even a hot bath can increase it by more than 10%. Even changes in blood pressure can alter the infusion rate. You'll need to closely and regularly monitor the patient's implanted pump to make sure he doesn't run out of drug.

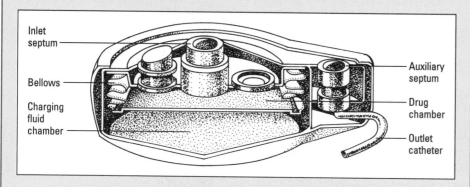

Inlet septum

Bellows

Charging fluid chamber

Auxiliary septum

Drug chamber

Outlet catheter

Danger zone

Vital VAP information

Use great care when you select a syringe and noncoring needle for a VAP. The larger the needle used, the shorter the life of the VAP. The smaller the syringe used, the greater the pressure created inside the device—pressure that can fracture the VAP or the attached catheter.

septum rather than cutting a chunk out of it. Thus, when you remove the needle, the septum can seal shut. (See *A close look at noncoring needles,* page 278.)

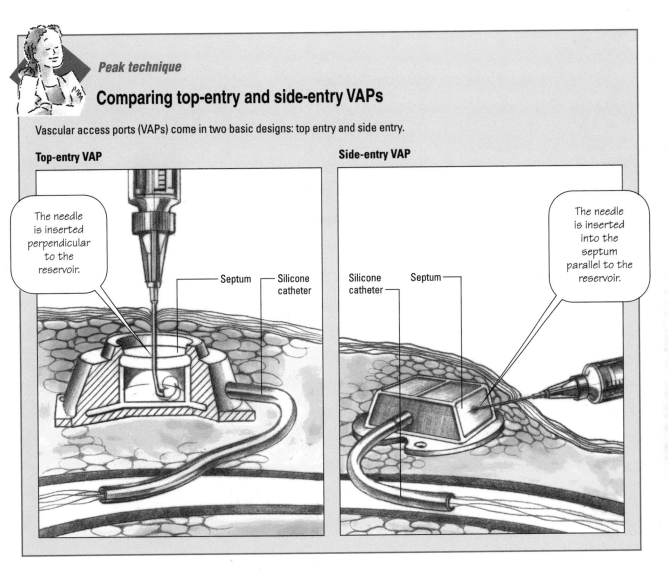

Peak technique

Comparing top-entry and side-entry VAPs

Vascular access ports (VAPs) come in two basic designs: top entry and side entry.

Top-entry VAP

The needle is inserted perpendicular to the reservoir.

Septum — Silicone catheter

Side-entry VAP

Silicone catheter — Septum

The needle is inserted into the septum parallel to the reservoir.

Gauging the situation

Noncoring needles typically come in 19G, 20G, and 22G sizes and are 1¼″ to 2″ long. Large, 14G and 16G noncoring needles are available for high-flow infusions and viscous fluids. Most VAPs are designed to withstand up to 2,000 punctures with a 22G noncoring needle. It's important to select the proper syringe and noncoring needle for your patient's VAP. (See *Vital VAP information.*)

Gear up!

A close look at noncoring needles

Unlike a conventional hypodermic needle, a noncoring needle has a deflected point, which slices the port's septum instead of coring it. Noncoring needles come in two types: straight and right angle.

Getting it right, getting it straight

Generally, expect to use a right-angle needle with a top-entry port and a straight needle with a side-entry port. When administering a bolus injection or continuous infusion, you'll also use an extension set.

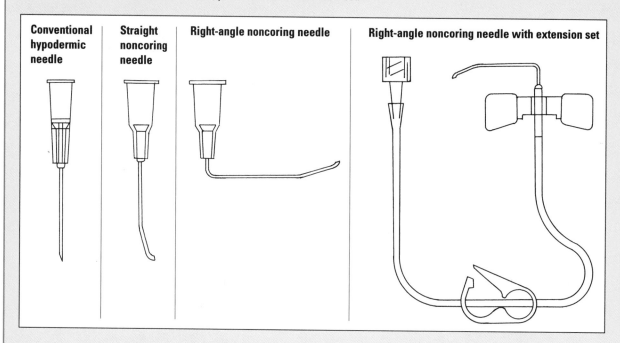

| Conventional hypodermic needle | Straight noncoring needle | Right-angle noncoring needle | Right-angle noncoring needle with extension set |

Giving a bolus using a VAP

With special training, you can safely administer drugs using a VAP. You may use a straight noncoring needle for bolus injections and a right-angled noncoring needle with an attached extension set for bolus injections or for infusions. In all cases, remember to use strict aseptic technique and to flush the device as specified in your facility's policy.

What you need

Prescribed drug ✳ noncoring needle of appropriate size ✳ three alcohol pads ✳ three povidone-iodine pads ✳ syringe with 3 to

5 ml of heparin solution (100 U/ml) ✳ 10-ml syringe with normal saline solution ✳ 7″ extension set (if needed) ✳ 2″ × 2″ sterile gauze dressing ✳ sterile towel ✳ tape ✳ mask ✳ sterile gloves

Getting ready

- Verify the order on the patient's chart.
- Identify the patient by checking his armband.
- Explain the procedure to the patient.
- Wash your hands.

How you do it

- Palpate to assess the depth and size of the VAP.

Ice might be nice

- If the patient is anxious or the port newly inserted, apply a topical anesthetic 60 minutes before the injection, or use an ice pack for 1 to 2 minutes just before the injection.
- Wash your hands again, set up your equipment on a sterile field, and put on sterile gloves.
- Attach the saline-filled syringe to the extension set and then to the noncoring needle.

Primed and ready

- Prime all air out of the system.
- Clean the site with the alcohol pads, then with the povidone-iodine pads. Start in the center and spiral outward about 2″ (5 cm). Let the povidone-iodine solution air-dry before you give the injection.
- Stabilize the VAP between your thumb and forefinger.

Take aim

- Hold the noncoring needle like a dart at a 90-degree angle over the VAP.
- Push the needle straight through the skin and septum until it hits the needle stop. Don't insert the needle at an angle; doing so may damage the septum.
- Verify correct needle placement by aspirating for blood. If you get no return, have the patient cough, turn, raise his arms, or take a deep breath. If you still get no return, remove the needle and try a different site. Repeated needle sticks in the same spot can cause skin erosion over the septum and possibly infection.

Here's a tip

- Steadily inject 5 ml of the saline flush solution. If you can't do this, the needle tip may not be in the correct position. Check that

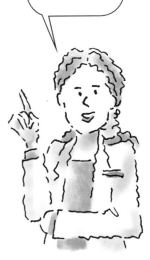

Remember to hold the noncoring needle like a dart at a 90-degree angle over the VAP.

the needle tip has advanced to the needle stop, and try to inject the solution again. (See *Flushing a VAP.*)
• After you've given the saline flush, clamp the extension tubing, remove the saline syringe, and attach the drug syringe. Then inject the prescribed drug.

Keep flushing

• Flush the tubing and port with 5 ml of normal saline solution after each drug injection to reduce the risk of drug incompatibility. Clamp the extension tubing each time you change syringes.
• Finally, flush the tubing with 3 to 5 ml of heparin solution according to your facility's policy.
• To remove the needle, stabilize the reservoir between your thumb and forefinger. Then grasp the needle and pull straight up and out. Don't twist or turn the needle.

Peak technique

Flushing a VAP

Flushing is part of the routine care of a vascular access port (VAP). See the illustrations below for a demonstration.

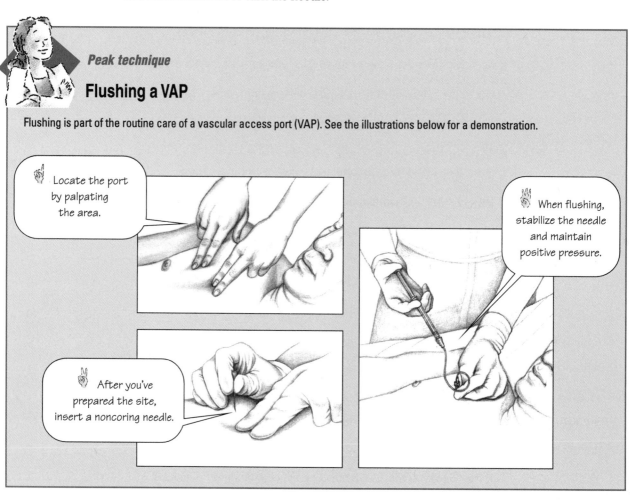

Locate the port by palpating the area.

After you've prepared the site, insert a noncoring needle.

When flushing, stabilize the needle and maintain positive pressure.

Caution

- You may meet resistance when removing a noncoring needle, which raises the risk that you'll stick yourself once the needle pulls free. Use caution or a protective device when removing a needle.
- After you have withdrawn the needle, you may note a slight serosanguineous discharge at the insertion site. Place a 2″ × 2″ sterile gauze dressing over the site.
- Discard used items according to standard precautions.

Practice pointers

- A patient with a VAP faces most of the same risks raised by traditional central venous catheters. Complications include hematoma, occlusion, infection, air embolism, extravasation, and VAP displacement.

Prone to precipitate

- Certain drugs, such as diazepam, calcium gluconate, and phenytoin, are prone to precipitate in the device and occlude the catheter. Some facilities use hydrochloric acid or sodium bicarbonate to break up the precipitate. Lipid occlusions can sometimes be cleared with ethyl alcohol.
- Erythema at the VAP site may be the first sign of infection. Preventing infection requires strict aseptic technique during both insertion and routine care.

Burn baby burn

- If the patient complains of burning at the port site, investigate thoroughly. (See *Uncovering extravasation.*)

What to teach

- Provide the patient with written material that includes a clear description of the port, including the type, brand name, location, gauge, length of catheter and access needles, insertion date, condition at discharge, and the environment in which the line was placed and by whom. Instruct the patient to keep this information handy and to present it to health care providers when necessary.
- Reassure him that a VAP won't restrict his activities and requires little maintenance except when the port is in use.

Have your patient hit bottom

- If the VAP is used at home for periodic infusions, make sure the patient or caregiver knows how to access the port. Stress that he should feel the needle hitting the reservoir bottom before he starts the infusion or injection.

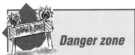

Danger zone

Uncovering extravasation

If the patient complains of burning at the port site, the needle may have dislodged from the port, causing extravasation. Look for edema under the patient's arm or in the neck area. Follow your facility's policy for treating extravasation. If you think the VAP is displaced, arrange for an X-ray to locate the tip.

• Teach the patient how to confirm correct needle placement with a blood return and how to change the dressing.
• Make sure he knows how and when to flush the VAP, how to recognize local and systemic complications, and when to report a complication.
• Urge him to carry identification that mentions the VAP.
• Tell the patient that he may need to take an antibiotic before undergoing dental work, surgery, or other invasive procedures.
• Warn him not to manipulate the VAP under his skin; doing so can displace the catheter or the port itself.

Giving an infusion with a VAP

A VAP can be used to infuse nutrition solutions, blood products, fluid replacement, and more. To keep the catheter attached, you'll need to use an infusion pump with a pressure rating lower than the pounds-per-square-inch rating of the VAP. Also, always use luer-lock connections to prevent the air embolism that could result from disconnected tubing.

What you need

Sterile gloves ✳ mask ✳ three alcohol pads ✳ three povidone-iodine pads ✳ 10-ml syringe that contains normal saline solution ✳ right-angled noncoring needle ✳ extension set with luer-lock and clamp (as needed) ✳ sterile towel ✳ prescribed I.V. solution and administration set ✳ infusion control device ✳ sterile adhesive strips ✳ 2″ × 2″ sterile gauze ✳ sterile transparent semipermeable membrane dressing

Getting ready

• Verify the order on the patient's chart.
• Identify the patient by checking his armband.
• Explain the procedure to the patient.
• Wash your hands.

Palpate the port

• Examine and palpate the access site and catheter track.
• Wash your hands again, assemble the solution container and tubing, and prime the tubing.

How you do it

• Using aseptic technique, prepare your sterile supplies on the sterile towel. Then put on a mask and sterile gloves.
• Prepare the site using alcohol and povidone-iodine pads. Let the skin air-dry.

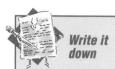

Documenting VAP bolus administration

Be sure to record:
• your assessment of the access site
• confirmation of patency
• each step taken to access a vascular access port (VAP) or remove a needle
• drugs or fluids infused
• needle size used
• dressing changes performed
• patient's response to the procedures
• patient teaching provided
• complications and the steps taken to handle them.

Peak technique

Stabilizing the VAP needle

Stabilize the needle at its hub using sterile adhesive strips. The right angle of the noncoring needle should sit as close to the skin as possible. Place a sterile 2" × 2" gauze pad under the needle for support, if needed, as shown in the first illustration below. Cover the needle with a transparent semipermeable membrane dressing, as shown in the second illustration below. Make sure the site is visible, and assess for edema, erythema, drainage, bleeding, or bruising.

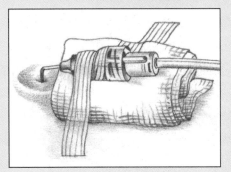

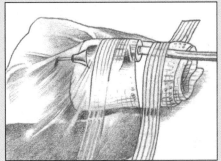

• Using aseptic technique, stabilize the port and insert the needle at a 90-degree angle until it touches the needle stop at the back of the port reservoir.
• Using the saline-filled syringe, aspirate for a blood return. When you get one, flush the catheter and clamp it. Maintain positive pressure in the VAP and tubing.

If at first you don't succeed...

• If aspiration or flushing proves difficult, reposition the patient and try again. Notify a doctor if aspiration and flushing fail to prompt a blood return.
• Stabilize the needle at its hub. (See *Stabilizing the VAP needle.*)
• Connect the I.V. tubing to the needle extension set.
• Unclamp the administration set and extension tubing, and begin the infusion. Tape the tubing and extension set securely to avoid placing tension on the tubing and accidentally dislodging the needle.

Keep watch

• During the infusion and at least every 8 hours, check for infiltration, especially when giving a vesicant drug.
• Discard used items according to standard precautions.

To prevent an air embolism caused by disconnected tubing, use luer-lock connections.

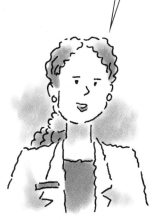

• If you're administering long-term therapy, change the noncoring needle and extension tubing at least every 7 days. Change the injection caps of a needleless system at the same time. Change the sterile occlusive dressing every 3 to 7 days (right away if it becomes loose, soiled, or wet) according to your facility's policy.

To flush (with heparin)...

• According to your facility's policy, regularly flush a dormant catheter with 5 ml of normal saline solution using the pulsing flush technique, which helps to clean fibrin residue from the lumen and reduces the risk of fibrin sheath formation. Afterward, use 3 to 5 ml of heparin flush solution (100 U/ml), according to your facility's policy.

...or not to flush?

• If the port is attached to a Groshong catheter, use 10 to 20 ml of normal saline solution, not heparin, as a flush. A *Groshong catheter* is a common tunneled catheter that has a pressure-sensitive valve in the catheter tip that keeps the lumen closed when not in use and opens inward during blood aspiration and outward during blood or fluid administration, eliminating the need to flush with heparin.
• If you're using one lumen of a two-lumen VAP, label the lumens carefully. Flush the dormant port according to your facility's policy. Rotating ports during prolonged therapy may increase the life of the septum.

Keep it together

• Don't use excessive pressure when flushing a two-lumen VAP because the catheter and VAP could separate.

Practice pointers

• A patient with a VAP faces most of the same risks raised by traditional central venous catheters. Complications include hematoma, occlusion, infection, air embolism, extravasation, and VAP displacement.
• Certain drugs, such as diazepam, calcium gluconate, and phenytoin, are prone to precipitate in the device and occlude the catheter. Some facilities use hydrochloric acid or sodium bicarbonate to break up the precipitate. Lipid occlusions can sometimes be cleared with ethyl alcohol.

Follow the signs

• Erythema at the VAP site may be the first sign of infection. Preventing infection requires strict aseptic technique during both insertion and routine care.

• If the patient complains of burning at the port site, the needle may have dislodged from the port, causing extravasation. Look for edema under the patient's arm or in the neck area. Follow your facility's policy for treating extravasation. If you think the VAP is displaced, arrange for an X-ray to locate the tip.

What to teach

• Provide the patient with written material that includes a clear description of the port, including the type, brand name, location, gauge, length of catheter and access needles, insertion date, condition at discharge, and the environment in which the line was placed and by whom. Instruct the patient to keep this information handy and to present it to health care providers when necessary.
• Reassure him that a VAP won't restrict his activities and requires little maintenance except when the port is in use.

On the home front

• If the VAP is used at home for periodic infusions, make sure the patient or caregiver knows how to access the port. Stress that he should feel the needle hitting the reservoir bottom before he starts the infusion or injection.
• Teach the patient how to confirm correct needle placement with a blood return and how to change the dressing.
• Make sure he knows how and when to flush the VAP, how to recognize local and systemic complications, and when to report a complication.
• Urge him to carry identification that mentions the VAP.
• Tell the patient that he may need to take an antibiotic before undergoing dental work, surgery, or other invasive procedures.
• Warn him not to manipulate the VAP under his skin; doing so can displace the catheter or the port itself.

Write it down

Documenting infusion through a VAP

Be sure to record:
• your assessment of the access site
• confirmation of patency
• each step taken to access a vascular access port (VAP) or remove a needle
• drugs or fluids infused
• needle size used
• dressing changes performed
• patient's response to the procedures
• patient teaching provided
• complications and the steps taken to handle them.

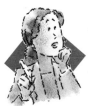

Quick quiz

1. When inserting an older adult's peripheral I.V. access, which of the following catheters would you use to avoid trauma?

    A.   18G
    B.   20G
    C.   22G
    D.   16G

Answer: C. To avoid trauma when inserting an older adult's peripheral I.V. access, use a 24G or 22G catheter.

2. Which of the following tunneled central venous (CV) catheters has the advantage of a valve that eliminates the need for Valsalva's maneuver, frequent flushing, and heparin?

    A.   Groshong
    B.   Hickman
    C.   Broviac
    D.   Per-Q-Cath

Answer: A. Groshong tunneled CV catheters have the advantage of a valve that eliminates the need for Valsalva's maneuver, frequent flushing, and heparin.

3. If your patient with a CV catheter in place developed dyspnea, chest pain, cyanosis, and decreased breath sounds on the same side as the catheter, which of the following complications would you suspect?

    A.   Pneumothorax
    B.   Thrombosis
    C.   Systemic infection
    D.   Catheter malposition

Answer: A. Dyspnea, chest pain, cyanosis, and decreased breath sounds on the same side as the CV catheter are signs and symptoms of pneumothorax, hemothorax, chylothorax, and hydrothorax.

4. Which of the following I.V. catheters is best to use to administer highly osmolar or caustic fluids?

    A.   Peripheral arterial catheter
    B.   Peripheral venous catheter
    C.   Midline catheter
    D.   Central venous (CV) catheter

Answer: D. A CV catheter can be used to administer highly osmolar or caustic fluids, because fluids and drugs are rapidly diluted in the large vena cava, thereby reducing the risk of chemical phlebitis.

Scoring

☆☆☆ If you answered all four questions correctly, superb! You truly belong in an I.V. League school!

☆☆ If you answered two or three correctly, great! You have no confusion when it comes to infusion!

☆ If you answered fewer than two correctly, it looks as if you have intermittent trouble with I.V. administration. For continuous success, review the chapter!

Specialized routes of administration

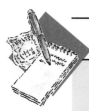

Just the facts

In this chapter, you'll learn:

♦ about specialized routes of administration

♦ how to administer drugs through specialized routes

♦ patient teaching associated with specialized routes

♦ how to document administration through specialized routes.

Understanding specialized routes of administration

Parenteral drugs aren't administered only into skin, muscles, and blood vessels. They can also be delivered into the:

- epidural space
- pleural space
- peritoneal cavity
- capsule of a joint
- interior of a long bone.

Going on special assignment

You may assist with drug delivery using these specialized routes or, after receiving special training, you may be able to deliver some of these drugs on your own. This chapter reviews the principles of drug delivery by these specialized routes, and it outlines the practices you should follow when using these routes.

Administering epidural drugs

Between the spinal cord and the ligamentum flavum that lines the vertebrae is the epidural space. To deliver drugs into the epidural space, you'll use an epidural catheter.

A doctor or nurse-anesthetist places an epidural catheter percutaneously into the epidural space after inserting a needle between two vertebrae. The catheter is then threaded through the needle and advanced into the epidural space. (See *Epidural catheter placement.*)

Pain prevention

Typically, you'll use the epidural route to give analgesic drugs. Opioids given by this route diffuse across the dura mater and mix with the patient's cerebrospinal fluid (CSF). They then bind with opiate receptors, blocking transmission of pain signals to the thalamus. Local anesthetics block pain signals moving from the dorsal root ganglion to the spinal cord.

Giving an opioid and a local anesthetic together may provide the analgesic effects of both drugs while allowing the use of lower doses, thus reducing the risk of adverse effects.

Race across the dura

Lipid-soluble drugs readily cross the dura mater and relieve pain rapidly. These drugs include:
- fentanyl
- sufentanil
- bupivacaine.

Epidural catheter placement

An epidural catheter enters the body between two vertebrae and extends into the epidural space, as shown in the illustration. It exits the body directly over the spine.

Body divisions
To produce analgesia for the chest and upper abdomen, the catheter is placed between the fifth and eighth thoracic vertebrae. To produce analgesia for the lower abdomen and legs, it's placed between the second and fourth lumbar vertebrae.

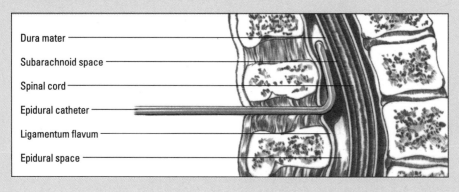

Dura mater

Subarachnoid space

Spinal cord

Epidural catheter

Ligamentum flavum

Epidural space

Water-soluble drugs cross the dura more slowly, resulting in pain relief of slower onset and longer duration. These drugs include:
• morphine
• hydromorphone.

Find another route

Don't give epidural drugs to a patient with:
• a low platelet count
• a coagulation disorder
• a local infection
• a diagnosed structural problem in the spinal column or epidural space
• spinal arthritis
• hypotension
• marked hypertension
• an allergy to the prescribed drug.

No preservatives!

All drugs administered into the epidural space must be preservative-free because preservatives can cause nerve damage.

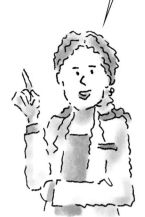

Remember, only preservative-free drugs can be given into the epidural space.

Giving an epidural drug

To give an epidural, drug follow the instructions below.

What you need

Povidone-iodine pads ✳ 5-ml syringe ✳ sterile gloves ✳ mask ✳ sterile 2″ × 2″ gauze pads ✳ transparent semipermeable dressing ✳ sterile, fenestrated drape ✳ infusion pump

Getting ready

• Verify the order on the patient's chart.
• Explain the procedure to the patient.
• Take the patient's vital signs.
• Wash your hands and put on sterile gloves and a mask.
• Drape the catheter area.
• Clean the injection cap with the povidone-iodine pads, and allow the solution to dry completely.

How you do it

• Insert the needle of the empty 5-ml syringe into the injection cap, and try to aspirate. If blood or CSF enters the syringe, stop the procedure and notify a doctor. If you don't aspirate blood or CSF, proceed with drug administration.

Gear up!

Changing injection caps and filters

The injection cap and filter on your patient's epidural catheter should be changed every 48 to 72 hours. To do so properly, follow these steps:
• First, gather a new injection cap, a new filter, povidone-iodine swabs, preservative-free normal saline solution, sterile gloves, and a mask.
• Wash your hands, and tell the patient what you're preparing to do.
• Put on sterile gloves and a mask.
• Connect the new injection cap to the new filter, and flush it with 3 ml of sterile, preservative-free normal saline solution.
• Clean the connection between the catheter and the filter with a povidone-iodine pad.
• Remove the old filter and injection cap.
• Using sterile technique, screw on the new filter and cap. Make sure they're attached securely.
• Dispose of all used equipment according to standard precautions.

Bolus dose

• For a bolus injection, replace the empty syringe with the drug-filled syringe, and then inject the drug into the catheter at the prescribed rate.

Continuous run

• For a continuous infusion, confirm the drug and the infusion rate. Then attach the tubing or filter to the drug container and purge all air from the system.
• Make sure you use a 0.2-micron filter without surfactant for epidural drug infusion. Also, always use luer-lock connections to the catheter.
• Attach the tubing to the infusion pump, and program the pump to deliver the drug at the prescribed rate.
• Begin the infusion at the prescribed rate.
• Label the drug container, tubing, and catheter FOR EPIDURAL USE ONLY to prevent medication errors.
• Coil the catheter and secure it with tape to prevent pulling on it.
• Dispose of all used equipment according to standard precautions.

Practice pointers

• Make sure you change the injection cap according to your facility's policy. (See *Changing injection caps and filters*.)

Danger zone

Headache alert!

When a patient is receiving drugs through the epidural route, it's important to monitor him closely for headache. If the patient develops a prolonged, pounding headache that worsens in a sitting or standing position, the catheter may have punctured the dura mater, which allows cerebrospinal fluid to leak from the epidural space and reduces pressure in the spinal canal. Notify a doctor immediately because the patient could receive an overdose of the ordered analgesic.

Patchwork

If the headache doesn't subside within 48 hours, the doctor may prescribe a blood patch, which involves withdrawing about 10 ml of the patient's blood from a peripheral vein and injecting it into the epidural space. As the blood clots, it typically seals off the leaking area, which relieves the headache.

• Assess the catheter exit site regularly, and clean it thoroughly with povidone-iodine pads according to your facility's policy. Using a circular pattern, start wiping at the exit site and move outward about 2″ or 3″ (5 to 7.5 cm). Let the povidone-iodine air-dry, and then apply a sterile gauze or transparent semipermeable dressing as prescribed.
• Don't use alcohol to clean the exit site because it could cause nerve damage if it gets into the epidural space.
• Check the position of the catheter by measuring its external length and, if your facility allows, by aspirating it. If you aspirate blood or CSF, notify a doctor. The catheter should be repositioned. (See *Headache alert!*)

Know your limits

• Policies and procedures for obtaining and delivering epidural drugs, discarding unused drugs, and documenting drug delivery vary by facility and by state nurse practice act. Make sure you know the requirements that apply to you.

What to teach

• Explain to the patient the purpose and effects of epidural analgesia, and the possible adverse effects of the analgesics used.

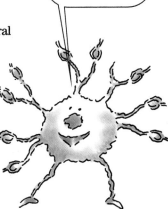

Hey, watch that alcohol! Cleaning the exit site of an epidural catheter with alcohol can cause nerve damage.

• Teach the patient additional ways to effectively manage his pain, and advise him to report continued pain. To help track changes in his pain, have him use a 0 to 10 scale in which 0 means no pain and 10 means the worst pain possible.

Administering intrapleural drugs

The pleural space is sandwiched between the visceral pleura that hugs the surface of the lungs and the parietal pleura that lines the chest cavity. Normally, this space contains a small amount of fluid that allows the pleural membranes to slide easily past each other during respiration.

Chemo and other concerns

Drugs may be delivered into the pleural space:
• to treat spontaneous pneumothorax
• to resolve pleural effusions
• to deliver chemotherapy. (See *Intrapleural drug administration.*)

For a patient with empyema, pleural effusion, or pneumothorax, intrapleural drugs are typically administered through a chest tube. For patients with other problems, delivery usually takes place through an intrapleural catheter.

When intrapleural is inappropriate

Some patients, such as those with fibrosis, adhesions, pleural inflammation, bullous emphysema, sepsis, or infection at the puncture site, shouldn't receive intrapleural drugs. Intrapleural delivery also isn't suitable for a patient receiving positive end-expiratory pressure because the treatment may worsen the patient's respiratory condition.

Giving an intrapleural drug

Usually, a doctor administers intrapleural drugs and a nurse assists.

What you need

Prescribed drug in a 60-ml syringe ✻ rubber-tipped clamp (for a chest tube) ✻ face shield ✻ gown ✻ sterile gloves ✻ sterile gauze ✻ povidone-iodine solution ✻ needles of appropriate size ✻ 1% lidocaine (if needed) ✻ dressings ✻ tape ✻ sterile drape

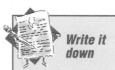

Write it down

Documenting the epidural route

Be sure to record:
• dates, times, and patient tolerance of all procedures (including site care)
• dose, volume, and rate of all drugs given
• type and amount of solution used to flush the catheter
• aspirate obtained
• degree of pain relief
• patient teaching
• complications
• nursing actions in response to complications.

Peak technique

Intrapleural drug administration

In intrapleural administration, a doctor injects a drug into the pleural space using a catheter. Before the procedure, help the patient lie on his side with the affected side up. The doctor then inserts a needle into the fourth to eighth intercostal space, 3″ to 4″ (7.5 to 10 cm) from the posterior midline. He advances the needle medially over the superior edge of the patient's rib through the intercostal muscles until it penetrates the parietal pleura at an angle, as shown below. The catheter is then advanced into the pleural space through the needle, which is subsequently removed.

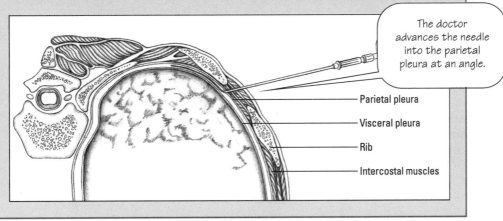

The doctor advances the needle into the parietal pleura at an angle.

Parietal pleura

Visceral pleura

Rib

Intercostal muscles

Getting ready

- Verify the order on the patient's chart.
- Confirm the drug and, if necessary, calculate the dose and dilute it with normal saline solution or other diluent, as ordered.
- Explain the procedure to the patient.
- Administer a narcotic analgesic or an antiemetic, if prescribed, 30 minutes before intrapleural administration.

How you do it

- Draw up the intrapleural drug in a 60-ml syringe.
- Position the patient with the affected side up.
- Help the doctor remove the dressing from the intrapleural catheter or chest tube, then clamp the chest tube.
- Provide antiseptic-soaked gauze so the doctor can disinfect the access port of the catheter or chest tube.
- Hand the syringe and drug vial to the doctor so he can verify the correct drug and dose before injecting the drug.

Practice pointers

• Check your state's nurse practice act and your facility's policy to see what role you should play in intrapleural drug administration.
• Assess the patient's respiratory status before, during, and every 15 minutes for 1 hour after intrapleural delivery.
• Monitor the patient during the procedure for adverse reactions.
• If the patient will be receiving a continuous infusion, label the solution bag FOR INTRAPLEURAL USE ONLY. Cover all injection ports so other drugs aren't accidentally injected into the pleural space.

Inflation index

• Keep rubber-tipped clamps at the bedside. If a commercial chest-tube system cracks or a tube disconnects, temporarily clamp the chest tube close to the insertion site. Watch the patient closely for signs of tension pneumothorax because no air can escape from the pleural space while the tube is clamped.
• Watch for complications of intrapleural drug delivery, such as pneumothorax, tension pneumothorax (if air accidentally enters the pleural cavity), chemical irritation of the pleurae and subsequent neutropenia or thrombocytopenia (or both), and infection at the insertion site. Meticulous skin preparation, strict sterile technique, and sterile dressings help to prevent infection.

Accidents happen

• If the chest tube accidentally dislodges, cover the site at once with a sterile air-occlusive dressing, and tape the pad in place. Have another nurse call a doctor and gather any equipment needed to reinsert the tube. Meanwhile, stay with the patient, monitor his vital signs, and assess carefully for evidence of tension pneumothorax, such as hypotension, distended neck veins, absent breath sounds, a tracheal shift, hypoxemia, dyspnea, tachypnea, diaphoresis, chest pain, and a weak, rapid pulse.

What to teach

• Keep the patient informed throughout the procedure. Provide comfort measures and instruct him to remain on the unaffected side for 10 to 30 minutes, as tolerated, to help make sure the drug circulates between the pleurae.

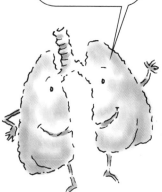

Cover the injection ports so other drugs aren't accidentally injected into the pleural space.

Administering intraperitoneal drugs

Drugs may be instilled into the peritoneal cavity for dialysis or chemotherapy. Catheters used for this type of administration include:
- short-term
- long-term
- implanted subcutaneous port.

Short and sweet

Short-term intraperitoneal catheters are rigid and designed for one-time or infrequent use, as when a patient receives chemotherapy only once a month. Each time it's used, a doctor inserts a new short-term intraperitoneal catheter. The device can be inserted at the bedside and used right away. It's less expensive and easier to remove than other intraperitoneal devices.

Short-term catheters can puncture organs, however, and may cause more pain than other devices. They're also more likely to leak and migrate out of the intraperitoneal cavity.

Take a long look at this

Long-term intraperitoneal catheters are made of silicone and polyurethane and usually have one or two cuffs that encourage tissue to grow around the catheter. The tissue stabilizes the catheter, blocks pathogens from entering, and prevents fluid from leaking.

This type of catheter offers a low risk of organ perforation and allows intermittent treatments over a long period, as may be needed for patients treated with chemotherapy. The catheter can be managed at home, and surgery isn't required for removal. (See *Tackling the Tenckhoff*, page 296.)

Getting under the skin

A subcutaneous intraperitoneal port is implanted under the skin of the patient's abdomen. A catheter tunneled through subcutaneous tissue leads from the port into the patient's peritoneal cavity. The body of the port has a drug reservoir and a self-sealing silicone septum that can withstand up to 2,000 needle punctures. Two cuffs anchor the catheter in place. The port itself may be made of stainless steel, titanium, plastic, polysulfone, or a combination of materials. Catheters are available in silicone or polyurethane and usually have radiopaque strips or tips that are visible under fluoroscopy.

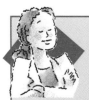

Peak technique

Tackling the Tenckhoff

To implant a Tenckhoff catheter (a peritoneal catheter that can be used for chemotherapy), the surgeon inserts the first 6 ¾″ (17 cm) of the catheter into the patient's abdomen. The next 2 ¾″ (7-cm) segment, which may have a Dacron cuff at one or both ends, is imbedded subcutaneously. Within a few days after insertion, the patient's tissues grow around the cuffs, forming a tight barrier against bacterial infiltration. The remaining 3 ⅞″ (10 cm) of the catheter extends outside the abdomen and has an adapter at the tip that connects to I.V. tubing.

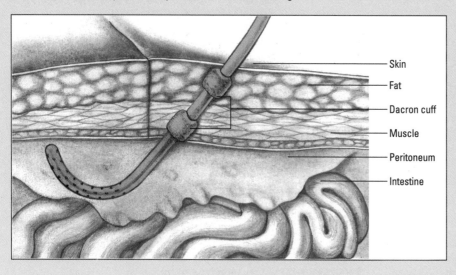

- Skin
- Fat
- Dacron cuff
- Muscle
- Peritoneum
- Intestine

User-friendly

These intraperitoneal ports tend to be more expensive than external catheters, and they don't allow high-pressure irrigation, forced irrigation, or manipulation to dislodge or loosen clots. However, because the port lacks an external catheter, it requires no special management after the patient goes home. It also offers a lower risk for infection and organ perforation than external catheters because the port is inserted during surgery.

What's im-port-ant to know

This type of port usually isn't appropriate for a patient who:
- has an infection
- has too little body tissue to anchor the device
- is obese (because of the difficulty in accessing the port)
- has had chest radiation or a mastectomy.

Giving a peritoneal infusion

Peritoneal infusions have three phases:
• During infusion time, the dialysate or chemotherapy drug flows into the peritoneal cavity.
• During dwell time, the instilled fluid remains in the peritoneal cavity.
• During drain time, the dialysate or chemotherapy drug flows out of the peritoneal cavity. (Some chemotherapy drugs may be left in the peritoneal cavity and absorbed into the portal circulation.)

What you need

Y-type dialysis administration set ✳ drainage bag ✳ warmed dialysate or chemotherapy drug ✳ povidone-iodine pads ✳ povidone-iodine solution ✳ two pairs of sterile gloves ✳ two or more masks ✳ a gown ✳ sterile 4″ × 4″ gauze pads ✳ tape ✳ two water-resistant sterile barriers or drapes ✳ normal saline solution ✳ antiseptic swabs

Getting ready

• To begin, explain to the patient what you'll be doing.
• Weigh the patient, obtain his vital signs, and measure his abdominal girth.
• Wash your hands, and put on a gown, a mask, and sterile gloves.
• Open the Y-type administration set and attach the single-output line to the drainage bag.
• Close the roller clamps on the tubing.
• Remove the cover from one tubing spike and insert this spike into the dialysate or other bag of solution.

Prime time

• Open the roller clamp between the dialysate or other solution and the patient. Prime the tubing. After you've expelled the air, close the roller clamp.
• Open the roller clamps to the drainage bag, and prime this section of tubing as well. Then close all clamps.
• Have the patient put on a mask.
• Next, create a sterile field using the sterile barrier or drape. Place the gauze pads and povidone-iodine solution and pads onto the sterile field.
• Place a second sterile barrier under the extension tubing leading from the catheter.
• Remove and discard your gloves according to standard precautions; then put on a new pair of sterile gloves.

How you do it

Here are instructions for administering a peritoneal infusion through a catheter and through an implanted port.

Administering an infusion through the catheter

- Using strict sterile technique, clean the catheter's connection site with povidone-iodine.
- Remove the cap from the extension tubing and connect the catheter tubing to the administration set.
- Secure the connection with adhesive tape. Also tape a loop of tubing to the patient's abdomen to prevent tension on the catheter.
- Open the clamp on the catheter extension tubing and on the administration set tubing so the dialysate or other solution can flow into the patient's peritoneal cavity. Record the time the infusion starts.
- Make sure the roller clamp on the drainage bag remains closed to keep infusate from accidentally flowing out of the peritoneal cavity and into the bag.
- When the solution has entered the patient's peritoneal cavity, close the clamps on the infusion line and the catheter extension tubing to keep air out of the tubing and the peritoneal cavity.

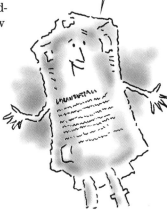

Close the roller clamp on the drainage bag or the infusate may accidentally flow into me! Yikes!

Positioning your patient

- Leave the solution in the cavity for the prescribed dwell time. As needed, turn the patient from side to side so the solution washes all surfaces in the peritoneum.
- At the end of the dwell time, drain the peritoneal cavity by opening the roller clamp that leads to the drainage bag and the catheter extension tubing. Reposition the patient as needed to help drain the fluid.
- As the fluid flows into the drainage bag, document its volume and color. Report abnormalities — such as grossly bloody fluid — to the doctor.

Do it again

- Repeat the infusion, dwell, and drain phases as prescribed.
- When you finish the full infusion, clean the catheter or tubing connection with povidone-iodine. Disconnect and discard the tubing according to standard precautions. Disinfect the open rim of the catheter, then place the sterile cap on it. Replace the dressing on the exit site, and secure the catheter.

Infusion through an implanted port

- First, locate the peritoneal port by palpating it through the patient's skin.

• Clean the skin over the port with antiseptic swabs, and allow the solution to air-dry.
• Put on sterile gloves, a mask, and a gown.
• Use your nondominant hand to hold the port steady, and then puncture the port with a noncoring needle that has been primed with normal saline solution and attached to an extension set or similar access device.

Anchors away

• Anchor the needle by placing sterile tape or adhesive strips across the hub of the needle and then wrapping the strips around the hub in a chevron pattern.
• Using a saline-filled syringe, verify the correct needle placement by trying to aspirate fluid. If you get no fluid return, then flush the port with normal saline solution.
• Connect the administration set to the extension tubing, and administer the infusion as you would through a catheter.

Practice pointers

• After an intraperitoneal catheter has been newly implanted for dialysis, flush the catheter according to your facility's policy or a doctor's order. For example, you may flush the catheter with 500 ml of a heparinized dialysate solution every 2 or 3 hours for 3 days. Then you'll fill the catheter with 5,000 U of heparin (1,000 U/ml) and cap it off. A healing period of 2 weeks allows the catheter to seal so it won't leak.
• Change the dressing daily until the site heals.

It's just routine

• Maintain the patency of an implanted port by routinely flushing it with 5 to 10 ml of normal saline solution. Also, flush it with 20 ml of a compatible solution before and after administering drugs through it.
• When removing a noncoring needle from a port, maintain positive pressure on the plunger.

Limit the pressure

• Don't exceed 40 pounds of pressure per square inch (psi) when delivering fluids through an intraperitoneal device. If you do, you may break the catheter or separate it from the body of the port. The infusion device should have a pressure setting, which will allow you to set an upper pressure limit.
• You may remove a short-term catheter as ordered. A doctor must remove a long-term catheter or an implanted port. (See *Removing a short-term catheter*, page 300.)

Removing a short-term catheter

If your patient has a long-term intraperitoneal catheter or an implanted port, a doctor will need to remove it at the end of therapy. If your patient has a short-term catheter, however, you may be asked to remove it. If so, follow these steps:

• Drain the peritoneal cavity, if indicated—after dialysis, for example.
• Wash your hands, and put on a mask and gloves.
• Remove the dressing and skin sutures, if present.
• Change to sterile gloves, and remove the catheter.
• If the exit site is large, apply adhesive strips to close it. If adhesive strips aren't sufficient, a doctor may need to close the site with a suture.
• Apply a topical antibiotic, if ordered, and a sterile dressing to the site.
• Inspect the site daily until it heals.

Documenting peritoneal infusion

Be sure to record:
• patient's vital signs, weight, and abdominal girth
• appearance of the exit site
• solution or drug administered, including the volume, dose, and rate
• drugs added to the dialysate
• color of the catheter drainage
• patient's response to the procedure
• patient teaching.

What to teach

• Teach the patient the purpose, use, and care of the catheter or port. Tell her not to take a shower or bath until the exit site is healed (about 4 to 6 weeks).

Helping with homework

• Explain how to perform intraperitoneal therapy at home, and discuss ways to help the fluid drain. For example, you may need to teach Valsalva's maneuver so the patient can use increased abdominal pressure to promote drainage. Also, show her how to flush the catheter or port.
• Explain the signs and symptoms of peritonitis, and tell the patient to report fever, chills, abdominal tenderness, anorexia, shortness of breath, nausea, and cloudy peritoneal drainage, as well as redness, swelling, tenderness, or drainage at the catheter exit site.

Administering intra-articular drugs

An intra-articular injection delivers a drug directly into the synovial cavity of a joint. This type of administration is used to:
• suppress inflammation
• relieve pain
• help preserve joint mobility

- prevent contractures
- delay muscle atrophy.

Drug profile

Drugs delivered most commonly by this route include cortico-steroids, anesthetics, and lubricants. These are usually intended to provide local, short-term treatment of rheumatoid arthritis, gout, systemic lupus erythematosus, osteoarthritis, or other joint disorders.

Intra-articular drugs must be absorbed into tissues or cells before they can exert an effect. Like other parenterally administered drugs, they have fewer barriers to overcome than oral drugs. However, doctors use the intra-articular route sparingly because of the greater risk of infection and the difficulty of delivering a drug into a synovial joint.

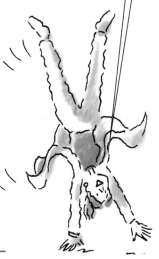

Intra-articular injections can be used to preserve joint mobility.

Not in this joint

The intra-articular route isn't appropriate for patients with:
- joint infection, instability, or fracture
- systemic fungal infection
- psoriasis around the injection site
- bacteremia
- bleeding disorders
- total arthroplasty.

Giving an intra-articular injection

To inject a drug into a synovial cavity, a doctor uses a standard needle and syringe. He may first aspirate fluid from the joint to relieve pain and inflammation and to improve the patient's range of motion.

What you need

18G 1½″ to 26G ⅝″ needle (depending on which joint is affected) ✳prescribed drug ✳3-ml and 5-, 10-, or 20-ml syringes ✳sterile towels ✳pillows ✳gauze pads ✳sterile gloves ✳emesis basin ✳ povidone-iodine or another antiseptic cleaning solution ✳drape ✳ 1% lidocaine, ethyl chloride, or other local anesthetic ✳adhesive bandage ✳test tubes for synovial fluid, along with appropriate additives and specimen labels ✳glass slides and cover slips (if necessary)

Getting ready

- Wash your hands.
- Draw the prescribed amount of drug into the 5- or 10-ml syringe. Label the syringe with the name and amount of drug inside.

• Take the medication container into the patient's room so the doctor can verify the contents of the syringe.

Positions, please

• Position the patient appropriately and stabilize the affected joint, supporting it with pillows, if necessary. Expose the joint.
• Using sterile technique, create a sterile field by opening a sterile towel. Place needles of appropriate size, syringes, and gauze pads on the towel.
• After putting on sterile gloves, the doctor picks up the gauze pads and holds them over the emesis basin. Pour the antiseptic cleaning solution over the gauze pads to saturate them.
• The doctor cleans the injection site with the gauze pads, and then drapes the site. He fills the 3-ml syringe with a local anesthetic while you hold the bottle upside down. Then he anesthetizes the skin and subcutaneous tissue at the injection site.

How you do it

• If the doctor will aspirate synovial fluid, place the sterile test tubes and slides in the correct order. The doctor withdraws fluid using a needle of appropriate size and a syringe, and then sets the syringe aside until after the procedure. He leaves the needle in the joint to inject the drug.

Fill 'er up

• After the doctor has aspirated synovial fluid, hand him the filled medication syringe so he can attach it to the needle that's still lodged in the joint. If he didn't aspirate fluid, then hand him the medication syringe with the appropriate needle attached. He then injects the drug into the synovial cavity.
• After the injection, apply pressure to the site and, if necessary, gently massage the area for 1 to 2 minutes to promote drug absorption. Then apply an adhesive bandage.

Practice pointers

• If the doctor has aspirated fluid, attach a needle to the specimen syringe and instill appropriate specimens into test tubes or onto slides. Appropriately label the test tubes or slides and send them to the laboratory. Aspirated fluid may be cultured or examined under a microscope to help diagnose joint effusion, infection, or trauma.

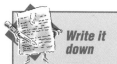

Write it down

Documenting intra-articular administration

Be sure to record:
• date, time, and site of the injection
• name of the doctor who administered the injection
• amount of synovial fluid aspirated (if any)
• all laboratory studies
• patient's tolerance of the procedure
• drug and dose given
• patient teaching.

What to teach

• As prescribed, tell the patient to rest the joint for 24 to 48 hours after the injection. Advise him to call his doctor if he develops a fever or redness, swelling, or persistent pain at the injection site.

Administering intraosseous drugs

The intraosseous route allows rapid administration of fluids and drugs into bone marrow. Fluid injected into bone marrow drains rapidly into the central venous channel and enters the systemic circulation through smaller veins.

Emergency!

Intraosseous infusion can be used for infants, children, or adults when emergency venous access can't be established within the first 2 minutes of care. It may also be used to administer regional anesthesia during treatment of certain orthopedic conditions in which venous access fails or isn't feasible. The intraosseous needle should be removed as soon as standard venous access has been established.

Needling remarks

The needle used to administer an intraosseous infusion varies with the patient's age and size. Some disposable needles are designed especially for intraosseous infusion. A sharp obturator protects the tip of the needle, and screw-type threads help the needle penetrate the bone. However, you may opt to use a steel hypodermic, spinal, trephine, sternal, or standard bone marrow needle as long as it has:
• a short shaft (to avoid accidental dislodgment)
• a stylet (to keep the needle from being plugged with bone)
• a large bore
• rigidity
• a handle that secures the stylet during insertion.

Bones to pick...or not to pick

Intraosseous infusion has a high success rate and few complications. However, it shouldn't be used in an infected area, in a bone in which intraosseous access has already been tried, or in a bone with an open fracture or a tumor. Also, avoid using this procedure if the patient has a bone disorder (such as osteoporosis).

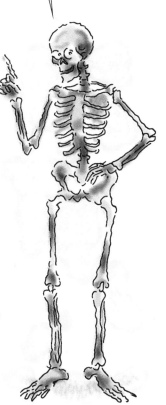

Avoid bones with open fractures or tumors when choosing a site for intraosseous infusion.

Giving an intraosseous infusion

Before you can insert an intraosseous needle, you'll need special training.

What you need

Device for needle insertion ✳intraosseous access needle and obturator of appropriate size ✳povidone-iodine pads ✳two pairs sterile gloves ✳3- to 5-ml syringe ✳1% lidocaine ✳normal saline flush solution ✳infusion syringe or I.V. administration set ✳medication and solution ✳sterile tape ✳sterile gauze or a transparent semipermeable membrane dressing ✳infusion pump, controller, or pressure infusion bag, as indicated

Getting ready

• Time constraints may severely limit your ability to properly prepare a patient for intraosseous infusion. However, preparation is important for a successful insertion. Begin by explaining the procedure to the patient or caregiver.

Map it out

• Determine the most appropriate site to insert the needle. (See *Intraosseous infusion sites.*)
• To find the proximal tibial site, measure one or two fingerbreadths below the tibial tuberosity on the anteromedial surface.
• Wash your hands.
• Set up a sterile field using sterile technique.
• If a limb will be used for the infusion, secure it in a comfortable, stable, dependent position. Restrain the limb if the patient is a child.
• Put on sterile gloves, and vigorously clean the skin over the site with povidone-iodine pads. Start in the center and work outward about 2″ (5 cm). Repeat, and allow the solution to air-dry.

How you do it

• Put on a fresh pair of sterile gloves.
• If ordered, anesthetize the skin with 1% lidocaine. Inject it down to the periosteum. Quickly advance the needle through the skin to the bony cortex. In some facilities, you'll use a bone injection gun to insert the needle. (See *Using a bone injection gun,* page 306.)
• If the patient is a child, angle the needle away from the joint space to avoid hitting the epiphyseal plate.

Ages and stages

Intraosseous infusion sites

Because bone marrow acts as a noncollapsible vein, drugs infused into the marrow cavity enter the circulation rapidly through an extensive network of medullary sinusoids, as shown to the right, top.

Child's site

An intraosseous site commonly recommended for use in children is the anteromedial surface of the proximal tibia, about 1″ (2.5 cm) below the tibial tuberosity, as shown to the right, bottom. Other sites that can be used in children are the distal tibia and the distal femur. Of the two, the distal tibia is preferred because of its thin covering of bony cortex and because it offers easier access on the flat area of bone proximal to the malleolus. The distal femur is more difficult because the bone is heavily padded with muscle and fat.

Sternal insertion isn't recommended for children because of the risk of penetrating the mediastinum. Also, don't insert an intraosseous needle into a child's epiphyseal plates.

Adults only

Recommended sites for adults include the iliac crest or sternum (except the upper anterior portion, where the injection could penetrate completely), the distal end of the radius, the proximal metaphysis of the humerus, and 1″ to 1½″ (2.5 to 3.5 cm) proximal to the distal tip of the lateral or medial malleolus. The needle can also be inserted into the ulnar styloid, the distal epiphysis of the second metacarpus, the distal epiphysis of the first metatarsus, the distal tibia, or the distal femur.

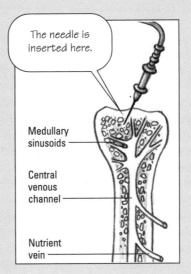

The needle is inserted here.

Medullary sinusoids

Central venous channel

Nutrient vein

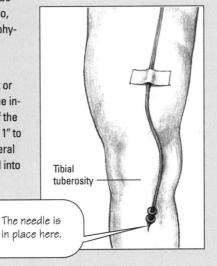

Tibial tuberosity

The needle is in place here.

• Insert the needle farther, into the marrow cavity, using firm pressure and a downward screwing or rotating motion. You'll feel the needle pass through the bony cortex and into a soft, hollow area — the spongy bone.

Gear up!

Using a bone injection gun

A bone injection gun—such as the B.I.G., manufactured by WaisMed Ltd.—can insert a 15G trocar needle (or an 18G needle for a child) rapidly and automatically into the bone of a patient. The needle is propelled by a powerful, charged coil.

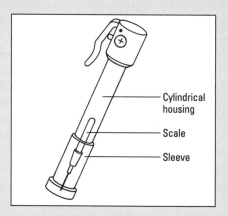

The gun starts in a locked position, as shown at right. First, set in centimeters the depth of penetration you need. In adults, injections into the proximal tibial metaphysis should penetrate to about 2.5 cm; into the medial malleolus, about 2 cm; into the lateral malleolus or distal metaphysis of the radius, about 1 to 1.5 cm.

After you've prepared the injection site, place the front of the gun perpendicular to and against the site. Hold the device firmly, pull out the safety latch, and trigger the B.I.G. by squeezing its two sides together. The housing will separate from the trocar-needle, as shown below, left.

Manually pull out the stylet trocar from the needle, leaving only the needle in the bone. After you've done so, attach either a syringe, as shown below, right, or standard I.V. tubing to the needle. Begin the infusion. Secure the needle, and apply dressings as for a standard intraosseous access needle.

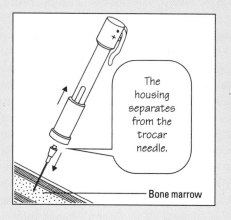

The housing separates from the trocar needle.

Bone marrow

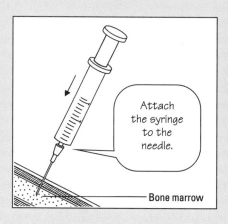

Attach the syringe to the needle.

Bone marrow

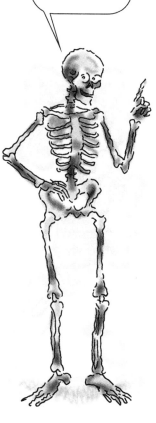

If you can't aspirate bone marrow or fluid doesn't infuse properly, the intraosseous needle may be obstructed.

Pop, you're in!

• When you feel a soft pop and a decrease in resistance, you've reached the bone marrow. The needle will stand upright without support when inserted into the bone.

• When you believe the tip of the needle is in the bone marrow, remove the obturator from the needle, attach a 5-ml syringe, and aspirate some bone marrow to verify the needle's placement.
• Replace the syringe with one that contains normal saline solution; then flush the cannula to clear it of blood and bone particles. If the needle is positioned correctly in the marrow, you should feel no resistance when flushing it.
• Remove the flush syringe and connect the needle to a standard syringe or I.V. administration set.
• Clean the site again with povidone-iodine pads.

Tight security

• Secure the needle with sterile tape. Also, securely tape the infusion syringe or I.V. tubing to keep the needle from rocking or being accidentally dislodged.
• Apply a sterile gauze or transparent semipermeable membrane dressing to the site.
• If the patient is conscious, minimize pain during the initial infusion by withdrawing 2 to 5 ml of bone marrow and then slowly injecting 2 to 5 ml of 1% lidocaine over 60 seconds.

If at first you don't succeed...

• If your first attempt to insert an intraosseous needle fails, use another bone for your second attempt. That way, you prevent infused fluid from leaking out of the original puncture site.

Practice pointers

• Drugs or fluids may be infused by gravity or infusion pump. The needle size and density and the size of the bone marrow cavity affect the rate of flow. Normal saline solution has been infused through a 13G intraosseous access needle by gravity at rates as high as 600 ml/hour and by an infusion pump at rates as high as 2,500 ml/hour.
• An intraosseous needle can become obstructed by pieces of bone marrow or blood clots, especially if the infusion is delayed or the needle isn't flushed after being inserted. Signs of obstruction include an inability to aspirate bone marrow and failure of the fluid to infuse properly. (See *Risky business.*)
• Don't use a bone injection gun if there's a skin infection, tumor, or fracture at the insertion site.

What to teach

• Explain to the patient the purpose, risks, and benefits of intraosseous infusion to the patient, parents, and family members. Doing so can help to allay their fears and encourage cooperation.

Danger zone

Risky business

The longer an intraosseous access needle is in place, the greater the risk of osteomyelitis. The risk also increases when the patient has another infection. Watch for signs of osteomyelitis, such as fever, pain, leukocytosis, and reduced movement in the affected limb.

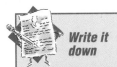

Write it down

Documenting an intraosseous infusion

Be sure to record:
• date and time of administration
• type and size of needle or cannula inserted
• site location and number of insertion attempts
• type and amount of flush solution
• drug or solution administered (including dose, volume, and rate)
• patient's response.

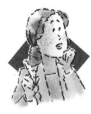

Quick quiz

1. You're unable to establish emergency I.V. access in a child who requires rapid fluid administration. You attempt intraosseous access. How do you know when you've reached the bone marrow?

    A.   Blood appears in the needle.
    B.   You feel a soft pop and a decrease in resistance.
    C.   You can aspirate fluid.
    D.   You feel an increase in resistance during aspiration.

Answer: B. When inserting an intraosseous needle, you'll feel a soft pop and a decrease in resistance when you've reached the bone marrow.

2. As you check the position of an epidural catheter, you aspirate blood. What should you do next?

    A.   Administer the prescribed medication.
    B.   Flush the catheter with a heparinized solution.
    C.   Reposition the catheter.
    D.   Notify the doctor immediately.

Answer: D. If you aspirate blood or cerebral spinal fluid, notify the doctor immediately. The catheter should be repositioned.

3. When delivering fluids through an intraperitoneal device, pressure shouldn't exceed:

    A.   20 psi.
    B.   40 psi.
    C.   60 psi.
    D.   80 psi.

Answer: B. Don't exceed 40 psi when delivering fluids through an intraperitoneal device.

Scoring

☆☆☆ If you answered all three questions correctly, excellent! Your specialty appears to be special routes of administration!

☆☆ If you answered fewer than three correctly, there's no reason to get bent out of joint. Review the chapter and you'll be back on the right route to success!

Part III   Specialized infusions

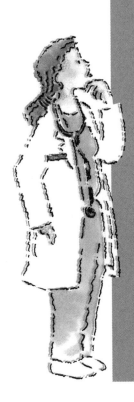

Chemotherapy infusions

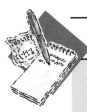

Just the facts

In this chapter, you'll learn:

♦ how chemotherapy works against cancer

♦ about the types of chemotherapeutic agents

♦ how to administer chemotherapy

♦ about the adverse effects of chemotherapy

♦ how to avoid dangerous exposure to chemotherapeutic drugs.

Understanding I.V. chemotherapy

Chemotherapy, surgery, and radiation are the mainstays of cancer treatment. Chemotherapy is most commonly administered I.V., using peripheral or central veins — although it's also administered by the oral, subcutaneous (S.C.), intrathecal, I.M., intra-arterial, and intracavitary routes. (See *Using an Ommaya reservoir*, page 312.)

Chemotherapy drugs may be administered in the doctor's office, an outpatient clinic, the patient's home, or a long-term care facility or hospital. Wherever treatments take place, the same basic principles of I.V. therapy apply. Because of rapid changes in health care delivery, leading to a rise in chemotherapy administration outside the hospital setting, there's an increased emphasis on patient teaching.

Precision is part of the decision

Suppressing rapidly dividing cancer cells with chemotherapy requires effective delivery of an exact dose of these toxic drugs. This can be achieved by I.V. chemotherapy. Additional benefits include complete absorption and systemic distribution.

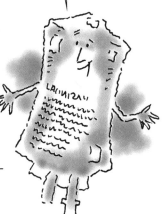

Once again, my ability to deliver an exact dose recommends me for the job.

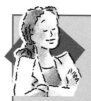

Peak technique

Using an Ommaya reservoir

If your patient has brain cancer, you may need to administer chemo-therapy by the intrathecal route — directly into the brain tissue — to cir-cumvent the blood-brain barrier.

You may use an Ommaya reservoir to administer a chemotherapy drug that can't cross the blood-brain barrier to reach its intended target in the brain. The device is inserted through a burr hole that's drilled into the patient's skull. A drug reservoir rests outside the skull under a scalp flap. A catheter extends from the reservoir through the patient's non-dominant frontal lobe and into the lateral ventricle. The drug reservoir is topped by a self-sealing silicone injection dome that forms a slight, soft bulge about the size of a quarter on the patient's head. You can inject drugs into this dome using a syringe, as shown.

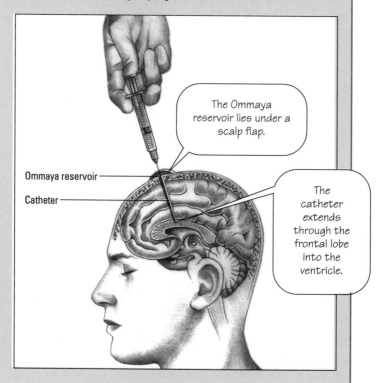

It attacks the healthy and cancerous alike

While chemotherapy is intended to control or eliminate cancer cells, it can also damage healthy cells. Healthy cells are attacked because the chemotherapy can't differentiate between healthy cells and cancerous ones. Chemotherapy attacks all rapidly growing cells. Two examples of rapidly growing cells are hair and nail follicles — this is why a patient loses his hair and his nails become brittle.

Frequent I.V. chemotherapy use can lead veins to be sclerotic. The patient can also be at risk for phlebitis or tissue necrosis due to certain chemotherapy drugs.

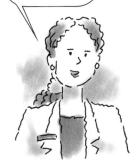

Cycle-specific drugs are effective only during a specific phase of the cell cycle...

How chemotherapy works

Healthy and cancerous cells pass through similar life cycles and are similarly vulnerable to chemotherapeutic drugs. Some of these drugs are cycle-specific — designed to disrupt a specific biochemical process, making them effective only during specific phases of the cell cycle. Other drugs are cycle-nonspecific, meaning their prolonged action is independent of the cell cycle, allowing them to act on reproducing and resting cells.

Covering all the bases

Because tumor cells are active in various phases of the cell cycle, chemotherapy typically employs more than one drug. This way, each drug can target a different site or take action during a different phase of the cell cycle.

Let's get specific...as well as nonspecific

During a single administration of a cycle-nonspecific chemotherapeutic drug, a fixed percentage of normal and malignant cells die, while a percentage of normal and malignant cells survive.

When cycle-specific chemotherapy is administered, cells in the resting phase survive. (See *The cell cycle and chemotherapeutic drugs*, page 314.)

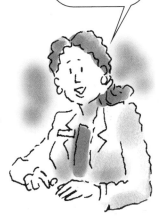

...cycle-nonspecific drugs act independent of the cell cycle.

Calculating collateral cost

The challenge is to provide a drug dose large enough to kill the greatest number of cancer cells but small enough to avoid irreversibly damaging normal tissue or causing toxicity. Given in combination, the drugs potentiate each other, and the tumor responds as it would to a larger dose of a single drug.

In addition, because different drugs work at different stages of the cell cycle or employ different mechanisms to kill cancer cells, using several drugs decreases the likelihood that the tumor will develop resistance to the chemotherapy.

The cell cycle and chemotherapeutic drugs

All cells cycle through five phases. Chemotherapeutic drugs that are active on cells during one or more of these phases are called cycle-specific. The illustration below tells what happens at each phase of the cell cycle and gives examples of cycle-specific drugs that are active during each phase.

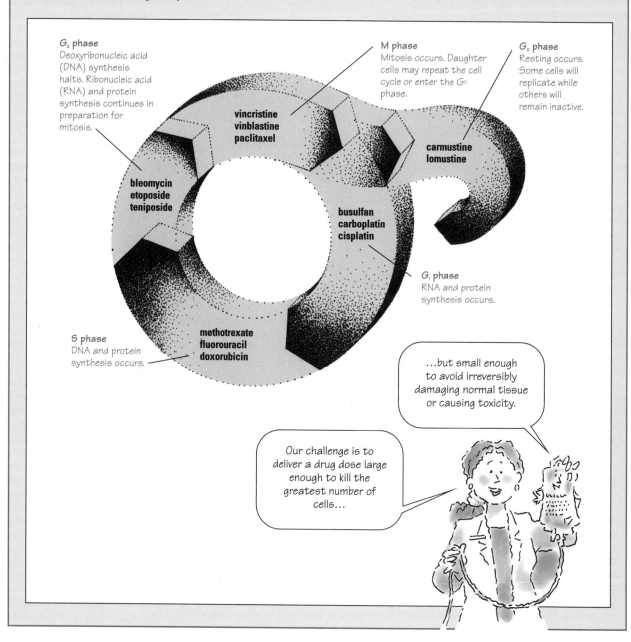

G_2 phase
Deoxyribonucleic acid (DNA) synthesis halts. Ribonucleic acid (RNA) and protein synthesis continues in preparation for mitosis.

M phase
Mitosis occurs. Daughter cells may repeat the cell cycle or enter the G_0 phase.

G_0 phase
Resting occurs. Some cells will replicate while others will remain inactive.

vincristine
vinblastine
paclitaxel

carmustine
lomustine

bleomycin
etoposide
teniposide

busulfan
carboplatin
cisplatin

G_1 phase
RNA and protein synthesis occurs.

S phase
DNA and protein synthesis occurs.

methotrexate
fluorouracil
doxorubicin

...but small enough to avoid irreversibly damaging normal tissue or causing toxicity.

Our challenge is to deliver a drug dose large enough to kill the greatest number of cells...

The selection process

Drug selection depends on the patient's age, overall condition, tumor type, and allergies or sensitivities as well as the stage of the cancer. Doctors strive to select the most effective drugs for the first round of chemotherapy because this is when cancer cells respond best. Second- or third-line chemotherapy drugs may have to be used depending on the patient's hypersensitivity reaction.

Going in cycles

Eradicating a tumor calls for repeated drug doses. This is considered a single course of chemotherapy and is repeated on a cyclic basis. The cycle can be repeated daily, weekly, every other week, or every three to four weeks. Treatment cycles are carefully planned so normal cells can regenerate. The timing of repeat treatment cycles depends on the cycle of the targeted cells and the return of normal blood counts.

Most patients require at least three treatment cycles before they show any beneficial response. However, every patient differs. Some patients show faster tumor response time than others and some don't respond at all.

Understanding chemotherapeutic drugs

Chemotherapeutic drugs are categorized according to their pharmacologic action as well as the way in which they interfere with cell production.

Dividing up the drugs

Cycle-specific drugs are divided into:
- antimetabolites
- vinca alkaloids.
  Cycle-nonspecific drugs are divided into:
- alkylating agents
- nitrosureas
- antineoplastics
- antibiotics
- miscellaneous.

Other drugs used to inhibit tumor cell growth include steroids, hormones, and antihormones. These drugs work in the intracellular environment. Steroids, which normally act as anti-inflammatory agents, make malignant cells vulnerable to damage from cell-specific drugs. Hormones alter the environment of cells by affecting the permeability of their membranes. Antihormones affect hormone-dependent tumors by inheriting the production of those hormones or neutralizing their effects. (See *Selected chemotherapeutic drugs*, page 316.)

Selected chemotherapeutic drugs

Compare the characteristics and toxic effects of these chemotherapeutic drugs.

Category	Characteristics	Toxic effects
Cycle-specific		
Antimetabolites (cytarabine, floxuridine, fluorouracil, hydroxyurea, methotrexate, thioguanine)	• Interfere with nucleic acid synthesis • Attack during S phase of cell cycle	• Effects on bone marrow (myelosuppression), central nervous system (CNS), and GI system
Plant alkaloids (vinblastine, vincristine)	• Prevent mitotic spindle formation • Cycle-specific to M phase	• Effects on CNS, GI system • Myelosuppression • Tissue damage
Enzymes (asparaginase)	• Useful only in leukemias	• Hypersensitivity reactions
Cycle-nonspecific		
Alkylating agents (carboplatin, cisplatin, cyclophosphamide, ifosfamide, thiotepa)	• Disrupt deoxyribonucleic acid (DNA) replication	• Infertility • Secondary carcinoma • Renal system
Antibiotics (bleomycin, doxorubicin, mitoxantrone, mitomycin)	• Bind with DNA to inhibit synthesis of DNA and ribonucleic acid	• Effects on GI, renal, and hepatic systems • Effects on bone marrow
Hormones and hormone inhibitors (androgens [testolactone], antiandrogens [flutamide], antiestrogens [tamoxifen], estrogens [estramustine], gonadotropin [leuprolide], progestins [megestrol])	• Interfere with binding of normal hormones to receptor proteins, manipulate hormone levels, and alter hormone environment • Mechanism of action not always clear • Usually palliative, not curative	• No known toxic effect
Folic acid analogs (leucovorin)	• Antidote for methotrexate toxicity	• Hypersensitivity reaction possible
Cytoprotective agents (dexrazoxane, mesna)	• Protect normal tissue by binding with metabolites of other cytotoxic drugs	• None

Multitasking drugs

Doctors order chemotherapeutic drugs to control cancer, to cure cancer, to prevent metastasis, or for palliation. Drugs may be given alone or in combinations called protocols.

Still hard at work

The search for new cancer treatments is ongoing. Each year, the National Cancer Institute screens about 15,000 potential new compounds for chemotherapeutic action. Specific areas of research include biological therapy and immunotherapy.

Understanding biological therapy

Biological therapy consists mostly of the administration of drugs known as biological response modifiers (BRMs), which alter the body's response to cancer. In addition to beneficial effects, some BRMs cause direct cytotoxicity.

Immunotherapy

In cancer immunotherapy, drugs are used to enhance the body's ability to destroy cancer cells.

Bringing up strong, healthy cells

Cancer immunotherapy seeks to evoke effective immune response to human tumors by altering the way cells grow, mature, and respond to cancer cells. Immunotherapy may include the administration of monoclonal antibodies and immunomodulatory cytokines.

Monoclonal antibodies

Monoclonal antibodies, which specifically target tumor cells, are a more recent form of biotherapy. Biotherapy is a unique approach because it manipulates the body's natural resources instead of introducing toxic substances that aren't selective and can't differentiate between normal and abnormal processes or cells.

All about antibodies

Antibodies are immunoglobulins produced by mature B cells or plasma cells in response to antigens—proteins found on the surface of normal and abnormal cells. Antibodies recognize specific

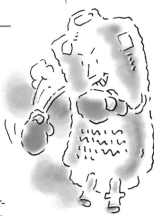

Some drugs try to pump up the immune system to help it destroy cancer cells.

antigens and bind exclusively to them; this process is referred to as a lock-and-key mechanism. When these antibodies attach to antigens, they can cause tumor-cell inactivation or destruction. A monoclonal antibody recognizes only a single unique antigen.

A monoclonal mix

Five monoclonal antibodies for cancer therapy, include:
- rituximab (Rituxan)
- trastuzumab (Herceptin)
- ibritumomab tiuxetan (Zevalin)
- gemtuzumab ozogamicin (Mylotarg)
- alemtuzumab (Campath).

Rituxan and Zevalin are specifically indicated for non-Hodgkin's lymphoma. Herceptin is beneficial against metastatic breast cancer. This monoclonal antibody may be used as a first-line treatment in combination with chemotherapy or as a second-line single agent. Mylotarg is indicated for the treatment of acute myeloid leukemia and Campath for B-cell chronic lymphocytic leukemia.

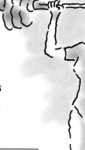

Biotherapy seeks to use the body's natural resources in combating cancer instead of bringing in toxic substances.

Immunomodulatory cytokines

Immunomodulatory cytokines are intracellular messenger proteins (proteins that deliver messages within cells). These proteins include:
- interferon
- interleukins
- tumor necrosis factor
- colony-stimulating factors.

Interferon

Interferon alpha is approved for treating chronic myeloid leukemia, hairy cell leukemia, and acquired immunodeficiency syndrome–related Kaposi's sarcoma. It's also used with low-grade malignant lymphoma, multiple myeloma, and renal cell carcinoma.

Interleukins

Interleukins are cytokines that primarily function to deliver messages to leukocytes. Interleukin-2 (IL-2) is an approved anticancer agent. IL-2 stimulates the proliferation and cytolytic activity of T cells and natural killer cells. High doses of IL-2 have been effective in a few patients with metastatic renal cell carcinoma and melanoma. The other interleukins remain under investigation for cancer therapy.

Tumor necrosis factor

Tumor necrosis factor (TNF) plays a role in the inflammatory response to tumors and cancer cells. In animal studies, TNF has sometimes produced impressive antitumor responses. This is considered to be an investigational drug.

Colony-stimulating factors

Colony-stimulating factors (CSFs) are substances that are naturally produced by the body. They stimulate the growth of different types of cells found in the blood and the immune system. CSFs have been helpful in the clinical care of patients receiving myelosuppressive therapy. Examples of CSFs include:

We're growing in numbers!

• Erythropoietin (Epogen) induces erythroid maturation (maturation of red blood cells [RBCs]) and increases the release of reticulocytes from the bone marrow—this stimulates the production of RBCs, which might reduce the number of blood transfusions needed by the patient.
• Granulocyte CSF (Neupogen) stimulates proliferation, differentiation, and functional activity of neutrophils, causing a rapid rise in white blood cell count. Granulocyte CSF is given to reduce the incidence of infection in patients receiving chemotherapy drugs.
• Granulocyte-macrophage CSF (Leukine) is indicated for older patients receiving chemotherapy for acute myelogenous leukemia, for patients undergoing bone marrow transplants, and for peripheral blood progenitor collection.

Preparing chemotherapeutic drugs

Many health care facilities use existing guidelines as a basis for their policies and procedures regarding chemotherapeutic drugs. Among the major sources for these guidelines are these agencies and associations:
• The American Society of Health-System Pharmacists (ASHP) has published guidelines for the preparation of chemotherapeutic drugs since 1990.
• The Occupational Safety and Health Administration (OSHA) published its revised standards for controlling exposure to chemotherapeutic agents in 1995, and needle-stick protection in 2001.
• The Oncology Nursing Society (ONS) published guidelines for nursing education, practice, and administration of chemotherapeutic agents in 1999.
• The Infusion Nurses Society (INS) published revised standards of practice for safe delivery of chemotherapeutic agents in 2000.

Certification required

At the local level, most health care facilities require nurses and pharmacists involved in the preparation and delivery of chemotherapeutic drugs to complete a certification program that covers the safe delivery of chemotherapeutic drugs and care of the patient with cancer.

Protective measures

Preparation of chemotherapeutic drugs requires adherence to guidelines regarding:
- drug preparation areas and equipment
- protective clothing
- specific safety measures.

Area and equipment

Drug preparation may be performed by a trained nurse, a pharmacist or, in states that allow it, a supervised pharmacy technician.

Prepare chemotherapeutic drugs in a well-ventilated workspace. Perform all drug admixing or compounding within a Class II Biological Safety Cabinet or a "vertical" laminar airflow hood with a HEPA filter, which is vented to the outside. The hood pulls the aerosolized chemotherapy drug particles away from the compounder. If a Class II Biological Safety Cabinet isn't available, OSHA recommends that you wear a special respirator.

Have close access to a sink, alcohol pads, gauze pads as well as OSHA-required chemotherapy hazardous waste containers, sharps containers, and chemotherapy spill kits.

Hazardous waste!

Hazardous waste containers should be made of puncture-proof, shatter-proof, leakproof plastic. Chemotherapy waste is usually identified with yellow biohazard labels. Use them to dispose of all chemotherapy contaminated I.V. bags, tubing, filters, and syringes. Red sharps containers are used to dispose all contaminated sharps such as needles.

Clothing

Essential protective clothing includes:

 cuffed gown

 gloves

 goggles and face mask or face shield.

The lowdown on gowns and gloves

Gowns should be disposable, water-resistant, and lint-free with long sleeves, knitted cuffs, and a closed front.

Gloves designed for use with chemotherapeutic drugs should be disposable and made of thick latex or thick non-latex material. They should also be powder-free because powder can carry contamination from the drugs into the surrounding air. Double gloving is an option when the gloves aren't of the best quality. Change gloves whenever a tear or puncture occurs. Wash your hands before putting on the gloves and after removing them.

Safety measures

Take care to protect staff, patients, and the environment from unnecessary exposure to chemotherapeutic drugs. Don't leave the drug preparation area while wearing the protective gear you wore during drug preparation. Eating, drinking, smoking, or applying cosmetics in the drug preparation area violates OSHA guidelines.

Laying the groundwork for safety

Put on protective gear before you begin to compound the chemotherapeutic drugs. Before preparing the drugs; clean the work area inside the cabinet with 70% alcohol and a disposable towel; do the same after you're finished and after a spill. Discard the towel into the yellow leakproof chemotherapy waste container.

Feeling exposed

If a chemotherapy drug comes in contact with your skin, wash the skin thoroughly with soap and water. This will prevent drug absorption into the skin. If the drug comes in contact with your eye, immediately flood the eye with water or isotonic eyewash for at least 5 minutes, while holding the eyelid open.

After an accidental exposure, notify your supervisor immediately. Your supervisor may send you to employee health, where you may receive treatment and the exposure event will be documented in your employee health record.

Better safe than sorry

Here are some other safety precautions to keep in mind:
- Use sterile technique when preparing all drugs.
- Use blunt-ended needles whenever possible.
- Use needles with a hydrophobic filter to remove solutions from vials.
- Vent vials with a hydrophobic filter or use the negative pressure technique to reduce the amount of aerosolized drugs.
- When you break ampules, wrap a gauze pad around the neck of the vial to decrease the chances of droplet contamination and glove puncture.

- Wear a face mask and goggles or face shield to protect yourself against splashes and aerosolized drugs.
- Place all contaminated needles in the sharps container, and don't recap needles.
- Use only syringes and I.V. sets that have a luer-lock fitting.
- Label all chemotherapeutic drugs with a yellow biohazard label.

Transport tactics

Transport the prepared chemotherapy drugs in a sealable plastic bag that's prominently labeled with a yellow chemotherapy biohazard label.

The spiel on spills

Make sure your facility's protocols for spills are available in all areas where chemotherapeutic drugs are handled, including patient care areas. Chemotherapy spill kits should be readily available.

If a chemotherapy spill occurs, follow your facility's protocol, which is probably based on OSHA guidelines. This protocol will likely instruct you to follow these steps:
- Put on protective garments, if you aren't already wearing them.
- Isolate the area and contain the spill with absorbent materials from the spill kit.
- Use the disposable dustpan and scraper to collect any broken glass or desiccant absorbing powder. Carefully place the dustpan, scraper, and collected spill in a leakproof, puncture-proof, chemotherapy-designated hazardous waste container.
- Prevent the aerosolization of the drug at all times.
- Clean the spill area with a detergent or bleach solution.

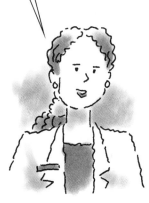

Put on your protective gear before you begin to do anything with chemotherapeutic drugs.

Administering chemotherapeutic drugs

Because dosage, route, and timing must be exact to avoid possible fatal complications, only chemotherapy-certified nurses should be involved in administering these drugs.

I.V. chemotherapy drugs can be administered in one of three ways:

 by direct I.V. push into the vein

 by indirect I.V. push through the side port of a running I.V.

 as a continuous infusion.

No matter which method of administration is ordered, flush the vein with normal saline solution between the administration of each drug.

What you need

Patient's medication order or record ✳ prescribed drugs ✳ I.V. access supplies, if necessary ✳ sterile normal saline solution ✳ transparent dressing ✳ chemotherapy gloves ✳ transparent dressing ✳ syringes and I.V. tubing with leur-lock fittings ✳ leakproof hazardous waste container labeled CAUTION: BIOHAZARDOUS WASTE ✳ chemotherapy spill kit ✳ extravasation kit

Getting ready

- Before administering a chemotherapeutic drug, verify the order with another chemotherapy-certified nurse.

Count on doing this

- Check the patient's blood count before beginning the chemotherapy infusion. Many facilities have nursing policies that require the nurse to notify the doctor for approval to administer the chemotherapeutic drug if the patient's blood count drops below a predetermined value.
- Check the patient's serum creatinine levels because some chemotherapeutic drugs are excreted through the kidneys, such as cisplatin and carboplatin.

Which drugs? Which route?

- Make sure you understand clearly which drugs are to be given and by which route. Check whether the drug is classified as a vesicant, nonvesicant, or irritant. (See *Risks of tissue damage.*)

Confirm and verify

- Confirm any written orders for needed antiemetics, fluids, diuretics, or electrolyte supplements to be given before, during, or after chemotherapy administration.
- Make sure that either the patient or a legally authorized person has signed an informed consent for each specific chemotherapy drug they're to receive and for the insertion of the I.V. device, if required.
- Selection of an intravenous route of administration, whether it's a peripheral route, an intermittent infusion device, or a central route, will be determined by the type of chemotherapeutic agent the patient will receive, as well as the condition of the patient's veins. Many patients requiring chemotherapy have a PICC or a central venous access device, such as a tunneled central venous catheter or an implanted port.
- Assemble the equipment you'll need for both insertion of the peripheral I.V. catheter, if necessary, and preparation for the drug administration. If you're administering a vesicant, the extravasation

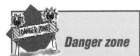

Danger zone

Risks of tissue damage

To administer chemotherapy safely, you need to know each drug's potential for damaging tissue. In this regard, chemotherapeutic drugs are classified as vesicants, nonvesicants, or irritants.
- Vesicants cause a reaction so severe that blisters form and tissue is damaged or destroyed.
- Nonvesicants don't cause irritation or damage.
- Irritants can cause a local venous response, with or without a skin reaction.

kit will need to be immediately available. A chemotherapy spill kit should be readily available as well.

Who's there?

- Check that you have the right patient. Call him by his first and last name, and ask for verification of his date of birth as a means of double-checking. Be sure to also check his identification band.
- Verify the patient's level of understanding of the treatment and adverse effects.
- Wash your hands and put on chemotherapy gloves.

How you do it

- Perform a new venipuncture proximal to an existing venous access site, if necessary, or access the existing PICC or central venous access device.
- Before administering a chemotherapeutic drug, connect an I.V. bag containing normal saline solution to the venous access.

A low-pressure situation

- Use a low-pressure infusion pump to administer vesicants through a peripheral vein, to decrease the risk of an extravasation. Central venous routes are more appropriate for continuous vesicant infusions. (See *Preventing infiltration.*)

Peak technique

Preventing infiltration

Follow these guidelines when giving vesicants:
- Use a distal vein that allows successive proximal venipunctures.
- Avoid using the hand, antecubital space, damaged areas, or areas with compromised circulation.
- Don't probe or "fish" for veins.
- Place a transparent dressing over the site.
- Start the push delivery or the infusion with normal saline solution.
- Inspect the site for swelling and erythema.
- Tell the patient to report burning, stinging, pain, pruritus, or temperature changes near the site.
- After drug administration, flush the line with 20 ml of normal saline solution.

Site-seeing encouraged

• Apply a transparent dressing if possible so that the venous access site can be observed at all times for early signs of infiltration, extravasation, and vein irritation.

Practice pointers

• Check for infiltration during administration as well as for signs of a hypersensitivity reaction. If swelling occurs at the I.V. site, the solution is infiltrating. Instruct the patient to report burning, stinging, or pain at or near the site. Sudden discomfort during drug administration or flushing could indicate infiltration.
• Observe around the site for streaky redness along the vein and other skin changes, which may indicate vein flare.

Finish with a flush

• After drug administration is complete, infuse at least 20 ml of normal saline solution through the venous access device before discontinuing the I.V. line. This flushes the medication from the infusion delivery set, preventing drug leakage and possible exposure if the venous access is to be removed.

• If the venous access device is removed, take the following steps:
• Dispose of all used needles and contaminated sharps in the red sharps container.
• Dispose of gloves in the yellow chemotherapeutic waste container.
• Dispose of unused medications, considered hazardous waste, according to your facility's policy.
• Wash your hands thoroughly with soap and water, even though you have worn gloves.
• According to facility policy and procedures, wear protective clothing when handling body fluids from the patient for 48 hours after the chemotherapy treatment.

What to teach

• To give the patient some sense of control in the face of overwhelming odds, explain each procedure you do and teach him strategies for dealing with fear, pain, and the adverse effects of chemotherapy.
• Make sure that the patient maintains a positive attitude and a strong emotional support system that will enable him to better endure — if not overcome — the disease and its treatments.

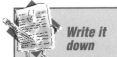

Write it down

Documenting chemotherapy administration

Be sure to record:
• sequence of drug administration
• site accessed
• gauge and length of catheter, and number of attempts if peripheral access was performed
• name, dose, and route of administered drugs
• type and volume of I.V. solutions
• adverse reactions and subsequent nursing interventions.

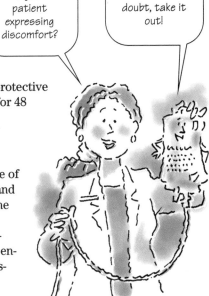

Is your patient expressing discomfort?

When in doubt, take it out!

Understanding the complications of chemotherapy

Complications resulting from chemotherapy can be categorized according to where or when exposure to the drug began. They're referred to as:
- infusion site related
- hypersensitivity or anaphylactic reactions
- short-term
- long-term.

Understanding infusion site-related complications

Infiltration, extravasation, and vein flare reactions are the most common infusion site-related complications.

How to prevent infiltration

Infiltration is the inadvertent leakage of a nonvesicant solution or medication into the surrounding tissue. The main signs are swelling around the venous access site — this swollen area will be cool to the touch — along with blanching and a change in the I.V. flow rate.

Compression and compartment

- Notify the doctor immediately if tightness in the patient's arm occurs. The patient will usually complain of numbness and tingling in the swollen area, which may be due to large quantities of I.V. solutions entering the tissue that indicates a nerve compression injury and can result in compartment syndrome.

Check, check, check

- Check for infiltration before, during, and after the infusion by flushing the vein with normal saline solution. In the event of an infiltration, remove the peripheral venous access catheter and insert it in a new location.

How to prevent extravasation

Extravasation is the inadvertent leakage of a vesicant (a drug that can cause tissue necrosis and sloughing) solution into the surrounding tissue.

Extravasation extra credit

When assessing the patient for extravasation, keep in mind:

Danger zone

Treatment of extravasation

If a vesicant has extravasated, it's an emergency! Quickly take the following steps, designed to limit the damage:
• Stop the infusion. Check your facility's policy to determine if the I.V. catheter is to be removed or left in place to infuse corticosteroids or a specific antidote. Treatment for extravasation should be in accordance with manufacturer's guidelines.
• Notify the doctor.
• Instill the appropriate antidote according to facility policy. Usually, you'll give the antidote for extravasation either by instilling it through the existing I.V. catheter or by using a 1-ml syringe to inject small amounts subcutaneously injected, then remove the I.V. catheter.
• Continue to visually monitor the site and document the site appearance and patient's response.
• Subsequent care of the extravasated area may include topical steroids or Silvadene cream.
• If the extravasation injury is severe, the patient may require skin debridement, skin grafts, or possibly, amputation.

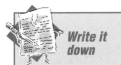

Write it down

Documenting infiltration, vein flare, or extravasation

Be sure to record:
• location of the infiltration, vein flare, or extravasation
• size of the swollen area or length of vein flare as well as other objective signs such as erythema
• name of drug and I.V. solution
• patient's complaints
• nursing interventions
• time you notified the doctor
• doctor's response and orders
• patient's response to treatment.

• Initial signs of an extravasation may resemble those of infiltration — swelling, pain, and blanching.
• Blood return is an inconclusive test and shouldn't be used to determine if the venous access device is correctly seated in the peripheral vein.
• To assess peripheral I.V. placement, flush the vein with normal saline solution and observe for site swelling.
• Remember, "When in doubt, take it out!"
• Symptoms can progress to blisters; to skin, muscle, tissue and fat necrosis; and to tissue sloughing. The outer surface of veins, arteries, and nerves can also be damaged. Depending on the drug and the concentration of the drug in the solutions, blistering can be apparent within hours or days of the extravasation.

How to prevent vein flare

• During infusion of an irritant into the vein, the patient may complain of burning pain or aching along the vein as well as up through the arm. A vein flare (a bright redness) may also appear in the vein along with blotches or hives on the affected arm.
• If the reaction is severe, injection of an I.V. steroid may be required. In some cases, the infusion of an irritant can result in damage to the lining of the vein wall, causing serious phlebitis or vein thrombosis.

Diluting the drug's effect

- If the patient complains of pain or burning during the infusion, increase the dilution of the infused medication, decrease the infusion rate, or restart the venous access in a different vein. (See *Treatment of extravasation*, page 327.)

Hypersensitivity or anaphylactic reactions

A hypersensitivity or anaphylactic reaction can occur at the initial dose of the drug or on subsequent infusions of the same drug. Some chemotherapeutic drugs put the patient at high risk for anaphylaxis.

Hypersensitivity reactions can occur at the beginning, middle, or end of the infusion. (See *Signs and symptoms of immediate hypersensitivity*.)

The specific treatment for a hypersensitivity reaction will depend on the severity of the reaction. Usually, you'll follow these five steps:

 Stop the infusion.

Begin a rapid infusion of normal saline solution to quickly dilute the drug.

Danger zone

Signs and symptoms of immediate hypersensitivity

An immediate hypersensitivity reaction to a chemotherapeutic drug will appear within 5 minutes after starting to administer the drug.

Organ system	Subjective complaints	Objective findings
Respiratory	• Tightness in chest, shortness of breath, "lump in the throat"	• Stridor, decreased breath sounds, wheezing, hoarseness
Skin	• Pruritus, sensation of burning or stinging	• Cyanosis, urticaria, angioedema, cold and clammy skin
Cardiovascular	• Chest pain, palpitations	• Tachycardia, hypotension, arrhythmias
Central nervous system	• Dizziness, anxiety	• Decreased sensorium, loss of consciousness

Check the patient's vital signs.

 Notify the doctor.

 Administer emergency drugs as ordered by the doctor.

What to give and when

Antihistamines are typically given first, followed by corticosteroids and bronchodilators. Epinephrine is given first in severe anaphylactic reactions. After you've administered the drug, monitor vital signs and pulse oximetry every 5 minutes until the patient is stable, and then every 15 minutes for 1 to 2 hours—or follow your facility's policy and procedures for acute treatment of allergic reactions.

Throughout the episode, maintain the patient's airway, oxygenation, and tissue perfusion. Life support equipment should be readily available in case the patient fails to respond to initial treatment. Document the drugs and dosage as well as the patient's response to the treatment.

Short-term adverse effects

The short-term adverse effects of chemotherapy include—but aren't limited to—the ones people commonly associate with the treatment, such as:
• nausea and vomiting
• hair loss (alopecia)
• diarrhea. (See *Managing short-term adverse effects of chemotherapy*, page 330.)

Additional short-term adverse effects include:
• myelosuppression
• stomatitis.

These effects are produced by damage to tissues with a large proportion of frequently reproducing cells—these tissues include bone marrow, hair follicles, and GI mucosa.

All patients are different; not all will experience these adverse effects, and some may not experience any of them.

Long-term adverse effects

Organ system dysfunction, especially in the hematopoietic and GI systems, is common after chemotherapy. These effects are usually temporary, but some systems suffer permanent damage that manifests itself long after chemotherapy. The renal, pulmonary, cardiac, reproductive, and neurologic systems all show a variety of

Danger Zone

Managing short-term adverse effects of chemotherapy

This chart identifies some common adverse effects of chemotherapy and offers ways to minimize them.

Adverse effect	Signs and symptoms	Interventions
Anemia	Dizziness, fatigue, pallor, and shortness of breath after minimal exertion; low hemoglobin (Hb) level and hematocrit (HCT); may develop slowly over several courses of treatment	• Monitor Hb level, HCT, and red blood cell count; report dropping values; remember that dehydration from nausea, vomiting, and anorexia will cause hemoconcentration, yielding falsely high HCT readings. • Be prepared to administer a blood transfusion or erythropoietin. • Instruct the patient to take frequent rests, increase intake of iron-rich foods, and take a multivitamin with iron as prescribed.
Leukopenia	Susceptibility to infections; neutropenia (an absolute neutrophil count less than 1,500 cells/μl)	• Watch for the nadir, the point of lowest blood cell count (usually 7 to 14 days after last treatment). • Be prepared to administer colony-stimulating factors. • Institute neutropenic precautions in the hospitalized patient. • Include the following information in patient and family teaching: good hygiene practices, signs and symptoms of infection, the importance of checking the patient's temperature regularly, how to prepare a low-microbe diet, and how to care for vascular access devices. • Instruct the patient to avoid crowds, people with colds or respiratory infections, and fresh fruit, fresh flowers, and plants.
Thrombocytopenia	Bleeding gums, increased bruising, petechiae, hypermenorrhea, tarry stools, hematuria, coffee-ground emesis	• Monitor platelet count: under 50,000 cells/μl means a moderate risk of excessive bleeding; under 20,000 cells/μl means a major risk and the patient may need a platelet transfusion. • Avoid unnecessary I.M. injections or venipunctures; if either is necessary, apply pressure for at least 5 minutes; then apply a pressure dressing to the site. • Instruct patient to avoid cuts and bruises, shave with an electric razor, avoid blowing his nose, stay away from irritants that would trigger sneezing, and not use rectal thermometers. • Instruct patient to report sudden headaches (which could indicate potentially fatal intracranial bleeding).
Alopecia	Hair loss that may include eyebrows, lashes, and body hair	• Minimize shock and distress by warning patient of the possibility of hair loss, discussing why hair loss occurs, and describing how much hair loss to expect. • Emphasize the need for appropriate head protection against sunburn and heat loss in the winter. • For patients with long hair, suggest cutting the hair shorter before treatment because washing and brushing cause more hair loss.

temporary and permanent dysfunctions from exposure to chemotherapy.

A devastating effect

One devastating long-term effect of chemotherapy is secondary malignancy. This can be caused by certain alkylating agents given for treatment of myeloma, Hodgkin's disease, and non-Hodgkin's lymphomas. A secondary malignancy can occur at any time. The prognosis is usually poor.

What to teach

- Inform the patient about the risks and benefits of therapy.
- Warn the patient about the adverse effects of each drug and how to minimize and manage them.
- Teach the patient ways to avoid infection and how to recognize the signs and symptoms and to report them immediately.
- Tell the patient about the signs and symptoms of abnormal bleeding and ways to help reduce the risk of injury.

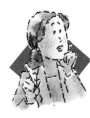

Quick quiz

1. The most commonly used route of administration for chemotherapy is the:

    A.   oral route.
    B.   intravenous (I.V.) route
    C.   Intra-arterial route.
    D.   Intracavity route.

Answer: B. Chemotherapy may be administered by many different routes, but is most commonly administered I.V. using peripheral or central veins.

2. Fluorouracil and methotrexate are examples of cycle-specific chemotherapeutic drugs that are active during which phase of the cell cycle?

    A. G_0 phase
    B. G_1 phase
    C.   S phase
    D.   M phase

Answer: C. Methotrexate and fluorouracil are active during the S phase of the cell cycle, when DNA and protein synthesis occur.

3. Erythropoietin (Epogen) is an example of which of the following immunomodulatory cytokines?

    A. Interferon
    B. Interleukins
    C. TNF
    D. CSFs

Answer: D. Erythropoietin (Epogen) is a CSF, which induces erythroid maturation and increases the release of reticulocytes from the bone marrow.

4. A cancer patient experiencing bleeding gums, petechiae, tarry stools, and hematuria is most likely experiencing which of the following short-term adverse effects of chemotherapy?

    A. Anemia
    B. Leukopenia
    C. Thrombocytopenia
    D. Alopecia

Answer: C. Bleeding gums, petechiae, tarry stools, and hematuria are signs of thrombocytopenia, an abnormal decrease in the number of blood platelets.

Scoring

✩✩✩ If you answered all four questions correctly, congratulations! Now treat yourself to some extra time in your resting phase.

✩✩ If you answered two or three correctly, not bad! You are getting into the flow of things.

✩ If you answered fewer than two correctly, don't get discouraged. Sometimes it takes a few learning cycles before the information starts taking effect.

Parenteral nutrition

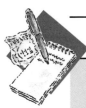

Just the facts

In this chapter, you'll learn:

♦ basic nutritional needs

♦ indications for parenteral nutrition

♦ nutritional solutions

♦ how to administer parenteral nutrition

♦ complications of parenteral nutrition.

Understanding parenteral nutrition

You may administer parenteral nutrition when illness or surgery prevents a patient from eating and metabolizing food. Common conditions that make parenteral nutrition necessary include:

• GI trauma
• pancreatitis
• ileus
• inflammatory bowel disease
• GI tract malignancy
• GI hemorrhage
• paralytic ileus
• GI obstruction
• short-bowel syndrome
• GI fistula
• severe malabsorption.

Critically ill patients may also receive parenteral nutrition if they're hemodynamically unstable or if GI tract blood flow is impaired.

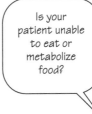

Is your patient unable to eat or metabolize food?

Then serve me up!

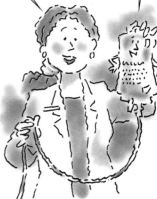

Nutritional needs

Essential nutrients found in food provide energy, maintain body tissues, and aid body processes, such as growth, cell activity, enzyme production, and temperature regulation.

Nutrients in food are essential for me to remain active.

Turning food into fuel

When carbohydrates, fats, and proteins are metabolized by the body, they produce energy, which is measured in calories (also called kilocalories). A normal healthy adult generally requires 2,000 to 3,000 calories per day. Specific requirements depend on an individual's size, sex, age, and level of physical activity.

A nutritional solution — in more ways than one!

A parenteral nutrition solution — also known as hyperalimentation, I.V. hyperalimentation, or I.V. feedings — may contain one or more of the following elements:
- dextrose
- proteins
- lipids
- electrolytes
- vitamins
- trace elements.

Depending on the type of therapy ordered, nutritional support solutions are administered through either a central venous (CV) or peripheral infusion device.

I offer calories and nutrients from dextrose, proteins, electrolytes, and more.

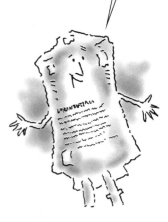

CV infusion

If a patient needs parenteral nutrition for more than 5 days, he usually requires total parenteral nutrition (TPN). TPN is delivered through a CV line, usually placed in the subclavian vein, with the tip of the catheter in the superior vena cava.

Peripheral infusion

Peripheral parenteral nutrition (PPN) — also called partial parenteral nutrition — is the delivery of nutrients through a catheter inserted into a peripheral vein. Generally, PPN provides fewer nonprotein calories than TPN because lower dextrose concentrations are used. A much larger volume of fluid must be infused for PPN to deliver the same number of calories as TPN. Therefore, most patients who require parenteral nutrition therapy receive TPN rather than PPN.

Benefits

Parenteral nutrition is an important support measure. Parenteral solutions can provide all needed nutrients when a patient can't take nutrients through the GI tract. This enables cells to function despite the patient's inability to take in or metabolize food.

Risks

Like all invasive procedures, parenteral nutrition incurs certain risks, including:
- catheter infection
- hyperglycemia (high blood glucose)
- hypokalemia (low blood potassium).

Complications of parenteral nutrition can be minimized with careful monitoring of the catheter site, infusion rate, and laboratory test results.

How did I survive when food intake stopped? Parenteral nutrition enabled me to keep functioning.

A matter of access

Another disadvantage of parenteral nutrition is the need for vascular access. If peripheral access isn't possible because of poor vasculature, central access may be necessary, perhaps requiring surgical intervention.

Price is a premium for PPN

Parenteral nutrition is expensive—about 10 times more expensive than enteral nutrition for the solutions alone. For this reason, it's used only when absolutely necessary.

Understanding nutritional deficiencies

The most common nutritional deficiencies involve protein and calories. Nutritional deficiencies may result from a nonfunctional GI tract, decreased food intake, increased metabolic need, or a combination of these factors.

Hunger strike

Food intake may be decreased because of illness, decreased physical ability, or injury. Decreased food intake can occur with GI disorders, such as paralytic ileus, surgery, or sepsis.

Metabolic activity up — need more calories!

Any increase in metabolic activity requires an increase in calorie intake. Fever commonly increases metabolic activity. The metabolic rate may also increase in victims of burns, trauma, disease, or stress; patients may require up to twice the calories of their basal metabolic rate (the minimum energy needed to maintain respiration, circulation, and other basic body functions).

Effects of protein-calorie deficiencies

When the body detects protein-calorie deficiency, it turns to its reserve sources of energy. Reserve energy is drawn from three sources:

First, the body mobilizes and converts glycogen to glucose through a process called glycogenolysis.

Next, if necessary, the body draws energy from the fats stored in adipose tissue.

As a last resort, the body taps its store of essential visceral proteins (serum albumin and transferrin) and somatic body proteins (skeletal, smooth muscle, and tissue proteins). These proteins and their amino acids are converted to glucose for energy through a process called gluconeogenesis. When these essential body proteins break down, a negative nitrogen balance results (which means more protein is used by the body than is taken in). Starvation and disease-related stress contribute to this catabolic (destructive) state.

Protein energy malnutrition

A deficiency of protein and energy (calories) results in protein energy malnutrition (PEM), also called protein calorie malnutrition. PEM refers to a spectrum of disorders that occur as a consequence of chronic inadequate protein or calorie intake or high metabolic protein and energy requirements.

PEM pals

Disorders that commonly lead to PEM include:
- cancer
- GI disorders
- chronic heart failure
- alcoholism
- conditions causing high metabolic needs such as burns.
    The consequences of PEM may include:
- reduced enzyme and plasma protein production
- increased susceptibility to infection
- physical and mental growth deficiencies in children
- severe diarrhea and malabsorption
- numerous secondary nutritional deficiencies
- delayed wound healing
- mental fatigue.

That's PEM!

PEM takes three basic forms:

 iatrogenic PEM

 kwashiorkor

 marasmus.

Iatrogenic

Commonly during hospitalization, a patient's nutritional status deteriorates because of inadequate protein or calorie intake, leading to iatrogenic PEM. Iatrogenic PEM affects more than 15% of patients in acute care centers. It's most common in patients hospitalized longer than 2 weeks.

Kwashiorkor

Kwashiorkor results from severe protein deficiency without a calorie deficit. It occurs most commonly in children ages 1 to 3. In the United States, it's usually secondary to:
• malabsorption disorders
• cancer and cancer therapies
• kidney disease
• hypermetabolic illness.

Marasmus

The third form of malnutrition, marasmus, is a prolonged and gradual wasting of muscle mass and subcutaneous fat. It's caused by inadequate intake of protein, calories, and other nutrients. Marasmus occurs most commonly in infants ages 6 to 18 months, after gastrectomy, and in patients with cancer of the mouth and esophagus.

Nutritional assessment

When illness or surgery compromises a patient's intake or alters his metabolic requirements, you'll need to assess the relationship between nutrients consumed and energy expended. A nutritional assessment provides insight into how well the patient's physiologic need for nutrients is being met. To assess nutritional status, follow these steps:
• Obtain a comprehensive health history, including dietary history.
• Perform a physical assessment.

- Obtain anthropometric measurements.
- Review the results of pertinent diagnostic tests.

Because poor nutritional status can affect most body systems, a thorough nutritional assessment helps you anticipate problems and intervene appropriately.

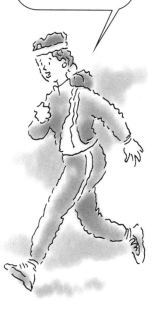

A nutritional assessment reveals the relationship between nutrients consumed and — whew! — energy expended.

Dietary history

When obtaining a dietary history, check for symptoms of decreased food intake, increased metabolic requirements, or a combination of the two. Also check usual daily intake, using either a 24-hour recall or diet diary. Note factors that affect food intake and changes in appetite. Ask the patient about dietary restrictions or supplements. Also ask if the patient consumes caffeine-containing beverages, such as coffee, tea, and cola drinks. Obtain a weight history.

When obtaining a health history, be sure to include:
- chief complaint
- present illness
- medical history, including previous major illnesses, injuries, hospitalizations, or surgeries
- allergies and history of intolerance to food and medications
- family history, including any familial, genetic, or environmental illnesses
- social history, including environmental, psychological, and sociologic factors that may influence nutritional status, such as alcoholism, living alone, or lack of transportation.

Physical assessment

The physical examination should focus on signs of nutrient deficiencies in the hair, skin, eyes, and oral cavity; loss of fat or muscle; and presence of edema or ascites. Also, be sure to observe for subtle signs of malnutrition. (See *Signs of poor nutrition.*)

Anthropometry

Anthropometry compares the patient's measurements with established standards. It's an objective, noninvasive method for measuring overall body size, composition, and specific body parts. Commonly used anthropometric measurements include:
- height
- weight
- ideal body weight
- body frame size
- triceps skinfold thickness
- midarm circumference

Signs of poor nutrition

When performing a physical assessment, note the patient's overall condition and inspect the skin, mouth, and teeth. Then look for these subtle signs:

- poor skin turgor
- abnormal pigmentation
- darkening of the mouth lining
- protruding eyes (exophthalmos)
- neck swelling
- adventitious breath sounds
- dental caries
- ill-fitting dentures
- signs of infection or irritation on the roof of the mouth
- muscle wasting
- abdominal masses and tenderness
- enlarged liver
- weight loss in adults; edema may mask weight loss
- failure to gain height and weight (in children).

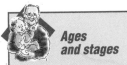

Ages and stages

Comparing anthropometric measurements

Because a patient's body composition changes with age, remember that comparing anthropometric measurements of elderly patients to standardized tables is less reliable than with younger patients. Most standard tables only show measurements in patients up to age 59.

- midarm muscle circumference. (See *Comparing anthropometric measurements*.)

Not up to 90%?

Any finding of less than 90% of the standard measurement may indicate a need for nutritional support.

Diagnostic studies

Evidence of a nutritional problem commonly appears in the results of a diagnostic test. Tests are used to evaluate:
- visceral protein status
- lean body mass
- vitamin and mineral balance.
    Diagnostic studies are also used to evaluate the effectiveness of nutritional support. (See *Detecting deficiencies*, page 340.)

Indications for TPN

A patient may receive TPN for:
- debilitating illness lasting longer than 2 weeks.
- deficient or absent oral intake for more than 7 days, as in cases of multiple trauma, severe burns, or anorexia nervosa.

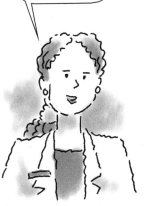

Use TPN when lengthy or chronic illness leads to patient weight loss and decreased calorie and protein intake.

Detecting deficiencies

Laboratory studies help pinpoint nutritional deficiencies by aiding in the diagnosis of anemia, malnutrition, and other disorders. Check out this chart to learn about some commonly ordered diagnostic tests, their purposes, normal values, and implications. Albumin, prealbumin, transferrin, and triglyceride levels are the major indicators of nutritional deficiency.

Test and purpose	Normal values	Implications
Creatinine height index • Uses a 24-hour urine sample to determine adequacy of muscle mass	• Determined from a reference table of values based on a patient's height or weight	• Less than 80% of reference value: moderate depletion of muscle mass (protein reserves) • Less than 60% of reference value: severe depletion, with increased risk of compromised immune function
Hematocrit • Diagnoses anemia and dehydration	• Male: 42% to 50% • Female: 40% to 48% • Child: 29% to 41% • Neonate: 55% to 68%	• Increased values: severe dehydration, polycythemia • Decreased values: iron deficiency anemia, excessive blood loss
Hemoglobin • Assesses blood's oxygen-carrying capacity to aid diagnosis of anemia, protein deficiency, and hydration status	• Older adult: 10 to 17 g/dl • Adult male: 13 to 18 g/dl • Adult female: 12 to 16 g/dl • Child: 9 to 15.5 g/dl • Neonate: 14 to 20 g/dl	• Increased values: dehydration, polycythemia • Decreased values: protein deficiency, iron deficiency anemia, excessive blood loss, overhydration
Serum albumin • Helps assess visceral protein stores	• Adult: 3.5 to 5 g/dl • Child: same as adult • Neonate: 3.6 to 5.4 g/dl	• Decreased values: malnutrition, overhydration, liver or kidney disease, heart failure, excessive blood protein losses such as from severe burns
Serum transferrin (similar to serum total iron-binding capacity [TIBC]) • Helps assess visceral protein stores; has a shorter half-life than serum albumin and, thus, more accurately reflects current status	• Adult: 200 to 400 µg/dl • Child: 350 to 450 µg/dl • Neonate: 60 to 175 µg/dl	• Increased TIBC: iron deficiency, as in pregnancy or iron deficiency anemia • Decreased TIBC: iron excess, as in chronic inflammatory states • Below 200 µg/dl: visceral protein depletion • Below 100 µg/dl: severe visceral protein depletion
Serum triglycerides • Screens for hyperlipidemia	• 40 to 200 mg/dl	• Increased values combined with increased cholesterol levels: increased risk of atherosclerotic disease • Decreased values: protein energy malnutrition (PEM), steatorrhea
Skin sensitivity testing • Evaluates immune response compromised by PEM	• Positive reaction within 24 hours for immunocompetent patients, marked by a red area of 5 mm or greater at the test site	• Delayed, partial, or negative reaction (no response): may point to PEM

Detecting deficiencies *(continued)*

Test and purpose	Normal values	Implications
Total lymphocyte count • Diagnoses PEM	• 1,500 to 3,000/µl	• Increased values: infection or inflammation, leukemia, tissue necrosis • Decreased values: moderate to severe malnutrition if no other cause, such as influenza or measles, is identified
Total protein screen • Detects hyperproteinemia or hypoproteinemia	• 6 to 8 g/dl	• Increased values: dehydration • Decreased values: malnutrition, protein loss
Transthyretin (prealbumin) • Offers information regarding visceral protein stores; should be used in conjunction with the albumin level (Prealbumin has a shorter half-life [2 to 3 days] than albumin. This test is sensitive to nutritional repletion.)	• 16 to 40 mg/dl	• Increased values: renal insufficiency; patient on dialysis • Decreased values: PEM, acute catabolic states, postsurgery, hyperthyroidism
Urine ketone bodies (acetone) • Screens for ketonuria and detects carbohydrate deprivation	• Negative for ketones in urine	• Ketoacidosis: starvation

• loss of at least 10% of pre-illness weight.
• serum albumin level below 3.5 g/dl.
• poor tolerance of long-term enteral feedings.
• chronic vomiting or diarrhea.
• continued weight loss despite adequate oral intake.
• GI disorders that prevent or severely reduce absorption, such as bowel obstruction, Crohn's disease, ulcerative colitis, short-bowel syndrome, cancer malabsorption syndrome, and bowel fistulas.
• inflammatory GI disorders, such as wound infection, fistulas, or abscesses.

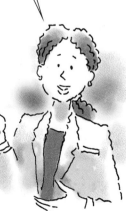

Use PPN to help the patient meet minimum calorie and protein requirements or to supplement oral or enteral feedings.

Indications for PPN

Patients who don't need to gain weight, yet need nutritional support, may receive PPN for as long as 2 to 3 weeks. It's used to help a patient meet minimum calorie and protein requirements. PPN therapy may also be used with oral or enteral feedings for a patient who needs to supplement low-calorie intake or who can't absorb enteral therapy.

Putting PPN on hold

PPN shouldn't be used for patients with moderate to severe malnutrition or fat metabolism disorders, such as pathologic hyperlipidemia, lipoid nephrosis, and acute pancreatitis caused by hyperlipidemia. In patients with severe liver damage, coagulation disorders, anemia, and pulmonary disease as well as those at increased risk for fat embolism, use parenteral nutrition cautiously.

Understanding parenteral nutrition solutions

The solution you administer depends on the type of parenteral nutrition and the patient's status.

Element roll call

Parenteral nutrition solutions may contain the following elements, each offering a particular benefit:
- *Dextrose* provides most of the calories that can help maintain nitrogen balance. The number of nonprotein calories needed to maintain nitrogen balance depends on the severity of the patient's illness.
- *Amino acids* supply enough protein to replace essential amino acids, maintain protein stores, and prevent protein loss from muscle tissues.
- *Fats*, supplied as lipid emulsions, are a concentrated source of energy that prevent or correct fatty acid deficiencies. These are available in several concentrations and can provide 30% to 50% of a patient's daily calorie requirement.
- *Electrolytes* and *minerals* are added to the parenteral nutrition solution based on an evaluation of the patient's serum chemistry profile and metabolic needs.
- *Vitamins* ensure normal body functions and optimal nutrient use for the patient. A commercially available mixture of fat- and water-soluble vitamins, biotin, and folic acid may be added to the patient's parenteral nutrition solution.
- *Micronutrients*, also called trace elements, promote normal metabolism. Most commercial solutions contain zinc, copper, chromium, selenium, and manganese.
- *Water* is added to a parenteral nutrition solution based on the patient's fluid requirements and electrolyte balance.

Depending on the patient's condition, a doctor may also order additives for the parenteral nutrition solution, such as insulin or heparin. (See *Understanding common additives*.)

Understanding common additives

Common parenteral nutrition solutions include dextrose 50% in water ($D_{50}W$), amino acids, and any of the additives listed here. The following additives are used to treat a patient's specific metabolic deficiencies:

- Acetate prevents metabolic acidosis.
- Amino acids provide protein necessary for tissue repair.
- Calcium promotes development of bones and teeth and aids in blood clotting.
- Chloride regulates the acid-base equilibrium and maintains osmotic pressure.
- $D_{50}W$ provides calories for metabolism.
- Folic acid is needed for deoxyribonucleic acid formation and promotes growth and development.
- Magnesium aids carbohydrate and protein absorption.
- Micronutrients (such as zinc, manganese, and cobalt) help in wound healing and red blood cell synthesis.
- Phosphate minimizes the potential for developing peripheral paresthesia (numbness and tingling of the extremities).
- Potassium is needed for cellular activity and tissue synthesis.
- Sodium helps regulate water distribution and maintain normal fluid balance.
- Vitamin B complex aids the final absorption of carbohydrates and protein.
- Vitamin C helps in wound healing.
- Vitamin D is essential for bone metabolism and maintenance of serum calcium levels.
- Vitamin K helps prevent bleeding disorders.

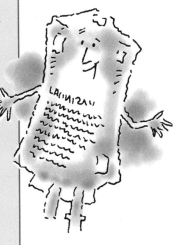

TPN solutions

Solutions for TPN are hypertonic, with an osmolarity of 1,800 to 2,600 mOsm/L. Electrolytes, minerals, vitamins, micronutrients, and water are added to the base solution to satisfy daily requirements. Lipids may be given as a separate solution or as an admixture with dextrose and amino acids.

The 3:1 solution

Daily allotments of TPN solution, including lipids and other parenteral solution components, are commonly given in a single 3-L bag, called a total nutrient admixture or 3:1 solution.

Maintaining glucose balance without adding insulin

Glucose balance is extremely important in a patient receiving TPN. Adults use 0.8 to 1 g of glucose per kilogram of body weight per hour. That means a patient can tolerate a constant I.V. infusion of hyperosmolar (highly concentrated) glucose without adding insulin to the solution. As the concentrated glucose solution infuses, a pancreatic beta-cell response causes serum insulin levels to increase.

To allow the pancreas to establish and maintain the necessary increased insulin production, start with a slow infusion rate and increase it gradually as ordered. Abruptly stopping the infusion may cause rebound hypoglycemia, which calls for an infusion of dextrose.

Glycemic imbalance may be caused by:

- sepsis
- stress
- shock
- liver or kidney failure
- diabetes
- age
- pancreatic disease
- concurrent use of certain medications, including steroids.

> For a patient receiving TPN, it's all about glucose balance — start off slow, then gradually increase.

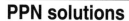

PPN solutions

Using an amino acid, dextrose, and lipid emulsion solution, PPN fulfills a patient's basic caloric needs without the risks involved in CV access. Because PPN solutions have lower tonicity than TPN solutions, a patient receiving PPN must be able to tolerate infusion of large volumes of fluid. Administer PPN through a peripheral vein.

PPN solutions usually consist of dextrose 5% in water (D_5W) to 10% dextrose and 2.75% to 4.25% crystalline amino acids. Alternatively, PPN solutions may be slightly hypertonic, such as dextrose 10% in water ($D_{10}W$), with an osmolarity no greater than 600 mOsm/L. Lipid emulsions, electrolytes, trace elements, and vitamins may be given as part of PPN to add calories and other needed nutrients.

Lipid emulsions

In an oral diet, lipids or fats are the major source of calories, usually providing about 40% of the total caloric intake. In parenteral nutrition solutions, lipids provide 9 kcal/g. I.V. lipid emulsions are oxidized for energy as needed. As a nearly isotonic emulsion, concentrations of 10% or 20% can be safely infused through peripheral or central veins. Lipid emulsions prevent and treat essential fatty acid deficiency and provide a major source of energy.

Patients requiring parenteral nutrition frequently receive I.V. lipids. Lipid emulsions call for special precautions. (See *Administering lipid emulsions.*)

Insulin insight

Because the synthesis of lipase (a fat-splitting enzyme) increases insulin requirements, the insulin dosage of a patient with diabetes may need to be increased as ordered. Insulin is one of the additives that may be adjusted in the formulation of the PPN solution.

> PPN solutions are less concentrated than TPN solutions...

> ...which means more fluid is needed to deliver nutrients.

Hormone hint

For a patient with hypothyroidism, you may need to administer thyroid-stimulating hormone (TSH). TSH affects lipase activity and may prevent triglycerides from accumulating in the vascular system.

Patient reports

Patients receiving lipid emulsions commonly report a feeling of fullness or bloating; occasionally, they experience an unpleasant metallic or greasy taste. Some patients develop allergic reactions to the fat emulsion.

Lipid letdowns

Early adverse reactions to lipid emulsion therapy occur in less than 1% of patients. These reactions may include:
- fever
- difficulty breathing
- cyanosis

Danger zone

Administering lipid emulsions

To safely administer lipid emulsions, follow these special precautions:
- Monitor the patient's vital signs and watch for adverse reactions, such as fever, a pressure sensation over the eyes, nausea, vomiting, headache, chest and back pain, tachycardia, dyspnea, cyanosis, and flushing, sweating, or chills. If the patient has no adverse reactions to the test dose, begin the infusion at the prescribed rate.
- Before the infusion, always check the parenteral nutrition with lipids for separation or an oily appearance. If either condition exists, the lipid may have come out of emulsion and shouldn't be used.
- Because lipid emulsions are at high risk for bacterial growth, never rehang a partially empty bottle of emulsion.

- nausea
- vomiting
- headache
- flushing
- sweating
- lethargy
- dizziness
- chest and back pain
- slight pressure over the eyes
- irritation at the infusion site.

Changes in laboratory test results may also reveal problems when a patient receives lipid emulsions, including:

- hyperlipidemia
- hypercoagulability
- thrombocytopenia.

Administering parenteral nutrition

You may deliver parenteral nutrition one of two ways:

 continuously

 cyclically.

Open for service 24 hours

With continuous delivery, the patient receives the infusion over a 24-hour period. The infusion begins at a slow rate and increases to the optional rate as ordered. This type of delivery may prevent complications such as hyperglycemia due to a high dextrose load.

En-cyclic-pedic knowledge

A patient undergoing cyclic therapy receives the entire 24-hour volume of parenteral nutrition solution over a shorter period, perhaps 10, 12, 14, or 16 hours. Home care parenteral nutrition programs have boosted the use of cyclic therapy. This type of therapy may be used to wean the patient from TPN. (See *Switching from continuous to cyclic TPN.*)

The dilution solution

Because TPN fluid has about six times the solute concentration of blood, peripheral I.V. administration can cause sclerosis and thrombosis. To ensure adequate dilution, the CV catheter is inserted into the superior vena cava, a wide-bore, high-flow vein. Usually, the catheter isn't advanced into the right atrium because of the risk of cardiac perforation and arrhythmias.

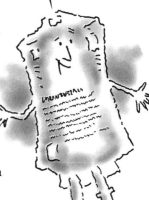

In continuous delivery, I have to work both day and night. In cyclic delivery, I get a few hours off.

Peak technique

Switching from continuous to cyclic TPN

When switching from continuous to cyclic total parenteral nutrition (TPN), adjust the flow rate so the patient's blood glucose level can adapt to the decreased nutrient load. Do this by reducing the flow rate by one-half for 1 hour before stopping the infusion. Draw a blood glucose sample 1 hour after the infusion ends, and observe the patient for signs of hypoglycemia, such as sweating, shakiness, and irritability.

TPN solutions must be infused in a central vein, using a central venous access device. Types of these devices include:
- peripherally inserted central catheters
- nontunneled percutaneous CV catheters
- tunneled CV catheters
- implanted ports.

In it for the long haul

Long-term therapy requires the use of one of the following:
- a tunneled CV catheter
- an implanted port.

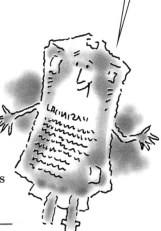

The TPN solution I'm filled with is highly concentrated. Infusion into a large vein ensures adequate dilution.

What you need

Parenteral nutrition solution ✳ lipid emulsion (if ordered) ✳ infusion pump ✳ appropriate administration set ✳ filter (if the administration set doesn't have an in-line filter) ✳ I.V. pole ✳ gloves ✳ 70% alcohol pads

Getting ready

- Before TPN administration begins, the doctor inserts a central venous access device. The location of the catheter tip is confirmed by X-ray prior to its use.
- Remove the parenteral nutrition solution from the refrigerator at least 1 hour before use so it can warm to room temperature.
- Double-check the solution label against the doctor's order to make sure it contains the correct components.
- Inspect the container for holes or cracks and the solution for turbidity, precipitates, and cloudiness. If the solution contains

lipids, look for separation, froth, and an oily appearance or a brown discoloration.
• Check the expiration date of the solution. If it has expired, or if you note any other problem with the solution, return it to the pharmacy.
• Gather the parenteral nutrition solution, a pump, an administration set with an appropriate filter, alcohol pads, gloves, and an I.V. pole. Be sure to wash your hands before preparing the parenteral nutrition solution for administration, and prepare the administration set in a clean area.
• Always use tubing with a filter when administering TPN. Filters are required by the Food and Drug Administration.

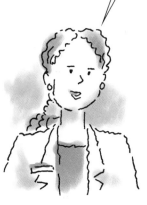

Check every solution for cloudiness, debris, or color changes.

How you do it

• Begin the infusion as ordered.
• Label the container with the time the solution was hung.
• Watch for swelling at the catheter insertion site. This may indicate extravasation of the parenteral nutrition solution, which can cause necrosis (tissue damage).

Practice pointers

• If the bag or bottle is damaged and you don't have an immediate replacement, you can approximate the glucose concentration until a new container is ready by hanging a container of dextrose 10% at the same rate prescribed for parenteral nutrition. This will prevent a significant hypoglycemic event.
• Maintain flow rates as prescribed, even if the flow falls behind schedule.
• Don't allow parenteral nutrition solutions to hang for more than 24 hours.
• Change the tubing and filter every 24 hours, using strict sterile technique. Make sure that all tubing junctions are secure. (See *Reducing the risk of infection.*)
• Perform I.V. site care and dressing changes according to your facility's policy and protocol—usually every 24 to 48 hours, more often if the dressing becomes wet, soiled, or nonocclusive.
• Check the infusion pump's volume meter and time tape every 30 minutes (or more often if necessary) to monitor for irregular flow rate. Gravity should never be used to administer parenteral nutrition solutions.
• Record vital signs when you initiate therapy and every 4 to 8 hours thereafter (or more often if necessary). Be alert for increased body temperature—one of the earliest signs of catheter-related sepsis.

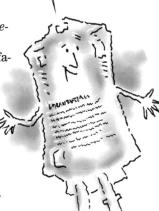

Need an emergency substitute for a damaged TPN bag? Try hanging a container of dextrose 10%.

• Monitor your patient's glucose levels as ordered using glucose fingersticks or serum tests.
• Accurately record the patient's daily fluid intake and output, specifying the volume and type of each fluid. This record helps assure prompt, precise replacement of fluid and electrolyte deficits.
• Assess the patient's physical status daily. Weigh him at the same time each morning (after voiding), in similar clothing, using the same scale. Suspect fluid imbalance if the patient gains more than 1 lb (0.45 kg) per day. If ordered, obtain anthropometric measurements.
• Monitor the results of routine laboratory tests, such as serum electrolyte, blood urea nitrogen, and glucose levels, and report abnormal findings to the doctor so appropriate changes in the parenteral nutrition solution can be made.
• Check serum triglyceride levels, which should be in the normal range during continuous parenteral nutrition infusion. Typically, alanine aminotransferase, aspartate aminotransferase, alkaline phosphatase, cholesterol, triglyceride, plasma-free fatty acid, and coagulation tests are performed weekly.
• Monitor the patient for signs and symptoms of nutritional aberrations, such as fluid and electrolyte imbalances and glucose metabolism disturbances. Some patients may require supplementary insulin throughout TPN therapy; the pharmacy usually adds insulin directly to the TPN solution.
• Provide emotional support. Keep in mind that patients commonly associate eating with positive feelings and may feel socially isolated when it's eliminated.
• Provide frequent mouth care for the patient.

A port of last resort

• Avoid using a parenteral nutrition infusion port for any other infusion.
• When using a single-lumen CV catheter, don't use the line to piggyback or infuse blood or blood products, give a bolus injection, administer simultaneous I.V. solutions, measure CV pressure, or draw blood for laboratory tests. In unavoidable circumstances, the TPN port may be used for electrolyte replacement or insulin drips because these infusions are commonly additives to the solution.
• Never add medication to a TPN solution container. Also avoid using add-on devices, which increase the risk of infection.

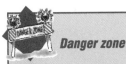

Danger zone

Reducing the risk of infection

Because a total parenteral nutrition (TPN) solution serves as a medium for bacterial growth and a central venous line provides systemic access, the patient receiving TPN risks infection and sepsis. To reduce the risk, always maintain strict sterile technique when handling the equipment used to administer therapy.

Gravity is great but not for controlling parenteral nutrition solutions. Always use an infusion pump and check it at least every half hour.

No place like home

Taking parenteral nutrition home

Understanding parenteral nutrition and its goals helps a home care patient assume a greater role in administering, monitoring, and maintaining therapy. When instructing a home care patient, focus your teaching on signs and symptoms of:
• fluid, electrolyte, and glucose imbalances
• vitamin and trace element deficiencies and toxicities
• signs and symptoms of catheter infection, such as fever, chills, discomfort on infusion, and redness or drainage at the catheter insertion site.

First and foremost
To help prevent glucose imbalance, teach the patient receiving his first I.V. bag of parenteral nutrition how to regulate the flow rate so he maintains the rate prescribed by the doctor. Explain that a gradual increase in the flow rate allows the pancreas to establish and maintain the increased insulin production necessary to tolerate this treatment. Once the goal rate of the parenteral nutrition infusion is met, there should be no reason to adjust the rate.

Review time
Finally, review the details of the administration schedule, the equipment the patient will use and, to avoid incompatibilities, the prescribed and over-the-counter medications he takes.

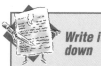

Write it down

Documenting parenteral nutrition administration

Be sure to record:
• type and amount of solution
• date and time solution was hung
• infusion rate
• administration equipment used
• location and condition of infusion site
• patient's tolerance and response to infusion
• monitoring performed
• complications, notification of doctor, interventions, and patient response
• patient teaching.

What to teach

• If the patient is to continue parenteral nutrition at home, teach him how to administer, monitor, and maintain therapy. (See *Taking parenteral nutrition home*.)

Complications of parenteral nutrition

Patients receiving parenteral nutrition therapy face many of the same complications as patients undergoing any type of peripheral I.V. or CV therapy. (See *Parenteral nutrition therapy hazards*.) Pediatric and elderly patients are also particularly susceptible to certain complications of parenteral nutrition therapy. (See *Patients with special needs*, page 352.)

Complications of parenteral nutrition therapy may result from problems that are:
• catheter-related
• metabolic
• mechanical.

Lipid low points

Prolonged administration of lipid emulsions can produce delayed complications, including enlarged liver or spleen, blood dyscrasia (thrombocytopenia and leukopenia), and transient increases in results of liver function studies. A small number of patients receiving 20% I.V. lipid emulsion develop brown pigmentation due to fat pigmentation.

Danger zone

Parenteral nutrition therapy hazards

Complications of total parenteral nutrition therapy can result from catheter-related, metabolic, or mechanical problems.

Catheter-related
• Clotted catheter
• Dislodged catheter
• Cracked or broken tubing
• Pneumothorax and hydrothorax
• Sepsis

Metabolic
• Hyperglycemia
• Hypoglycemia
• Hyperosmolar hyperglycemic nonketotic syndrome
• Hypokalemia
• Hypomagnesemia
• Hypophosphatemia
• Hypocalcemia
• Metabolic acidosis
• Liver dysfunction
• Hyperkalemia

Mechanical
• Air embolism
• Venous thrombosis
• Too rapid an infusion
• Extravasation
• Phlebitis

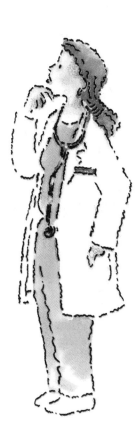

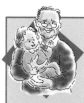

Ages and stages

Patients with special needs

Your pediatric and elderly patients have special needs when receiving parenteral nutrition. For example, pediatric and elderly patients are susceptible to fluid overload. With these patients, be careful to administer the correct volume of parenteral nutrition solution at the correct infusion rate.

The following are additional special considerations to keep in mind.

Considerations for children
Children have a greater need than adults for certain nutrients. This is an important consideration in accurately calculating solution components for pediatric patients. Overall, a child has a greater need for:
- protein
- carbohydrates
- fat
- electrolytes
- micronutrients
- vitamins
- fluids.

Administering PPN with lipid emulsions in a premature or low birth-weight neonate may lead to lipid accumulation in the lungs. Thrombocytopenia (platelet deficiency) has also been reported in neonates receiving 20% lipid emulsions.

As with adults, children receiving TPN should be evaluated carefully by the nurse, doctor, and nutritional support team. Keep the following factors in mind when planning to meet children's nutritional needs:
- age
- weight
- activity level
- size
- development
- caloric needs.

Considerations for adults
An elderly patient may have an underlying clinical problem that affects the outcome of treatment. For example, he may be taking medications that can interact with the components in the parenteral nutrition solution. For this reason, ask the pharmacist about possible interactions with any other drug the patient is taking.

Elderly patients are subject to fluid overload and drug interactions. It's always something.

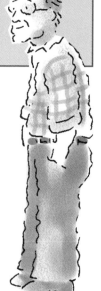

Discontinuing therapy

One major difference exists between the procedures for discontinuing TPN and PPN therapy. A patient receiving TPN should be weaned from therapy and should receive some other form of nutritional therapy such as enteral feedings.

When to wean and when not to wean

When the patient is receiving PPN, therapy can be discontinued without weaning because the dextrose concentration is lower than in TPN. When discontinuing TPN therapy, you should wean the patient over 24 hours to prevent rebound hypoglycemia.

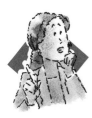

Quick quiz

1. Which form of protein energy malnutrition results from a prolonged and gradual wasting of muscle mass and subcutaneous fat?

    A.   Iatrogenic
    B.   Kwashiorkor
    C.   Marasmus
    D.   Hypermetabolic

Answer: C. Marasmus is a prolonged and gradual wasting of muscle mass and subcutaneous fat. It's caused by inadequate intake of protein, calories, and other nutrients. It occurs most commonly in infants ages 6 to 18 months, after gastrectomy, and in patients with cancer of the mouth and esophagus.

2. Which of the following serum laboratory studies has a shorter half-life than serum albumin, and is a sensitive indicator of nutritional repletion?

    A.   Transferrin
    B.   Hemoglobin
    C.   Transthyretin (prealbumin)
    D.   Total iron binding capacity

Answer: C. Transthyretin (prealbumin) has a shorter half-life than serum albumin, a sensitive indicator of nutritional repletion.

3. Which of the following is added to parenteral nutrition solutions to help prevent metabolic acidosis?

    A.   Acetate
    B.   Calcium
    C.   Folic acid
    D.   Vitamin K

Answer: A. Acetate is added to parenteral nutrition solutions to help prevent metabolic acidosis.

4. Which of the following complications of parenteral nutrition therapy can result from a mechanical problem?

    A.   Hyperglycemia
    B.   Air embolism
    C.   Metabolic acidosis
    D.   Liver dysfunction

Answer: B. Air embolism, as well as venous thrombosis, extravasation, phlebitis, and rapid infusion, are complications of parenteral nutrition therapy that can result from a mechanical problem.

Scoring

⭐⭐⭐ If you answered all four questions correctly, feel fulfilled. You've metabolized the chapter components and converted them to cerebral energy.

⭐⭐ If you answered two or three questions correctly, sit back and digest. Your mind has been well nourished.

⭐ If you answered fewer than two questions correctly, have a snack and review this book. There's nothing wrong with enhancing your diet of knowledge with a fact-filled supplement.

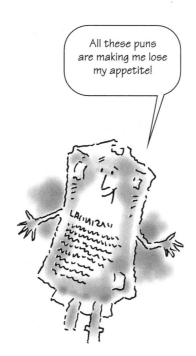

All these puns are making me lose my appetite!

Index

A

Absorption, factors that affect, 12, 13i, 14
Additive interaction, 27t
Administer versus dispense, 48
Administration guidelines, 73-74
Administration procedures, 66-76
Administration sets, drip factors of, 94-95
Administration times, standardized, 70
Adsorption, I.V. drug administration and, 29
Adverse reactions
    drug action outcome and, 25-26
    lipid emulsions and, 345-346, 351
    reporting, 106
Age, effect of, on drug action and effect, 17
Agonist, 22
Alcohol use as drug history component, 38
Alkylating agents, 316t. *See also* Chemothera-
    peutic drugs.
Allergic reactions, 26. *See also* Hypersensitivity
    reaction to chemotherapeutic drug.
Allergies, obtaining data about, in patient
    assessment, 32-33
Alopecia as chemotherapy adverse effect, 330t
Ambiguous drug order, clarifying, 50
Ambulatory infusion pump, 263
Anal ointment application, 202-203
    documenting, 203
    patient teaching for, 203
Anaphylactic reaction. *See* Hypersensitivity
    reaction to chemotherapeutic drug.
Anemia as chemotherapy adverse effect, 330t
Antagonist, 23
Antagonistic interaction, 27t
Anthropometric measurements, comparing, 339
Antibiotic antineoplastics, 316t. *See also*
    Chemotherapeutic drugs.
Antimetabolites, 316t. *See also* Chemothera-
    peutic drugs.
Antineoplastics that alter hormone balance,
    316t. *See also* Chemotherapeutic drugs.
Apothecaries' measurement system, 84-85
    measures used in, 85
Assessment as nursing process step, 32-41
Automated drug delivery system, 75, 76
Autonomy of patient, respect for, 57
Avoirdupois measurement system, 85

B

Bedside medications for self-administration,
    orders for, 74
Beneficence as moral principle, 57
Binding of drug to plasma proteins, drug
    distribution and, 14
Bioavailability of drug, 12, 14
Biological therapy, 317-319
Biotransformation, 199. *See also* Metabolism.
Blood level of drug, dosing regimen and, 18-19
Body surface area, pediatric dosage calculation
    and, 98-100
Body weight, pediatric dosage calculation
    and, 98
Bolus injection, administering, 248-255
    directly into vein, 253-255
    documenting, 255
    through peripheral line, 248-249, 251
    through saline lock, 251-253
    through vascular access port, 278-282
Bone as drug storage compartment, 15
Brand name of drug, 4
Bronchodilators, cardiac patient and, 159
Broviac catheter, 271i
Buccal administration, 177-178
    documenting, 178
    drug placement in, 176i, 177
    patient teaching for, 178
Buccal route, 7

C

Cancer immunotherapy, 317
Capsule, administering, 183, 184-186
    documentation of, 186
    patient teaching for, 186
Care plan, developing, 41-43
Cell cycle, chemotherapeutic drugs and,
    313, 314i
Central venous catheter, 270
    documenting drug administration through, 274
    how to use, 272-274
    types of, 271t
Central venous therapy
    administering, 272-274
    catheters used for, 270, 271t
    documenting, 270
    in home setting, 274
    risks of, 273

Chemical name of drug, 3, 4
Chemotherapeutic drugs. *See also* Chemo-
    therapy.
    administering, 322-325
    categories of, 315, 316t
    cell cycle and, 313, 314i
    guidelines for preparing, 319-322
    methods of administering, 322
    selection of, 315
Chemotherapy, 311, 313. *See also* Chemo-
    therapeutic drugs.
    adverse effects of, 329, 331
    documenting administration of, 325
    hypersensitivity reactions and, 328-329, 328t
    infusion site–related complications of, 326-328
    managing adverse effects of, 330t
    mechanics of, 313, 314i, 315
    safe administration of, 323, 324
    treatment cycles and, 315
    using Ommaya reservoir for, 312i
Cigarette smoking, drug metabolism and, 16
Clinical status of patient as assessment com-
    ponent, 40-41
Cognitive barriers, presence of, as assessment
    component, 39-40
Collagen shields, 5
Colony-stimulating factors, 319
Combining drugs
    in cartridge-injection system, 224-225
    in syringe
        from multidose vial and ampule, 223
        from two ampules, 224
        from two multidose vials, 222-223
Compliance aids for injectable drug
    therapy, 233i
Comprehensive Drug Abuse Prevention and
    Control Act, 48
Conditions that affect drug action and effect,
    16-17
Conflicting drug regimens, detecting, 35-36
Continuous infusion, administering
    with infusion pump, 262-264
        documenting, 264
    with vascular access port, 282-285
Continuous secondary infusion, administering,
    256, 257-258
Controlled substances, legal responsibility
    for, 48

i refers to an illustration; t refers to a table.

i refers to an illustration; t refers to a table.

i refers to an illustration; t refers to a table.

i refers to an illustration; t refers to a table.

i refers to an illustration; t refers to a table.

i refers to an illustration; t refers to a table.

Notes